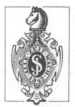

The complete five-volume set consists of

A. Berenstein   P. Lasjaunias

Surgical Neuroangiography

4 Endovascular Treatment
of Cerebral Lesions

With 203 Figures in 735 Separate Illustrations

Springer-Verlag
Berlin Heidelberg New York
London Paris Tokyo
Hong Kong Barcelona
Budapest

ALEJANDRO BERENSTEIN, M.D.
Professor of Radiology and Neurosurgery
Director of Surgical Neuroangiography Service
New York University and Bellevue Medical Center
560 First Avenue, New York, NY 10016, USA

PIERRE LASJAUNIAS, M.D., Ph.D.
Professeur des Universités en Anatomie
Professor of Radiology and Neurosurgery (Adj.) New York University
Service de Radiologie, Hôpital de Bicêtre
Université Paris XI, 78 Rue du Général Leclerc
94275 Le Kremlin Bicêtre, France

Library of Congress Cataloging-in-Publication Data (Revised for volume 4 and 5). Lasjaunias, Pierre L.
Surgical neuroangiography. Includes bibliographies and indexes. Contents: v. 1. Functional anatomy of
craniofacial arteries − v. 4. Endovascular treatment of cerebral lesions − v. 5. Endovascular treatment of
spine and spinal cord lesions. 1. Nervous system − Blood-vessels − Radiography. 2. Nervous system −
Blood-vessels − Surgery. 3. Angiography. I. Berenstein, Alex, 1947− . II. Raybaud, C. III. Title. [DNLM:
1. Angiography. 2. Neuroradiography. WL 141 L344s] RD594.2.L37 1987 616.8 86-26028

ISBN-13: 978-3-642-71866-3   e-ISBN-13: 978-3-642-71864-9
DOI: 10.1007/978-3-642-71864-9

Production editor: Meike Seeker, Heidelberg
Reproduction of the figures: Gustav Dreher GmbH, Stuttgart
Typesetting: K+V Fotosatz GmbH, Beerfelden

27/3130-5 4 3 2 1 0 − Printed on acid-free paper

To Josee, Pascale, Erica, Estelle, Vanessa, Aude and Colin. To the team of technicians and nurses of both New York University and Bicêtre, for their invaluable assistance. To Norman E. Chase, M.D., and Irvin I. Kricheff, M.D., for their support. To Joseph Ransohoff, M.D., Professor and chairman in the department of Neurosurgery at N.Y.U., we would like to express a special thanks for his trust, encouragement, intellectual and moral guidance, that was fundamental in the formation of our specialty. His vision and enthusiasm has been a guidance and inspiration from the onset. And to all our coworkers and referring physicians for placing their trust in us.

Preface

In Volume 4 of *Surgical Neuroangiography* we will discuss indications and approaches for endovascular treatment of disorders affecting the cerebral circulation. Our approach requires integration of knowledge concerning functional vascular anatomy, lesion angioarchitecture, and the relationship between normal and pathological circulations.

In AVMs these features are considered as they relate to the clinical presentation, progression, and natural history of the lesion. All these factors must then be combined with an understanding of technical capabilities to formulate a pretherapeutic plan designed to favorably affect the long term outcome in the individual patient.

In brain AVMs, endovascular surgery may be the sole form of treatment, or may be combined with other therapeutic modalities including microsurgery or radiosurgery. A multidisciplinary approach is therefore essential for decision making to best accomplish the desired objectives. Embolization of deep supply to a malformation, closure of high flow fistulas, etc. prior to surgical excision for example, may significantly facilitate the operation. In the same way, reduction of the volume of a large inoperable lesion will often convert the abnormality to one that can be safely and effectively treated by radiosurgery.

Although the aim of any intervention is to eliminate the abnormality, a significant number of patients referred for endovascular surgery (primarily BAVMs), cannot presently be cured by either embolization alone or in a combination of treatments. In such patients, our approach aims to intervene at specific points of weakness of the vascular system to arrest the progression of symptoms or to decrease the potential for future complications of the disease. Our experience in more than 10 years and over 500 treated patients with BAVMs, utilizing such strategy, suggests that this plan is effective in providing protection to such patients. Furthermore, treatments may be carried out over a long period of time, permitting technical limitations that could not be initially overcome to be resolved later thanks to either technological improvements or hemodynamic alterations.

As our technical capabilities for cerebral navigation are improving, and we are able to enter aneurysms and mechanically dilate spastic vessels, a major revolution in the management of SAH is quickly developing, and will be dealt with in Vol. 5.

Catheterization of normal distal vessels, with a high degree of precision in a safe, reproducible, and expeditious manner represents a magnificent means of access to the human body. It permits us for example, to reach selective small volumes of cerebral tissue via its circulation. Functional mapping can then be performed using CNS *depressants* such as sodium amytal to test the function of a specific neuronal population, or xylocaine to test axonal function. Non toxic substances that *stimulate* CNS function may be introduced that will reveal or enhance neural function.

Immediate clinical possibilities for pharmacological manipulation in the CNS include functional mapping of memory centers to aid in the management of epilepsy, and determination of speech, motor, or sensory function locations prior to BAVM surgery.

Endovascular operations for the management of ischemic disease, utilizing mechanical and/or chemical recanalizations promises to become one of the most intense and potentially important areas for *Surgical Neuroangiography*, and are reviewed in Vol. 5. Redistribution of cerebral blood flow utilizing more than one catheter can easily be accomplished, and may play an important role in the future of intravascular embolization or infusion.

The administration of short acting, or rapidly metabolized agents may be best accomplished by a highly selective transarterial route for maximal efficacy. Conceivably such agents as monoclonal antibodies, or "killer" RNA, that would be metabolized prior to action if introduced any other way may become clinically practical.

The field of Neuroendocrinology, at the functional or molecular level may represent an other fertile area for future research, to either measure neurotransmitters (superselective venous sampling), or stimulate the release of neurotransmitters.

Superselective percutaneous venous catheterization in the cerebral circulation can now be accomplished in all age groups in a safe, reliable, and reproducible manner. Retroperfusion of ischemic tissues, or retroperfusion chemotherapy in neoplastic or degenerative-metabolic diseases may become an important therapeutic modality in the future.

These are only some of the new horizone opening to *Surgical Neuroangiography*, and therefore we believe that future applications are limited only be imagination and by our ability to provide sufficient human resources to explore the full potential of endovascular surgery. As we commented in the preface of Volume 1 and 2, *Surgical Neuroangiography*, where the adjective "surgical" refers to the use of hands and tools in treatment.

Knowledge of functional arterial and venous vascular anatomy is increasing rapidly, driven by and aided by technical improvements in catheterization techniques. This rapid knowledge expansion combines with the requirement for full understanding of the clinical feature, pathophysiology, and therapeutic options for the increasing number of diseases that can be approached by endovascular means demand that individuals involved in *Surgical Neuroangiography* no longer be "part time", or "occasional" participants in this subspecialty. For proper performance and future advancement, full dedication and commitment is imperative. Proper training in *Surgical Neuroangiography* requires expertise in radiological knowledge, i.e. fluoroscopy, radiation physics and radiobiology. In addition, a solid clinical background is essential in dealing with the various disease entities, their effect on the CNS and the body, as well as with complications that may result from either the abnormality or from treatment. Previous experience in some aspects of diagnostic Radiology is advantageous, but knowledge of barium enemas or mammography are, for example not a prerequisite for proper performance. Training in Neurosurgery also has advantages, but the ability to perform craniotomies or disc removals is again of only limited value in the practice of *Surgical Neuroangiography*. Cooperation between Radiology and Surgery i.e. Neuroradiology and Neurosurgery is essential to properly train individuals interested in *Surgical Neuroangiography* and indeed represents a responsibility both to our patients and to society. Of all recent advances, few have the potential of *Surgical Neuroangiography* to impact so dramatically on so many aspects to medicine from efficacy, to cost effectiveness. This impact already demonstrated, can be expected to increase significantly in the future.

We hope that these 5 volumes of *Surgical Neuroangiography* will be a useful tool for those involved in this fascinating and rewarding specialty. However, the series *Surgical Neuroangiography* is not intended as a replacement for proper training.

March 1992   A. BERENSTEIN and P. LASJAUNIAS

Acknowledgements

We would like to acknowledge the following for their help in providing illustrations: I. S. Choi, M.D., Ch. Kerber, M.D., G. Debrun, M.D., K. Terbrugge, M.D., and Duvrnua, M.D.

We also wish to thank Robert Hurst, M.D., for his language editing assistance.

We are particularly grateful to Jill Scott for typing the manuscript and its multiple revisions, and to Angel Arce, Martha Helmers, and Tony Jalandoni for the technical and photographic expertise.

Contents

Chapter 4

Technical Aspects of Surgical Neuroangiography

Chapter 5

Arteriovenous Fistulas of the Brain

CHAPTER 1

Classification of Brain Arteriovenous Malformations

I. Incidence of Brain Arteriovenous Malformations

The prevalence of brain arteriovenous malformations (BAVMs) in a given population is difficult to estimate. It is believed that between 0.14% and 0.8% of the population may present with a BAVM in a given year (Garretson 1985; Jellinger 1986). These varying figures result from studies of disparate populations, ranging from the residents in a small community (Mohr 1984) to autopsy series (Jellinger 1986). Overall, however, the incidence of symptomatic BAVMs in adults appears to represent about one-tenth the frequency of intracranial arterial aneurysms. Various neurosurgical series comparing the relative incidence of symptomatic BAVMs to that of brain tumors also show considerable variability, with figures ranging from 0.59% – 7.9% (Yasargil 1987). This reflects different referral patterns and the introduction of ever more sensitive diagnostic tools.

Table 1.1 shows the incidence of each type of cerebral vascular malformation (CVM) in a review of a general autopsy series. Jellinger (1986) reviewed the various published autopsy series from 1945 (Courville) to 1985 (Linz Hospital experience). A comparison of the overall incidence in the general autopsy series to the incidence of CVM in those autopsies performed specifically for cerebral hemorrhage within the same material suggests the bleeding potential of each type of CVM by its association with a lethal bleeding episode.

The accuracy of the reported incidence and number of telangiectasias in relation to other CVMs in an autopsy series may be questioned, since, when telangiectasias have not bled, they cannot usually be found at autopsy.

Despite this caveat, AVMs and telangiectasias are encountered 18–20 times more frequently in autopsies for cerebral hemorrhage. Cavernomas and "venous angiomas" show a tenfold and a threefold increase, respectively, in their incidence. The increased incidence of the venous angiomas is not statistically significant and supports the view that the incidental discovery

Table 1.1. Incidence of cerebral vascular malformations

	General autopsy series ($n = 45464$)	Autopsy series for cerebral hemorrhage ($n = 1529$)
Cerebral vascular malformations	6%	7%
Arteriovenous malformations	0.15%	3% ($\times 20$)
Cavernomas	0.05%	0.5% ($\times 10$)
Venous angiomas	0.25%	0.8% ($\times 3$)
Telangiectasias	0.15%	2.7% ($\times 18$)

From Jellinger 1986.

Table 1.2. Overall distribution of CVMs regardless of type[a]

CVM	Distribution (%)
Cerebral hemisphere and corpus callosum	64.8 – 70
Intraparenchymatous and deep-seated	8.5 – 9
Brainstem	13 – 16.1
Cerebellum	11.8 – 17

CVM, cerebral vascular malformation. (From McCormick and Rosenfield 1973; Jellinger et al. 1968).
[a] Autopsy series; $n = 1019$.

of most such lesions is a normal finding (see Vol. 3, Chap. 7, Developmental Venous Anomalies). BAVMs and telangiectasias are equally present in both the general population (0.15%) and in autopsies of patients with cerebral hemorrhage (3%). This suggests the overall fatal outcome of both types of lesions; however, there is some discrepancy between autopsy findings (Table 1.2) and their discovery in clinical series (Table 1.3).

In clinical series the percentage of supratentorial CVMs is higher than in autopsy series (9% – 20%). The opposite is true in infratentorial CVMs, where the percentage in autopsy series is higher than in clinical series (two to five times). Telangiectasias, however, are significantly more frequent in the posterior fossa (60% – 70%) and occur mainly in the brainstem (Table 1.4). They have not been described in children below 5 years of age. In addition, they are usually silent until they bleed. This difference in preferential location, favoring the brainstem, combined with the fact that infratentorial hemorrhages are, in general, more lethal than supratentorial bleeding, explains the discrepancy between clinical and autopsy results.

Attempts to understand the incidence of CVM from reviewing the literature are often disappointing and misleading. Various names are given to the same lesions, and different lesions are collected under the same labels. The normal character of the venous angiomas, which represent vascular anomalies and not malformations, further alters the reliability of the numbers given.

Classification of CVMs often carry significant limitations. There are often uncertainties if data are derived only from pathology specimens. Conclusions are a posteriori, and only a portion of the lesion is reviewed. The specimen is not seen in vivo, missing the often critical hemodynamic factors

Table 1.3. Overall distribution of CVMs regardless of type[a]

CVM	Distribution (%)
Cerebral hemisphere and corpus callosum	76.6 – 90
Intraparenchymatous and deep-seated	2 – 8
Brainstem	2.6 – 7
Cerebellum	5 – 9.6

CVM, cerebral vascular malformation. From Morello and Borghi 1973; Krayenbühl 1972; Berry 1966; Perret and Nishioka 1966.
[a] Clinical series; $n = 1320$.

Table 1.4. Topographic repartition per type of CVM[a]

	Supratentorial (%)	Infratentorial (%)
Arteriovenous malformations	70 – 76	24 – 30
Cavernomas	61 – 74	26 – 39
"Venous angiomas"	57 – 60	40 – 43
Telangiectasias	30 – 37	63 – 70

CVM, cerebral vascular malformation. From McCormick and Rosenfield 1973; Jellinger 1986.
[a] Autopsy series; $n = 854$.

of a vascular lesion. Therefore, the true clinical significance of the lesion and its actual biological behavior are often obscured (Tables 1.4, 1.5). Topographic and morphological descriptions are hindered by poor anatomical analysis, incomplete angiographic studies, and misunderstanding or overlooking of unusual vascular variations or dispositions, thereby making the description and interpretation of many lesions inaccurate.

Surgical classifications are technically oriented (Drake 1979; Forster et al. 1972; Luessenhop 1977; Wilson et al. 1979; Parkinson and Bachers 1980; Shi and Chen 1986; Spetzler and Martin 1986) and are frequently based on surgical skill. Such classifications promote techniques more than an understanding of the pathophysiology of the disease and its epidemiology. It is often assumed that the behavior of the vascular tree is identical from one patient to the other and remains so throughout life. Most surgical series are difficult to compare as interseries differences or inconsistencies occur. Surgical series may overlook potentially important features such as arterial aneurysms, venous pouches, anatomical variations (30% of Yasargil and 24% – 32% of Willinsky's series), collateral circulation, or specific topographic localization. Spetzler and Martin (1986) assumed "eloquent cortical regions occupy their normal locations", whereas Crawford et al. (1986) claimed that "the lobes of the brain involved in the arteriovenous malformation did not influence the mode of presentation". Few reports of surgical series refer to clinical and anatomical comparisons (Laine et al. 1981; Waltimo 1973b). Spetzler's classification (Spetzler and Martin 1986) incorporates the size of the AVM, the pattern of venous drainage, and the neurological "eloquence" of brain regions adjacent to the AVM. It permits the comparison of various surgical series and is intended for use when a deci-

Table 1.5. Distribution by type of CVM[a]

CVM	Distribution (%)
Arteriovenous malformations	13 – 57
Cavernomas	9 – 16
"Venous angiomas"	15.4 – 59.3
Telangiectasias	12 – 20.6
Varix	1.2 – 2.3
Multiple lesions	2 – 3.5

CVM, cerebral vascular malformation. From McCormick 1968; Jellinger 1986.
[a] Autopsy series; $n = 1019$.

sion has already been made to surgically treat the patient. The assessment of surgical risk is the major objective, this derived risk then being compared to the assumed natural history of all AVMs as a group. In addition, such comparisons assume that the surgical skills are identical within the neurosurgical community.

To compare the natural history of, for example, a temporal AVM with that of a deep-seated lesion, one should be precise as to the location of each lesion, its arterial supply, and its venous drainage. The same need for precision applies within the group of deep-seated lesions, where different lesions are topographically regrouped, e.g., thalamic, choroid, plexus, pineal, tectum, vein of Galen AVM. All of the latter can look very similar but do not represent the same disease or the same challenge for treatment. Some of them can easily be cured, others are unreachable.

II. Principles of Classification

Several types of BAVM classifications have been proposed. The various schemes listed below reflect an evolution in our knowledge and the techniques available to study or treat the lesions:

1. Pathological classifications (macroscopic and microscopic) relate to the era of visual description.
2. Demographic classifications enhance subpopulations or specific groups (pediatric, adult, neurological, neurosurgical, etc.).
3. Topographic classification and the concept of eloquent areas refer to modern radiology and open surgery.
4. Hemodynamic and morphological classifications express the interests of modern surgery and neuroanesthesiology in hemodynamic problems (the "perfusion breakthrough" phenomenon).
5. Anatomoclinical and radiological classifications introduce the biological behavior of the normal and abnormal vascular system.

Although all classifications have their limitations, a need exists to have some common basis of understanding. Therefore, we will attempt to set forth a classification that meets a number of goals. Such a classification should aid in the comparison of clinical series, first by establishing common terminology to better communicate features of CVMs and second by considering known mechanisms of lesion evolution and symptom production to emphasize pathophysiologic features. The goals of a useful classification should also include enhancement of significant differences between apparently identical lesions or patients, prediction of clinical outcome, and prediction of the natural history of CVMs prior to treatment planning. Our contribution to the understanding of CVMs is based on a fundamental principle: *Both the vascular system and the vascular malformation are evolving entities.* Both exhibit change with aging, following angioectatic or angiogenetic stimuli, and stenotic phenomena and other constraints. Thus, when confronted with a vascular malformation, one must simultaneously analyze the net result of two dynamic situations: (1) a congenital defect (the malformation) and (2) its effect (and consequent response) on the remaining vascular system.

The congenital defect depends on the embryonic stage at which the disorder has occurred. In that sense, the embryologic classification of vascular malformations could be universal. At present, it is based on the fundamental work of Woolard (1904) on capillary maturation (see Vol. 2, Chap. 8). As already seen for the maxillofacial region, some significant restrictions have to be introduced in relation to the specificity of development of brain vessels. Nevertheless, even in the CNS, the broad categories of vascular malformations remain: arterial, arteriovenous, capillary, and venous. Fundamentally, all correspond to a defect or a dysfunction of the embryonic capillary maturation process. Pathological study has helped in characterizing these different broad categories of CVM. Confusion and contradictions occurred when the pathology of secondary effects (representing the vascular system's response to the lesion) was considered for the purposes of precision and completeness. We shall keep the basic part of the pathological classification (primary classification) and outline the specific, additional, pathological response of the system as secondary changes.

The effects on the surrounding vessels are acquired; such effects correspond to the reaction and adaptation of the vascular tree both to the congenital defect and to the hemodynamic alterations that it produces. Nonetheless, the acquired effects will influence the differences in clinical presentations and outcome. As seen in clinical practice, the same apparent lesion can produce major symptoms in one patient and none in another. Conversely, some vascular malformations with vastly different architecture may create the same clinical problems. These facts outline the importance of the response of the host. Similar lesions may present in different ways in patients of different ages. Interpretation of natural history may therefore lead to completely opposite therapeutic discussions and decisions. Conversely, the apparent clinical or therapeutic consensus on some lesions, e.g. the vein of Galen aneurysmal malformation (VGAM), is misleading and erroneous (see Chap. 5).

The reaction of the vascular tree starts immediately, i.e., in utero, following establishment of the flow abnormalities (anatomical adaptation). The reaction persists or evolves with age (and development of thrombosis, steal, kinking, vessel wall defects, collateral circulation, etc.) or following acute events (rupture of the malformation, surgery, radiation therapy, embolization, etc.). Many of these acquired features are reversible. Some express a weakness of the system (high-flow angiopathy), others its compensatory nature (spontaneous thrombosis, anatomical dispositions, collateral circulation, etc.). Appreciation of both the weaknesses and the adaptability of the system may allow us to predict the biological effect of a malformation in a specific host and not merely a statistically probable event in a given population. The concept of response and/or adaptation of the host (carried out by the vascular system) has always been ignored and therefore not considered in the natural history of the specific lesion.

The location of a malformation is best assessed by magnetic resonance imaging (MRI) and/or computerized tomography (CT). Angiography, however, permits the anatomical identification of the arterial feeders and the draining veins. These features confirm and delineate with accuracy the topography of a lesion and reveal associated vascular lesions. Complete analysis is possible only if proper knowledge of the functional anatomy, including significant arterial and venous variations, is mastered (see Vol. 3,

Chaps. 4, 5 and 6). Poor angiographic studies will make the identification of the vascular anatomy or its comparison within a given series or other reports impossible or unreliable. Based on our experience in the analysis of over 900 CVMs using high quality imaging techniques, we propose a practical classification of CVMs. Proper description of a CVM includes analysis of three different but interconnected aspects which we will consider separately for clarity: (1) What is the lesion? (2) Where is it located? and (3) How has it evolved? In the following chapter we will discuss how it produces symptoms.

III. Classification of CVMs

Four major types of primary defects or malformations of the vascular systems can be individualized (Table 1.6) *arterial, arteriovenous, capillary, and venous*. For each of them, different effects on the remaining vascular system can be encountered (Table 1.7).

We consider the arteriovenous and venous malformations separately. The venous angiomas are actually developmental venous anomalies (Saito and Kobayashi 1981; Yasargil 1987; Valavanis 1983; Lasjaunias et al. 1986). They have been discussed in Vol. 3, Chap. 7 and will not be the subject of further discussions here.

Table 1.6. Classification of CVMs

Arterial
Aneurysms
Arteriovenous
Malformations
Fistulas
Capillary
Telangiectasias
Venous
Cavernous malformations

CVM, cerebral vascular malformation.

1. Arteriovenous Shunts

Arteriovenous shunts correspond to an abnormal capillary bed with a shortened arteriovenous transit time. Their exact location has been somewhat controversial, whether they lie either intrapially or subpially depends on the theory that prevails for the relationships between pia mater and cortical vessels. We favor Hutching's (1986) (see Vol. 3) description that places all BAVMs subpially and consequently does not differentiate (as far as the meningeal space) between the pure cortical and the "intraparenchymatous" (deep-seated) ones. All arteriovenous lesions can therefore be viewed as a homogeneous group, including those involving the spinal cord (see Vol. 5, Chap. 1). The concept of intra- vs extracerebral location refers only to the surgical management of these lesions. All BAVMs can be regarded as being primarily extraparenchymatous, even though they may be buried in the depth of the neural tissue (Yasargil 1987).

2. General Appearance of Arteriovenous Shunts

Schematically, two broad categories of arteriovenous shunts can be recognized: the AVMs and the arteriovenous fistulas (AVFs). The AVMs are characterized by a network of abnormal "channels" (nidus) between the arterial feeder(s) and the draining vein(s). They may be small (micro-AVMs) with "normal" sized artery(ies) and draining vein(s) and a nidus smaller than 1 cm in diameter (Fig. 1.1). Macro-AVMs, in contrast, have arteries and veins that are usually larger than normal; the size of the nidus is larger than 1 cm in diameter (Fig. 1.2).

Table 1.7. Primary classification of the cerebral vascular lesions

Arteriovenous shunts
  Single
    Micro AV shunts (mAVM or mAVF)
    Macro AV shunts (compartmented nidus or mAVF)
  Multiple (nonfamilial)
    Systemic (Wyburn-Mason)
    Nonsystemic (multiple separate niduses or "separated" compartment within one nidus)
  Multiple (familial)
    Systematized (Rendu-Osler-Weber)
    Nonsystematized (multiple separate niduses with or without AVF

Associated vascular variants
  Arterial or venous

Secondary vascular changes
  Angiogenesis, kinking, and dolichoid vessels
  Arterial aneurysms, venous ectasias, and pouches
  Venous and arterial stenoses or thrombosis
External carotid supply; dural AV
  shunting (remote)
  Arterial and venous collateral circulation
  Pseudoaneurysms (hematomas)

Secondary morphological changes
  Hydrocephalus, cerebral atrophy, cavities
  Perivascular ischemia, calcification
  Bone hypertrophy

Associated vascular tumors

AV, arteriovenous; mAVM, microarteriovenous malformation; mAVF, micro-arteriovenous fistula; AVF, arteriovenous fistula.

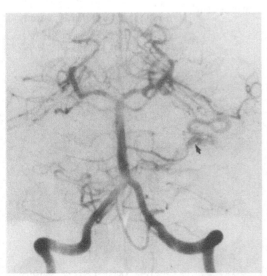 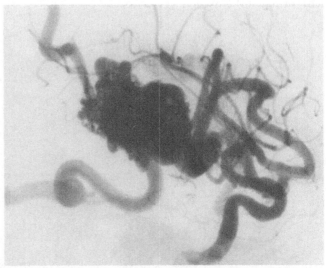

1.1   1.2

Fig. 1.1. Vertebral angiography in frontal view. Microarteriovenous malformation at the level of the left flocculus (*arrow*)

Fig. 1.2. Right internal carotid injection in lateral view. Temporal (T-2) arteriovenous malformation draining into cortical veins

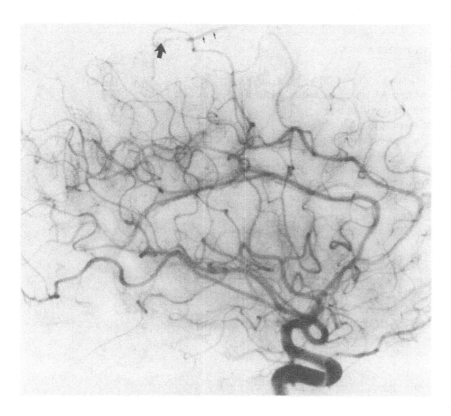

Fig. 1.3. Right internal carotid injection in lateral view. Micro-arteriovenous fistula of the upper frontal convexity (*arrow*). Note the normal sized draining vein (*small arrows*)

Compartments can be observed within the lesions either during angiography or surgery (see "Multiple BAVMs"). AVFs may also be of the micro- (Fig. 1.3) or macrotype (Fig. 1.4). In the same lesion one may find both micro-AVFs or macro-AVFs and micro-AVMs and macro-AVMs (Fig. 1.5).

AVMs and AVFs represent the two basic forms of arteriovenous shunts that can be encountered throughout the CNS. Theoretically, all combinations of types, sizes, flow patterns, and topographies can be seen, but AVFs (micro- or macro-) have only been encountered on the brain or spinal cord

Fig. 1.5. **A** Right internal carotid injection in lateral view. **B, C, and D** three separated superselective injections into the corresponding feeders to the arteriovenous malformation. Note the different types of arteriovenous shunts within the same nidus: **B** direct supply (*arrowhead*), **C** indirect supply and shunt (*double arrowhead*), and **D** direct fistula (*triple arrowhead*)

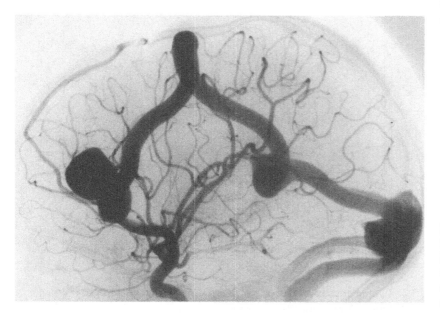

Fig. 1.4. Left internal carotid injection in lateral view. Single-hole pial arteriovenous fistula draining into a medial hemispheric vein and the straight sinus

surfaces. AVFs are relatively rare and were seen in only 2% of our patients (Berenstein et al. 1990), mainly in children (see Chap. 5).

Association of the different types of CVMs (arterial, arteriovenous, capillary and/or venous), mentioned by Rubinstein to be present at pathology, has not been seen by us.

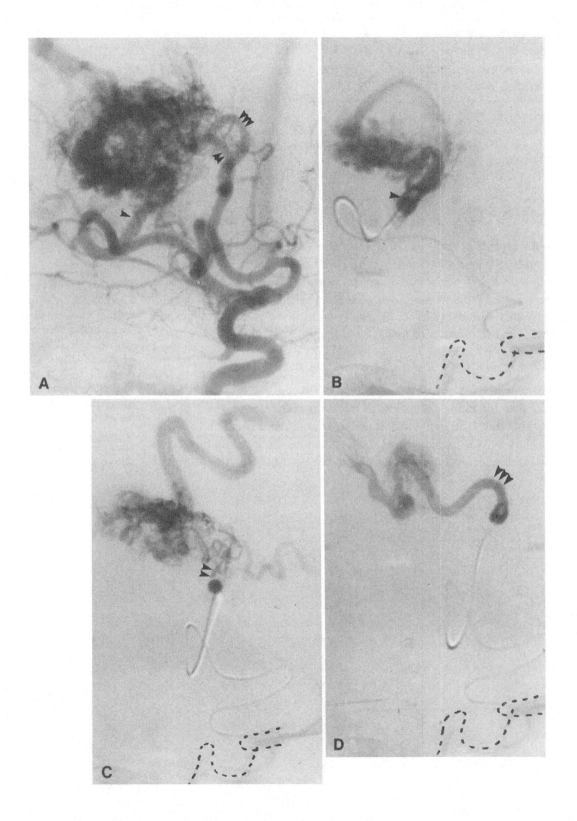

Table 1.8. Multifocal AVMs

Population	All ages (n = 390)			Children only (n = 98)	
Multiple AVMs	Incidence		Repartition	Incidence	
	n	%	%	n	%
Rendu-Osler-Weber disease	9	2.3	25.7	1	0.8
Wyburn-Mason syndrome	4	1	11.4	3	3.1
Dural shunt (remote pial shunts)	3	0.8	8.6	3	3.1
Unclassified, multifocal	19	4.9	44.3	8	8.2

Arteriovenous malformation.
If 40 patients with vein of Galen aneurysmal malformations (VGAMs) are excluded the incidence of multifocal AVMs in children rises to 25.8%. From Bicêtre 1980–1990 (unpublished data).

3. Multiple BAVMs (Table 1.8)

The occurrence of multiple BAVMs is rare (3% among 500 patients in Yasargil's 1987 series). Willinsky et al. (1990a) found a 10% incidence of multiple AVMs, in our population of patients. In this heterogeneous group three types of patients were identified (Table 1.7): (a) those with Rendu-Osler-Weber disease (ROW), (b) those with Wyburn-Mason syndrome (WMS), and (c) those with unclassified multiple lesions.

a) Rendu-Osler-Weber Disease

ROW represents 25% of the multifocal AVMs in our series. These are predominantly young patients (half of them less than 16 years of age) presenting with CNS symptoms related to arteriovenous shunt and a family history of ROW. Angiography of the CNS lesions disclosed multiple areas of shunting and, most of the time, multiple AVFs of the high-flow type with

Fig. 1.6 A, B. Multiple, single-hole, high-flow arteriovenous fistulas (AVFs) in a child presenting with a familial history of Rendu-Osler-Weber disease. **A** Right and **B** left internal carotid injections. Each posterior cerebral artery supplies a high-flow AVF (*single and double arrowheads*) and each drains into a separate ectatic venous pouch
▼

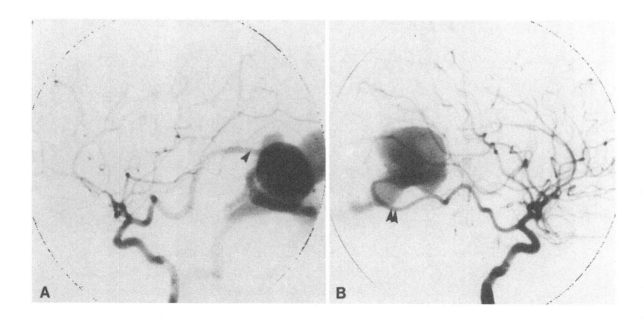

Fig. 1.7. Vertebral artery injection in lateral view in a patient presenting with a familial history of Rendu-Osler-Weber disease. Note the three micro- and macro-niduses (*arrows*). Previous surgical clips indicate direct surgical approach to cerebral abscess related to septic emboli from an associated pulmonary arteriovenous shunt

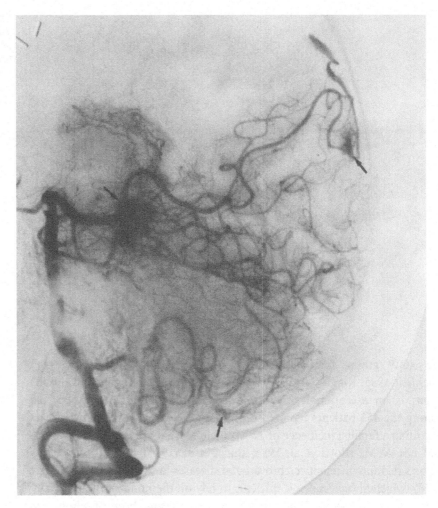

venous pouches (Boynton and Morgan 1973) (Fig. 1.6). The remaining CNS vascular lesions were of the small (<3 cm) nidus type (Fig. 1.7). Few patients had presented with a history of nose or GI bleeding. None of our patients evaluated for ROW with epistaxis developed a CVM during follow-up. CVMs in systemic diseases were seldom symptomatic, as well as other locations in multifocal AVMs. All CNS AVMs were discovered during the initial workup in these patients. Roman et al. (1978) found that 28% of ROW patients had cerebral AVMs, whereas 8% had spinal cord lesions.

The diagnosis of ROW in a patient with single or multifocal AVMs is not based on the CNS location or angioarchitectural characteristics. BAVMs in ROW patients look exactly like those in other patients with single or multiple lesions that do not present with the remaining ROW systemic and familial manifestations (Fig. 1.8). Therefore, the diagnosis is based on the family history and/or the cutaneous and mucous membrane manifestations (see Vol. 2, Chaps. 9, 10). There is no hereditary transmission of the specific lesion topography: ROW families with one member having multifocal CNS AVMs do not have a significantly higher incidence of identical CNS lesions in other generations. Furthermore, based only on clinical history, it is impossible to differentiate between an acute complication of a pulmonary AVF and an acute manifestation of an associated cerebral AVM. Outside

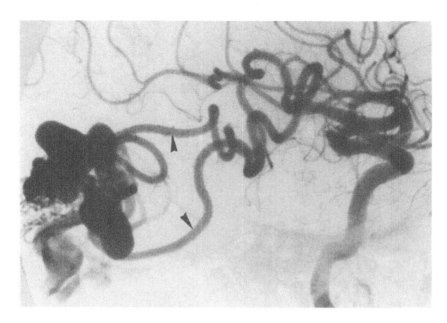

Fig. 1.8. Right internal carotid injection in lateral view. Patient presented with a familial history of Rendu-Osler-Weber disease. Note the high-flow type of lesion, with converging fistulas (*arrowheads*) into a posterior temporal draining vein

the ROW group, familial incidence of cerebral AVM(s) (Zellem and Buchheit 1985; King et al. 1977) remains a controversial issue and, in any event, is an exceptional situation since no familial incidence occurred among the 453 patients reported on by Perret et al. (1966). Many reports regarding a familial incidence of AVMs include what are in fact cavernomas and not AVMs (Boyd et al. 1985; Bucci et al. 1986). In addition, many reports regroup different cerebrovascular diseases in the same family (Barre 1978), which always makes it difficult to rely on the nonangiographic confirmation of the AVM. Similarly, we saw two cousins, both of whom had VGAMs (Lasjaunias et al. 1989), but one died 15 years ago in the neonatal period and complete records are missing, making firm conclusions impossible. We have also seen two monozygotic twins, one has a VGAM, and the other has not (Berenstein 1989, presented at the ASNR 1989).

Finally, in our experience of patients with multifocal lesions either with or without ROW, a CNS AVM in the same family was probably fortuitous. Specifically, in ROW patients, it is not even obvious that the CNS AVMs are part of the telangiectatic disease; they could be either an associated type of vascular lesion or represent early (in utero) expression of the disease. Therefore treatment of these AVMs or AVFs should be undertaken as if no additional lesion was to appear. Incidentally, the few patients with recurrent AVMs in other locations were not those with ROW. The secondary development of telangiectasias corresponds to a hereditary disorder of capillary angiogenesis, revealing with age an abnormal capillary regeneration which is often (but not always) symptomatic.

b) Wyburn-Mason Syndrome

Wyburn-Mason (1943a) or Bonnet's syndrome is an AVM of one or both sides of the brain. It associates ipsilateral or bilateral AVMs with vascular anomalies of the retina and multiple cutaneous nevi. Theron et al. (1974) reviewed a series of 25 such patients and referred to this entity as a unilateral retinocephalic vascular malformation. The lesion in all but three of his patients involved the optic nerve. The AVM closely follows the visual pathways and extends to the thalamus and hypothalamus. The nidus may be compact or separated by noninvolved normal brain, constituting multifocal AVMs along the optic pathways (Fig. 1.9). Treatment is particularly challenging (Morgan et al. 1985). We have managed six patients with WMS, two of whom were blind.

Different types of lesions can be described depending on the amount of territory involved (from face to calcarine fissure) but not on the continuity of the nidus. Symptoms are the same as in other single AVMS (hemorrhage, seizures, etc.). Other multifocal AVMs which associate facial and cerebral AVMs in a less systematic fashion (Haniech et al. 1981; Smith and Donat 1981) probably constitute a transitional form between ROW and WMS (polymorphic involvement in the vascular system and multifocality in the craniocerebral region; Fig. 1.10). However, this group should be distinguished from AVMs with associated arterial aneurysm. In such patients, almost three-quarters of the aneurysms are flow-related. The remaining one-quarter of arterial aneurysms that are not flow-related (Lasjaunias et al. 1988; Voigt et al. 1973; Noterman et al. 1987) are difficult to relate to any known dysplasia (vide infra).

c) Nonsystematized Multifocal CNS AVMs

Multiple AVMs are the subject of numerous case reports and a few series (Willinsky et al. 1990a). Despite the frequency with which the subject is mentioned, the anecdotal data and confusing descriptions make review of these cases laborious. The difficulty is particularly acute in ascertaining the association, if any, between CNS AVMs and other cryptic, occult, or dural lesions (Schlachter et al. 1980; Tada et al. 1986; Hash et al. 1975). Indeed, the capacity to diagnose multifocal lesions depends largely on the quality of the imaging protocol performed, its completeness, and the selectivity achieved. High standards of imaging are required particularly to disclose micro-AVMs (Nakayama 1989; Willinsky et al. 1990a). Although the ability of MRI to discern additional lesions is higher than that of CT, it has been our observation that most lesions not seen on CT were also MRI occult and were only demonstrated by high-quality angiography (Fig. 1.11). The association between spinal cord and BAVMs in adults or children is rare; even in ROW it is unusual (Mazza et al. 1989; Parkinson and West 1977; Hoffman et al. 1976).

The association between tumors and AVMs (Goodkin et al. 1990; Chovanes and Truex 1987) raises the question of the role of growth factors and angiogenic activity. Furthermore, are some or all of the so-called congenital cerebral AVMs actually acquired? If so, can some of them develop after birth?

It is difficult today to answer these questions but the existence of false multifocal AVMs may contribute to this discussion. The only feature on which diagnosis of AVM depends is evidence of an arteriovenous shunt. Depending on the imaging modality chosen and skill of the diagnostician, the diagnosis of an AVM, especially if small, can become a difficult exercise in evaluation. Gabrielsen and Heinz (1969) showed that cortical arteriovenous shunts may open following venous thrombosis. We have observed such AVM-like shunting several times, either at the dural level or at the pial or transcerebral venous level (Willinsky et al. 1990a) (Fig. 1.12). In addition to

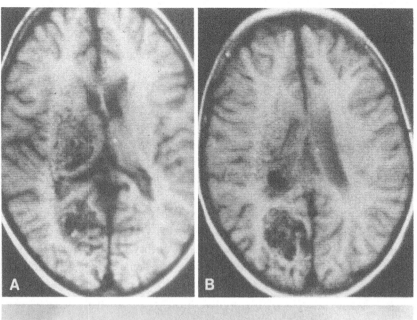

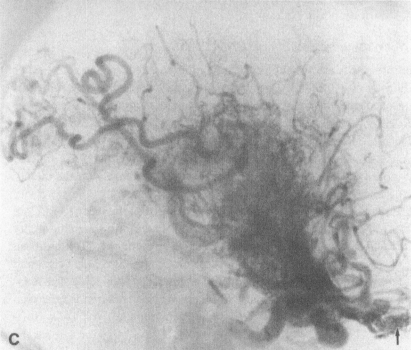

Fig. 1.9 A–E. Arteriovenous malformation in a child with Wyburn-Mason syndrome. **A** and **B** T1-weighted MRI, axial cuts, demonstrating the apparent discontinuity between the diencephalic and occipital location of the lesion. **C** Right internal carotid injection in early and **D** late phases. Note the extensive aspect of the diencephalic nidus, the optic nerve location (*arrow* in **C**), and the separate precuneus nidus. **E** Vertebral injection in lateral view. Note the separate supply of the thalamic and occipital lesions

lesions which may mimic AVMs, one can postulate that some multifocal AVMs may have both a hereditary and an acquired nidus. Further study of such a presumed association may not be possible and the pathological nature and evolution of the secondary arteriovenous shunt unknown. False multifocal lesions may also correspond to compartmented AVMs. A careful search for specific venous drainage and an interval of normal tissue will eliminate most of these mimics of multifocal AVMs.

Finally, the association of AVMs with cavernomas remains possible, as seen in some reported cases. Cryptic lesions and occult malformations refer to an unclear concept which cannot be properly covered here (see Occult and Cryptic Malformations). The association of an AVM with a DVA is

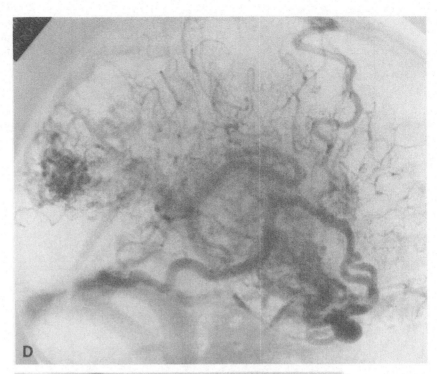

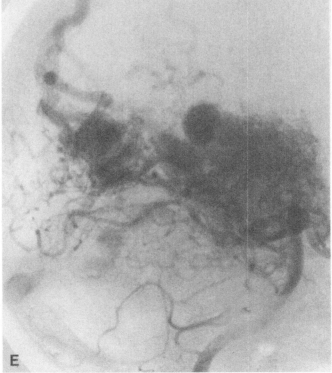

equivalent to any association of an AVM and another vascular anomaly (see Vol. 3, Chap. 7). Several case reports have pointed to so-called recurrent AVMs in different locations. Unfortunately, the angiographic analysis prior to surgery was often incomplete. Therefore one can postulate that most cases involved either misdiagnosed multiple AVMs or incompletely removed AVMs.

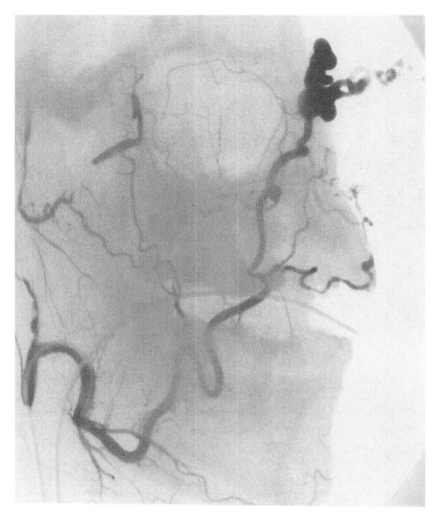

Fig. 1.10 A–C. Associated facial and cerebral arteriovenous malformation (AVM). **A** Right facial artery injection. **B** Left and **C** right internal carotid artery angiograms in lateral view. The hypothalamic AVM (*arrows*) drains into the basal vein (*curved arrows*)

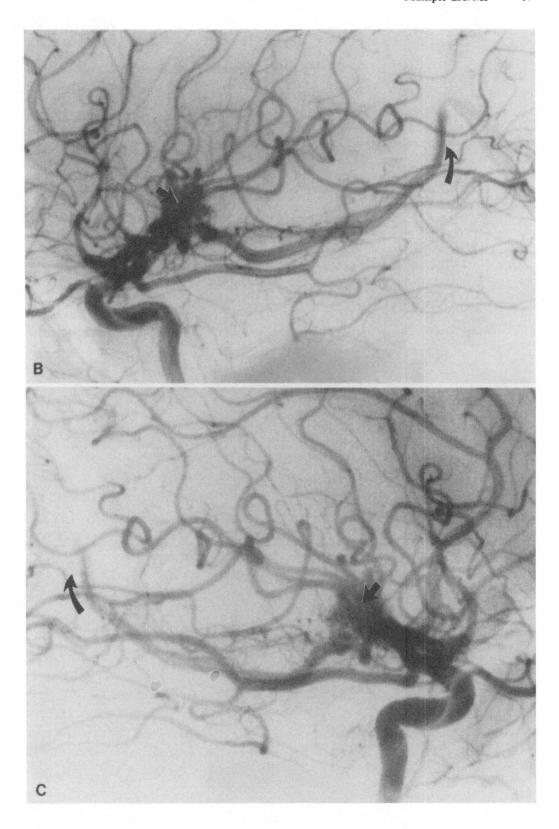

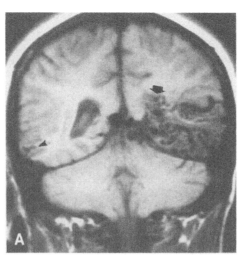

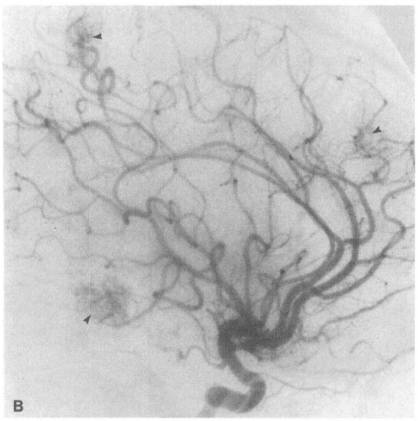

Fig. 1.11 A, B. Multiple arteriovenous malformations (AVMs) in a child presenting with a protein S deficiency. **A** Coronal MRI demonstrating a large, left temporal, AVM (*arrow*) and a small right temporal lesion (*arrowhead*). **B** Right internal carotid injection demonstrates three cordical AVMs (*arrowheads*) that were MRI occult; a total of six separate AVM nidi were demonstrated during angiography

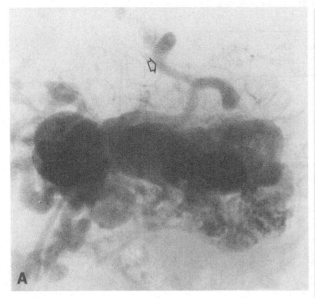

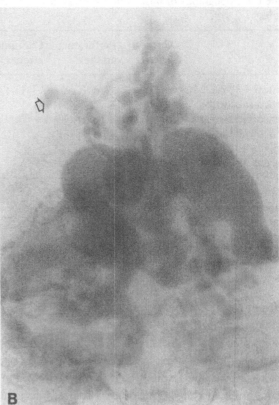

Fig. 1.12 A–D. Temporal arteriovenous malformation (AVM) with multiple venous constraints. (Same patient as in Fig. 2.5.) **A** Right internal carotid artery injection in lateral and **B** frontal projections in a patient with a large, temporal AVM with multiple venous constraints. Bilateral ectatic veins reroute the venous drainage into the transcerebral venous system (*open arrow*)

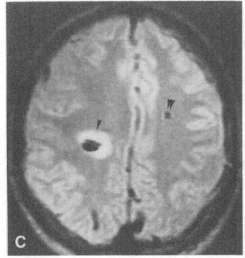

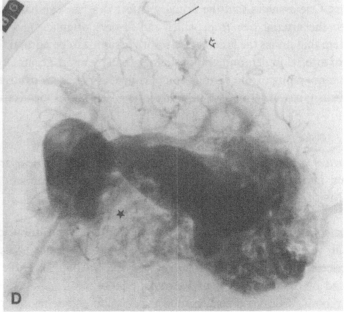

C Axial MRI demonstrates the enlarged transcerebral venous drainage on the left (*arrowhead*) and the perivenous increased signal on the right (*double arrowheads*). **D** Right internal carotid injection in midarterial phase following partial embolization of the AVM. Decrease of the venous congestion has led to disappearance of several venous pouches (*star*) and decrease of the transcerebral venous drainage. Note the associated arteriovenous shunt (*open arrow*) draining into a small transcerebral vein (*arrow*) previously not visualized during the screening angiogram. This shunt could not be demonstrated in a follow-up study and was therefore felt to correspond to a secondary nonmalformed arteriovenous communication

Table 1.9. Topography of intracranial arteriovenous lesions and gross vascular territories

	Cortical arteries	Perforating arteries	Choroidal arteries	Deep veins	Superficial veins
Cortical	+	−	−	−	+
Cortico-subcortical	+	−	−	− [b]	+
Cortico-ventricular	+	+ [a]	+ [a]	+	+
Cortico-callosal	+	−	+ [a]	+	+
Deep-seated	+ [c]	+	−	+	+ [b]
Choroid plexus	−	+ [a]	+	+	+ [b]

+, Involved; −, noninvolved.
[a] Subependymal arterial anastomosis or branches can be seen.
[b] Can be recruited via transcerebral veins.
[c] Insular and cerebellar.

4. Topographic Analysis

Topographic location of an AVM (Table 1.9) is best assessed by combining the information conveyed by angiography and MRI and/or CT. Some additional angiographic findings help in determining the different types of lesion and in increasing suspicion of associated or acquired changes. Lesions in most locations recruit predictable arterial feeders and specific draining veins. One assumes that the primary defect is at the capillary level. Thus, both the arterial tree from which the feeders originate and the venous system that drains the lesion are, a priori, assumed to be normal. The analysis of arterial feeders and venous drainage can therefore accurately delineate the topography of the various compartments or niduses involved. Several general types of lesion can be differentiated based on localization.

a) Lesions That Reach the Cortex

Cortical arteriovenous lesions are exclusively fed by cortical arteries and drain into superficial veins. These lesions (Fig. 1.13) represent the sulcal AVMs of Valavanis (1990, personal communication).

Cortico-subcortical lesions recruit cortical arteries and drain into superficial veins but may also drain into the deep venous system if the transcerebral venous system is patent (see Vol. 3, Chap. 7). These are represented by the gyral AVMs of Valavanis (1990).

In both cortical and cortico-subcortical lesions, some regions of the cortex drain to deeply located veins that should not be considered as truly part of the "deep venous system". Such vessels include the medial veins of the temporal lobe and the basal vein, the veins of the cerebellar vermis, and the precentral vein (see Vol. 3, Chap. 7) (Fig. 1.14).

Cortico-ventricular arteriovenous lesions correspond to the classical pyramidal shaped malformation, reaching the ventricular wall at their apex. Feeding arteries are both perforating and cortical. Draining veins are also deeply and superficially located (Fig. 1.15).

Fig. 1.13. Right internal carotid artery injection in lateral view in a patient with a temporopolar arteriovenous malformation draining into cortical veins

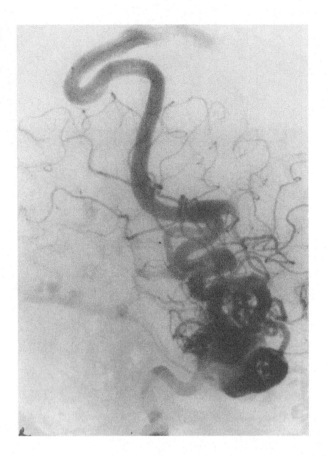

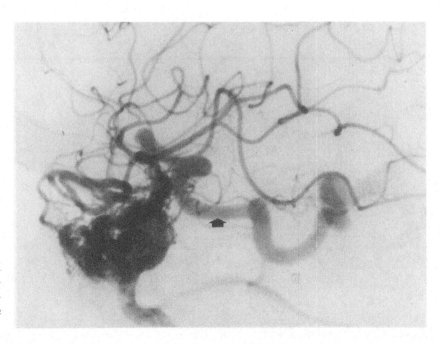

Fig. 1.14. Left internal carotid injection in lateral view in a patient with a cortical temporomedial lesion draining into the basal vein (*arrow*)

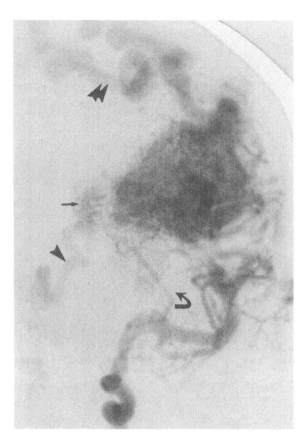

Fig. 1.15. Cortico-ventricular arteriovenous malformation (AVM). Left internal carotid injection in frontal view. Note the ventricular extension (*arrow*). The lesion is fed by cortical and lenticulostriate arteries (*broken arrow*) and drains into both cortical (*double arrowhead*) and subependymal and ventricular veins (*arrowhead*)

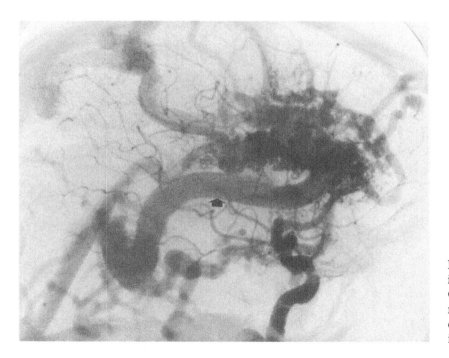

Fig. 1.16. Right internal carotid injection in lateral projection. Corpus callosum arteriovenous malformation draining into medial cortical vein and septal and internal cerebral veins (*arrow*)

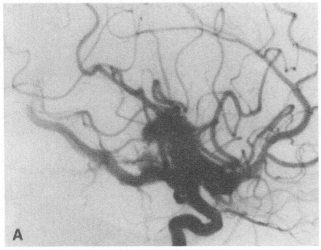

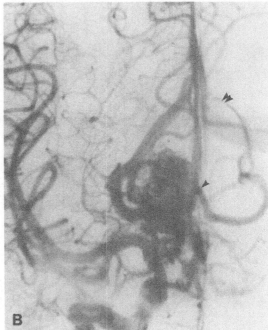

Fig. 1.17A, B. Ventral thalamic and hypothalamic arteriovenous malformation (AVM). **A** Lateral and **B** frontal projections of the right internal carotid artery. The AVM is draining into the basal vein on the right side, and on the left side via the anterior communicating vein (*arrowhead*). Note the tentorial sinus on the left side (*double arrowhead*). Also see Fig. 1.10

Cortico-callosal lesions belong to the cortico-ventricular group, as they present the same venous characteristics but do not recruit "perforating" arteries. They drain into the subependymal veins and later into the deep venous system (Fig. 1.16). The arterial supply to the corpus callosum is linked to the cortical arterial network, even though it may simulate perforating arterial channels (in the supraoptic region), and to choroidal arteries at the splenium.

b) Deep-Seated Arteriovenous Lesions

Deep-seated lesions can be located supra- or infratentorially in the depth of the telencephalon, diencephalon, brainstem, or cerebellum (Fig. 1.17). Their niduses involve the deep nuclei and the long fiber tracts with their arterial and venous connections. They recruit exclusively perforating arteries and drain into the deep venous system. They may use transcerebral veins if patent, either as a direct venous outlet (Fig. 1.18) or as a collateral pathway. Transcortical arteries from the insular branches of the middle cerebral artery and the hemispheric collaterals of the cerebellar arteries can be involved in lenticulostriate nucleus and in dentate nucleus arteriovenous lesions, respectively (Fig. 1.19). Prior to angiography, MRI usually allows differentiation of these deep-seated lesions from cortico-subcortical lesions, particularly since the dominant supply of the intracerebrally located deep lesions arises from the perforators. Therefore, except for the above mentioned locations, a cortical arterial supply is not seen in the deep-seated lesions.

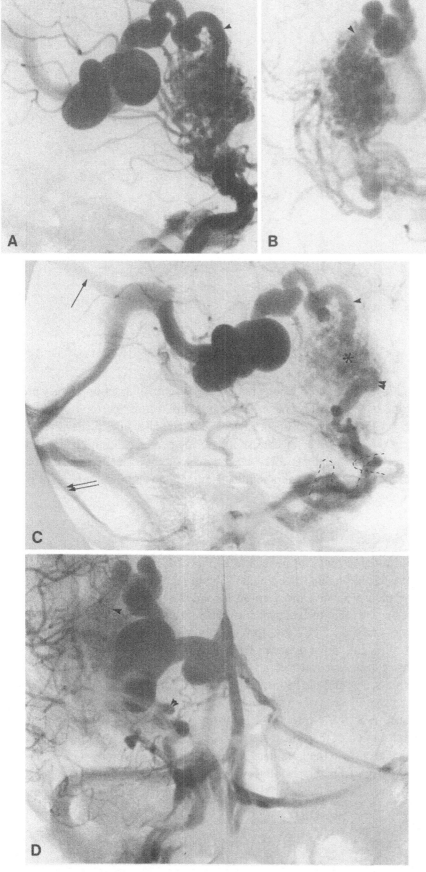

Fig. 1.18 A–D. Lenticular nucleus arteriovenous malformation (AVM). **A** Lateral and **B** frontal views of the right internal carotid artery in early phase. **C** Lateral and **D** frontal projections in venous phase. Lenticular nucleus AVM (*asterisk* in **C**) fed by lenticulostriate arteries and insular perforators. The lesion is seating on the interstriate draining system. It drains into the superior striate (*arrowhead*) and atrial veins, inferior striate vein (*double arrowhead*), and into the deep middle cerebral vein and cavernous sinus inferiorly. Note the venous ectasias at the subependymal junction and the persistence of falcine (*arrow*) and occipital (*double arrow*) sinuses

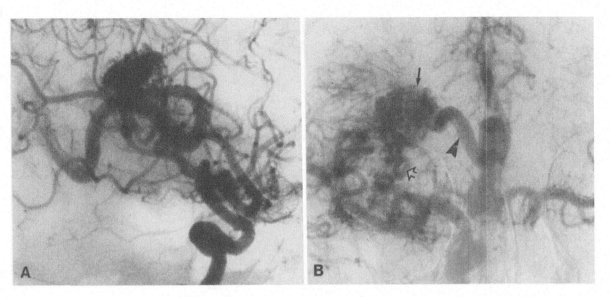

Fig. 1.19 A, B. Deep-seated arteriovenous malformation (AVM). **A** Lateral and **B** frontal views of the right internal carotid artery injection. Deep-seated AVM (*arrow*) supplied by lenticulostriate arteries (*open arrow*) and draining exclusively into thalamostriate and internal cerebral veins (*arrowhead*)

c) Choroid Plexus Arteriovenous Lesions

Choroid plexus AVMs are difficult but important to recognize due to their extracerebral nature and their surgical accessibility (Fig. 1.20). They are fed primarily by choroidal arteries and subependymal arterial feeders arising from the circle of Willis, including arteries arising from the basilar tip and coursing through the walls of the third ventricle to reach its roof and the choroid fissure (Fig. 1.21). Drainage is via ventricular veins, with occasional recruitment of transcerebral veins when patent. A cortical arterial supply is excluded in this type of lesion.

5. Angioarchitecture

Analysis of the angioarchitecture (Table 1.10) of BAVMs permits anatomical study of the various portions of the lesion (arteries, nidus, and veins) and shows how these portions relate to the rest of the circulation. It discloses their original disposition and outlines some of the differences between the primary defect and acquired features. From these uni- or multifocal, developmental, vascular malformations, additional arterial and venous patterns will be grafted onto the remaining vascular system (host) in response to the chronic shunting. Some of the vascular patterns are due to associated anatomical variations that provoke a predictable change (dural agenesis and vein of Galen ectasias) (Fig. 5.22); others are acquired and are related either to the high-flow character of the lesion (kinking, plications, arterial aneurysms, etc.) or the development of secondary obstacles (stenosis, venous ectasias) (Fig. 1.18) or both (Fig. 1.28). The high-flow hemodynamics or decreased tissue perfusion associated with AVM shunting can stimulate nonsprouting angiogenesis (Folkman 1986) and development

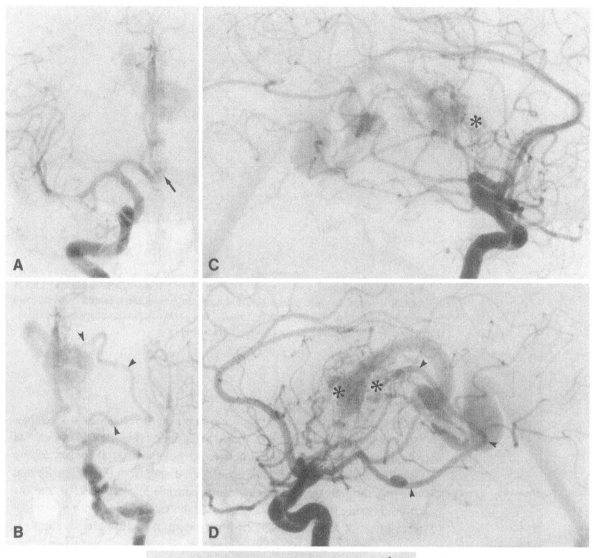

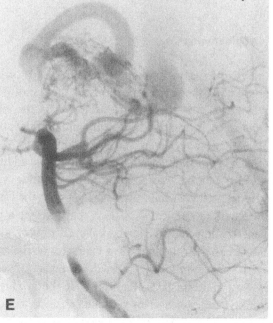

Fig. 1.20 A–E. Third ventricle choroid plexus arteriovenous malformation (AVM). **A** Frontal and **B** lateral views of the right internal carotid artery. **C** Frontal and **D** lateral projections of the left internal carotid artery. **E** Vertebral artery injection in lateral view. Third ventricle choroid plexus AVM (*asterisks*) draining into the choroidal vein and vein of Galen. All choroidal arteries participate in the supply to this lesion, including subependymal perforators arising from the circle of Willis, anterior communicating hypothalamic perforators (*arrow*), and the anterior choroidal artery (*arrowheads*)

Fig. 1.21 A–C. Transmesencephalic supply in a tectal arteriovenous malformation (AVM). **A** Axial MRI study demonstrates the transmesencephalic supply (*arrowhead*) to a tectal AVM. **B** Frontal and **C** lateral views of the left vertebral artery injection in a different patient, demonstrating a thalamo-perforating artery supplying a thalamic AVM and projecting above the mesencephalic region (*double arrowhead*)

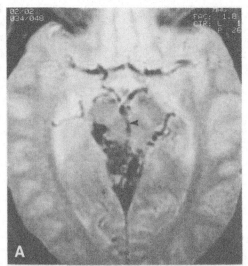

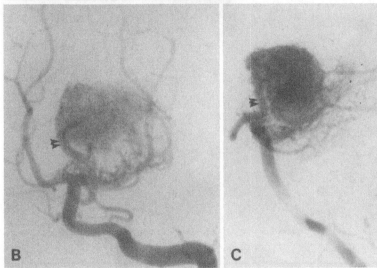

Table 1.10. Cerebral arteriovenous malformations: elements of angioarchitecture

Arteries	Nidus	Veins
Direct feeder	Size	Variations: cortical and
Indirect feeder	AV communication	dural types
Stenotic segments	Pouches	Stenosis
Dural supply		Thrombosis
Leptomeningeal anastomoses		Kinkings
Variations		Ectasias
Aneurysms		Calcifications
Flow-related		
Dysplastic		

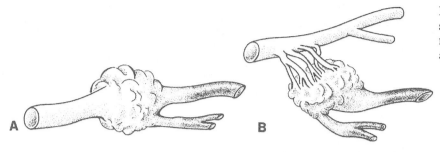

Fig. 1.22. Two types of arterial supply to an arteriovenous malformation nidus: **A** direct and **B** "en passage"

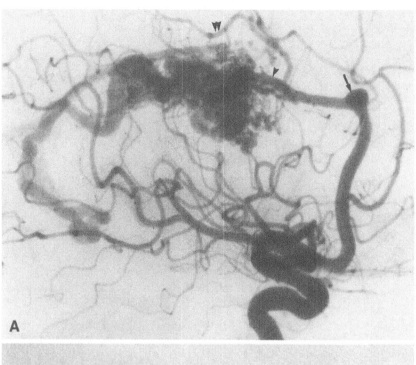

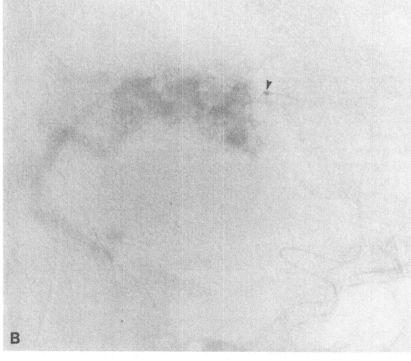

Fig. 1.23. Left internal carotid injection before (**A**), during (**B**), and after (**C**) partial embolization with IBCA. Note the preexisting direct (*arrowhead*) and indirect (*double arrowhead*) supply, and the proximal, flow-related, arterial aneurysm (*arrow*). Following embolization (**C**), the nidus is partially excluded. The "en passage" supply is well demonstrated. The shape of the aneurysm is slightly different. Further embolization will later exclude the lesion entirely. The aneurysm will not be treated and will disappear completely. The overall procedure was uneventful

of collateral circulation with morphological changes which may be reversible after elimination of the shunt (Fig. 1.24). Additional local or regional rearrangements are observed in the evolution of complications (hemorrhagic or ischemic). Thrombosis of a draining vein at the time of bleeding (Fig. 1.50), development of external carotid supply (Fig. 1.37), or intralesional pouches may be present (Fig. 1.42) at a specific moment. Full evaluation requires the understanding of various factors, including angiogenic reactions, recanalization of thrombosed channels, and organization of hematomas (Figs. 1.48, 1.52–1.54). These and other factors can result in misinterpretation of the size of the malformation and its topography if not properly considered. Some other factors are more difficult to comprehend, for example, progressive arterial stenosis reproducing a moyamoya disease type disposition, and will be dealt with in detail in the section.

Associated parenchymal and CSF space changes (Figs. 1.67, 5.4) may express location distortion caused by the abnormal hydrodynamic conditions or mechanical stress from vascular outlets of the lesion (Figs. 1.30, 5.5).

It is in allowing the anticipation of potential biological behavior and in aiding establishment of an ideal therapeutic objective (see Chap. 3 and Chap. 4), that this angioarchitectural analysis will show its full advantages. This will be discussed further in the following chapter.

a) Arterial Supply

Arterial feeders in arteriovenous shunts can be of different types: (1) *direct* feeders supply the shunting area as a "terminal" branch. (2) *Indirect* feeders supply the shunting area "en passage," i.e., they predominantly supply the normal territories and only secondarily the shunt (Fig. 1.22). Indirect feeders may arise from the chronic "sump" effect of the lesion. As the sump effect increases, indirect feeders can become more involved in the AVM

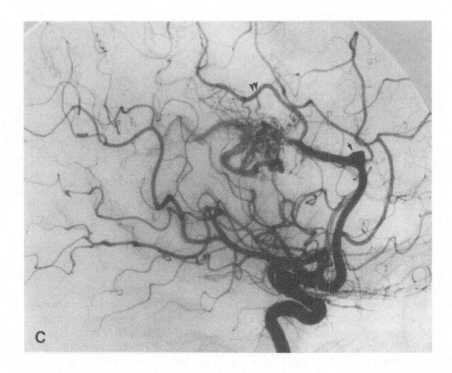

c

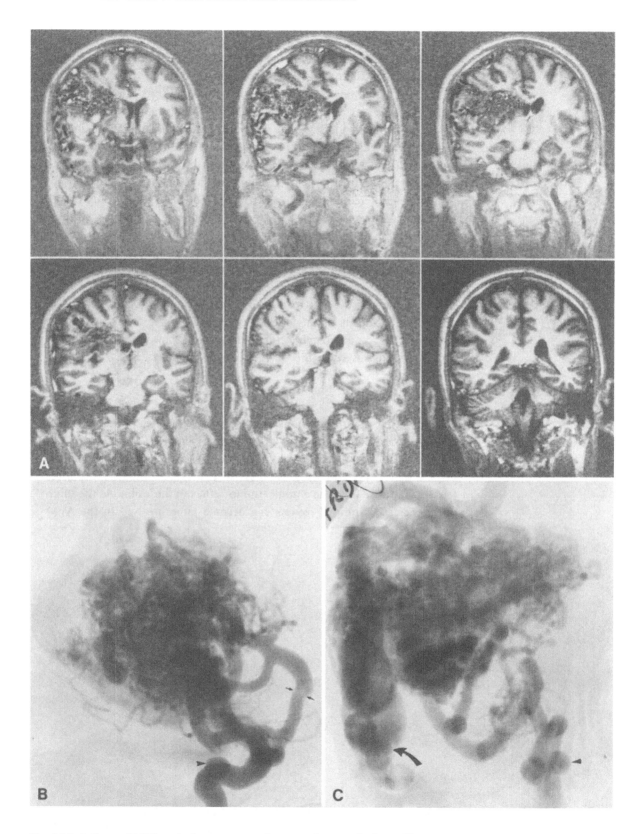

Fig. 1.24. A Coronal MRI study demonstrates a large cortico-ventricular malformation in the upper convexity of the right hemisphere, with deep extension and mass effect on the ventricular system. Note the absence of an arteriovenous malformation (AVM) in the anterior-middle cerebral watershed area. **B** Lateral and **C** frontal views of the right internal carotid artery. **D** Frontal and **E** lateral projections of the left internal carotid artery. Note the architecture of this large frontal AVM of the cor-

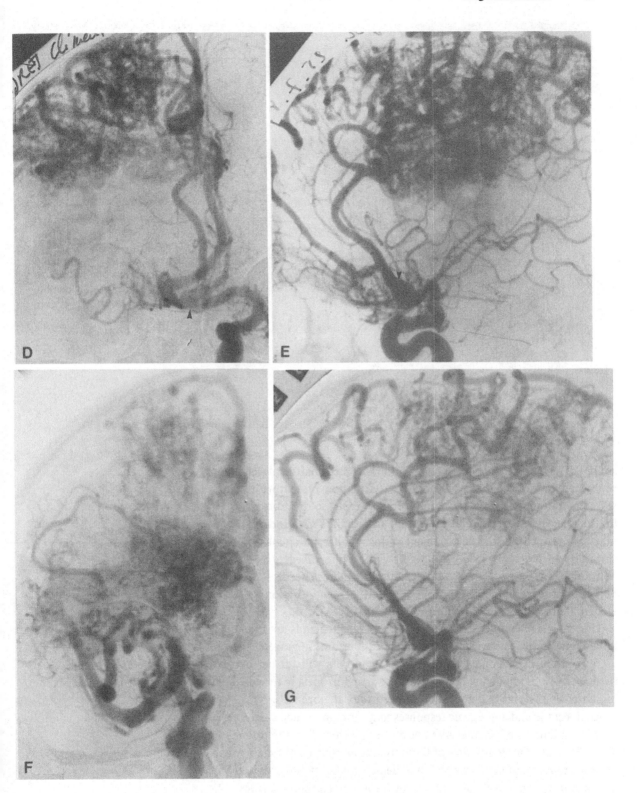

tico-ventricular type, with multiple flow-related changes: arterial stenosis (*arrows*) and aneurysms (*arrowhead*), venous ectasia (*curved arrow*), opposite side non-sprouting leptomeningeal angiogenesis with no evidence of arteriovenous communication in the upper frontal region (**D** and **E**). **F** Frontal and **G** lateral views of the left internal carotid after embolization of the right cortical feeders, with significant reduction of the nidus. Note the regression in the leptomeningeal circulation. It demonstrates that the upper frontal network did not correspond to an extension of the nidus but to a secondary regressive phenomenon (nonsprouting angiogenesis) which responded favorably following diminution of the pathological shunt

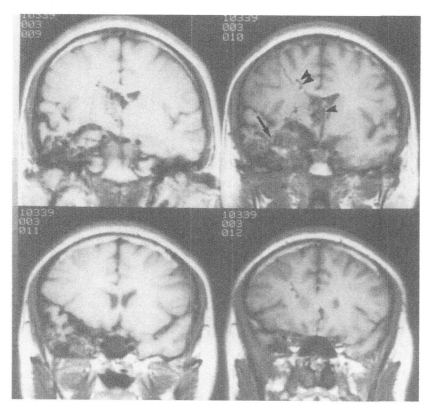

Fig. 1.25. Coronal MRI study in a patient with a temporal lobe arteriovenous malformation (AVM) (*arrow*). Note the intraventricular nidus (*arrowhead*) associated with the temporal lesion which is not in continuity. Note the transcerebral venous drainage (*double arrowhead*) of this additional arteriovenous shunting zone. This associated "lesion" was felt to correspond to a posthemorrhagic subependymal and intraventricular sprouting angiogenesis. Although speculative, this aspect of the nidus did not correspond to any of the architecture usually demonstrated in brain AVMs, even in multiple lesions

supply. They will then be responsible for the proximal displacement of watershed areas. Both direct and indirect feeders may present with stenotic segments (although apparently more often in the case of indirect feeders) that further increase collateral circulation around the AVM. Indirect supply may also result from the development of local collateral circulation (nonsprouting angiogenesis) reconstituting flow into a direct feeder (see Chap. 5, Vein of Galen Aneurysmal Malformation). Indirect feeders may also become more prominent following ligation or embolization of direct feeders if the nidus is not completely occluded (Fig. 1.23).

The various phenomena that increase rheologic demands are fundamentally angioectatic. These same phenomena can become angiogenic as soon as they produce ischemia. Stenosis of AVM feeders will further decrease tissue perfusion, producing or aggravating existing hypoxia in the surrounding parenchyma and thereby stimulating further angiogenesis.

Angioectatic and angiogenic responses may develop to such a degree that they can mimic an additional AVM or an "enlargement" of the primary lesion (Fig. 1.24). Differentiation of these conditions may be difficult. Angiogenesis (nonsprouting) is observed in ischemic regions at pathology and are also a normal feature of an organizing thrombus (sprouting) (Figs. 1.25, 1.52). Yasargil (1987), quoting Virchow and Hamby, observed perilesional angiogenesis. Dobbelare et al. (1979) and Laine et al. (1981) noted that both evolving and recurrent AVMs often present with the same architectural aspect, a dense capillary bed with no special venous character. Although the changes seem related to neovascularization, there is no in vitro growth.

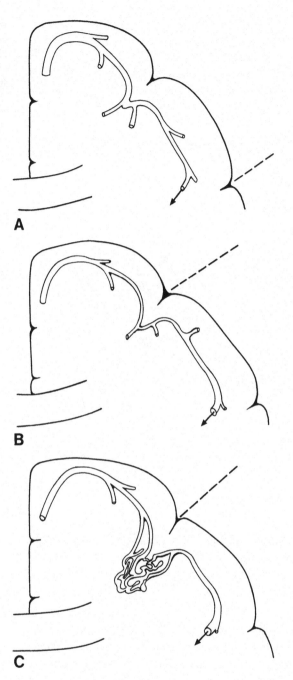

Fig. 1.26 A–C. Watershed transfer in brain arteriovenous malformations (BAVMs). The three stages in the transfer of the watershed (*interrupted line*) in cerebral BAVMs. **A** Congenital transfer of the watershed, as demonstrated by the harmonious decrease in the caliber of the cortical arteries (see Fig. 1.27). **B** Secondary transfer of the watershed demonstrated by the decrease and increase in cortical artery caliber (see Fig. 1.28). **C** Secondary transfer of the watershed zone with postischemic nonsprouting angiogenesis (see Figs. 1.24 and 1.29) at the watershed level

A

B

C

Arterial Enlargement

Arterial enlargement is a purely hemodynamic phenomenon that stimulates natural (anatomically preexisting) channels to supply both the lesion itself and adjacent territories (Figs. 1.26–1.29). Within the CNS, such enlargement corresponds to recruitment of leptomeningeal and subependymal anastomoses. The hemodynamic demands of the lesion interfere with the development of an arterial supply to normal brain and may result in the persistence of embryonic vascular arrangements (see Chap. 5, Vein of Galen, Aneurysmal Malformation).

Adventitial capillary proliferation is part of the constellation of findings constituting "the high-flow angiopathy" (Pile-Spellman et al. 1986) (Table 1.11). Some of these features of "induced" angiogenesis can regress

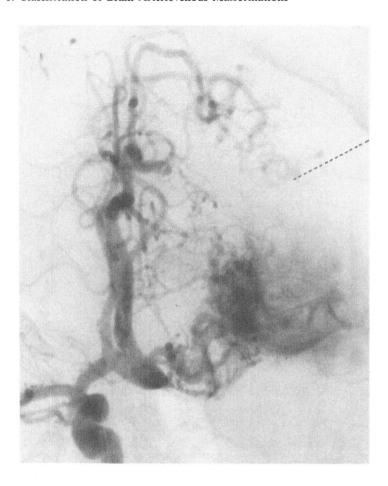

Fig. 1.27. Right internal carotid artery injection in frontal view. High-flow left frontal arteriovenous malformation demonstrating congenital transfer of the watershed area of the anterior-middle cerebral artery territories (*interrupted line*)

following occlusion of the dominant shunt (Fig. 3.26). However, this benefit is hardly predictable. Failure to completely occlude a dominant shunt will most often transform such an accessory supply into a significant supply.

Stenotic Changes

Stenosis of feeders to vascular malformations is also seen as part of the high-flow angiopathy (Table 1.11). Any quantitative relationship between the degree of stenosis and that of the shunt is, however, difficult to establish. Changes of concentric narrowing by intraluminal protrusion of the endothelial cells, mesenchymal cell proliferation, and thinning of the wall may result in intraluminal stenosis (Fig. 1.28). MacCormick (1962–1966) described arteries with wall thinning to the extent that it was possible to directly visualize blood flowing through them (commonly observed at surgery). In our series (Willinsky 1988), there was a 17% incidence of arterial stenosis.

Rarely, arterial stenosis is extrinsic (bony or dural compression, venous compression, etc.). Stenosis can be reversible if the external mechanical constraint is relieved. Extrinsic narrowing is usually encountered in high-flow lesions with mass effect (Fig. 1.30).

"Spontaneous" rupture of an AVM during diagnostic angiography has been reported (Tsementzis et al. 1984) and observed once in our series.

Other caliber irregularities, creating a pseudoectatic configuration, can

Fig. 1.28. A Right and **B** left internal carotid injection in frontal views in a patient presenting with a high-flow frontal arteriovenous malformation (AVM). Note the secondary transfer (*arrows*) of the watershed area between the anterior-middle cerebral artery territories (*interrupted line*). Also note the middle cerebral arterial stenosis (*arrowhead*) proximal to the lesion (**B**) secondary to the high-flow angiopathy, therefore testifying to the secondary transfer of the watershed junction distal to the AVM

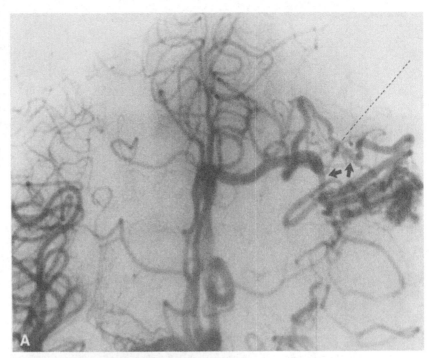

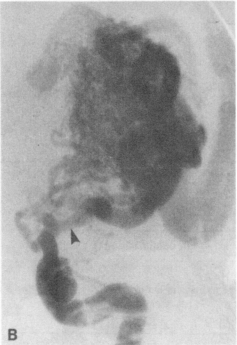

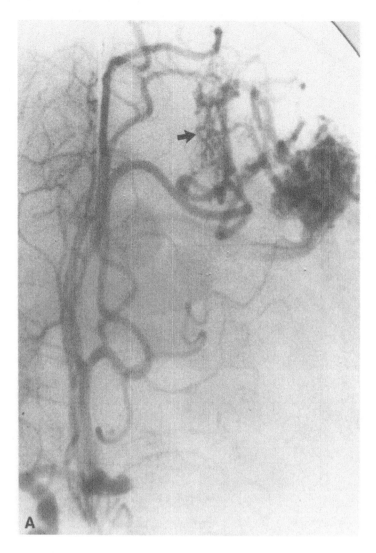

Fig. 1.29. A Frontal internal carotid angiogram. Sulcal arteriovenous malformation with secondary transfer of the anterior-middle cerebral watershed area, representing leptomeningeal nonsprouting angiogenesis (*arrow*). **B, C, D,** and **E** Coronal MRI confirms the absence of a true malformed nidus in that region. Note the absence of venous drainage at the level of the secondary angiogenesis

Table 1.11. High-flow angiopathy in the rabbit

Luminal protrusion of the endothelial cells with desquamation
Smooth muscle vacuolization
Mesenchymal cell proliferation
Corrugation and destruction of the internal elastic lamina
Capillary proliferation in the adventitia
Fenestrated and leaky endothelial junctions

From Pile-Spellman et al. 1986.

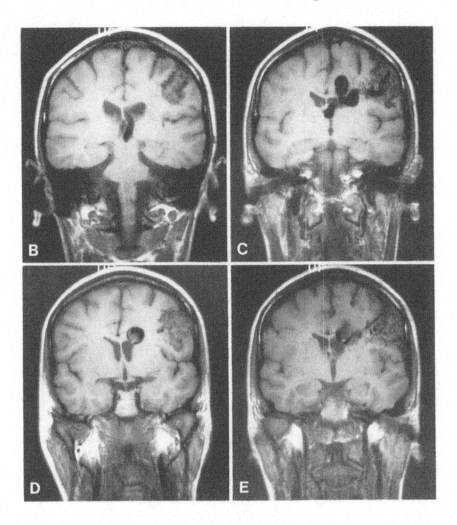

be seen following embolization (Fig. 1.31), surgical excision of the AVM, or during the evolution of a "stenotic process." The apparent increased diameter of the opacified lumen, however, actually remains within the size of the direct feeder in its initial state. Moyamoya patterns in AVMs are rare (Kayama et al. 1986), yet they can be encountered usually in young patients (Fig. 1.32). This arrangement does not seem to be reversible. It is not known if such an arrangement corresponds to true vascular proliferation, to progressive local response to arterial narrowing, or to a combination of factors (Figs. 1.33, 1.34). Aoki and Mizutani (1985) reported a stenosis that reopened after surgery. Mawad et al. (1984), in reviewing 13 patients with a moyamoya phenomenon, associated with BAVM, postulated the development of an acquired dysplasia linked with the AVM. The proximal "turbulence" would create the moyamoya appearance at the base of the brain. Furthermore, Mawad et al. (1984) felt that moyamoya might protect an AVM from bleeding. In Suzuki's series of patients with moyamoya without an associated BAVM, however, there was a 4% incidence of hemorrhage in those with the juvenile form, which rose to 43% in those with the adult form, hardly suggesting a protective effect of such a small vessel network. Suzuki also reports a 3% incidence of moyamoya associated with BAVM. Yasargil (1987) discussed only three cases of associated moyamoya and BAVM, corresponding to a 0.3% incidence in his experience.

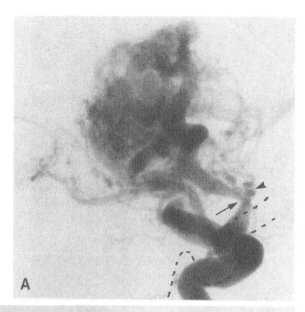

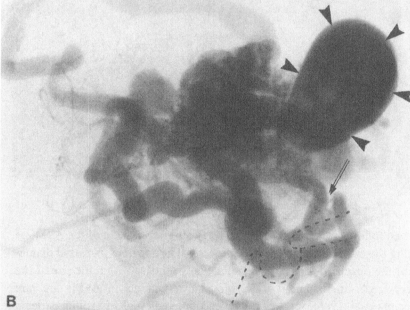

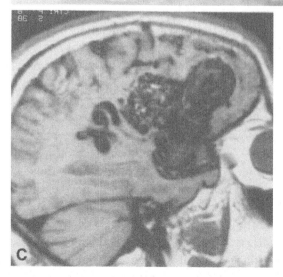

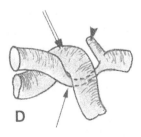

Fig. 1.30. A Early and **B** late phases of the right internal carotid injection in lateral view. **C** Sagittal MRI study. Deep frontal arteriovenous malformation fed by stenotic frontal branches from the ipsilateral middle cerebral artery (*arrow*). Note the presence of a large, deep-seated, venous ectasia (*arrowheads* in **B**) which, in conjunction with the remaining nidus and congested medullary vein, is producing a mass effect on the stenosed arterial feeder. Note the apparent "strangulation" of the feeder around the vein (*double arrow*) and the mass effect on the sphenoid ridge (*single arrowhead* in **A**). The changes associated with the high-flow angiopathy can also be advocated to explain this stenotic aspect. **D** The mechanism of arterial stenosis produced by venous dilatation

Fig. 1.31. A Left vertebral artery injection in lateral view before embolization, **B** after partial treatment in a patient presenting with a cerebellar and vermian arteriovenous malformation. 3 months following the first session of embolization of the posterior inferior cerebellar artery, note the caliber changes in the proximal aspect of the vessel mimicking an aneurysm (*arrow*)

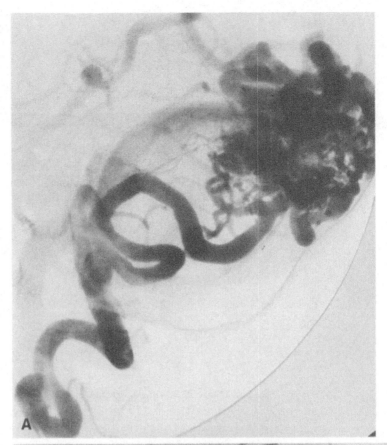

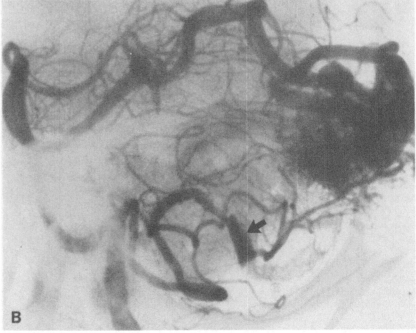

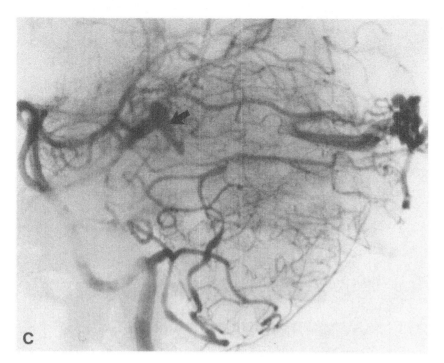

Fig. 1.31. C After additional embolization of the antero-superior cerebellar artery contribution to the lesion, note similar changes onto the artery embolized. The remaining nidus was removed surgically. **D** The progressive and irregular changes in vessel caliber that may occur proximal to the occlusion. The regression of the increased caliber may occur with or without associated acrylic deposition and proximal intraluminal clot resorption. Additional regression will bring the feeding artery into an almost normal aspect as demonstrated on the last vertebral control angiogram (**C**). These irregularities do not carry any risk of rupture, despite their pseudoaneurysmal aspect

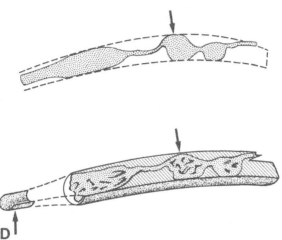

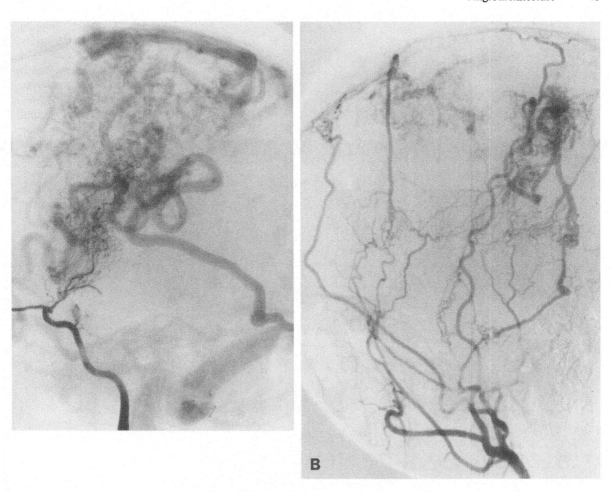

Fig. 1.32 A, B. Moyamoya type of supply to a brain arteriovenous malformation (BAVM). **A** Left internal carotid and **B** internal maxillary injections in lateral view. Moyamoya type supply to a frontal AVM, interpreted as the final evolution of the high-flow angiopathy. Note the transdural supply into what was considered to be normal cortical territories (**B**)

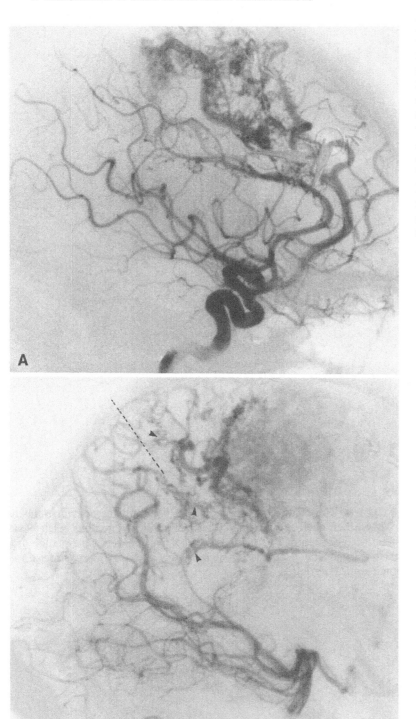

Fig. 1.33. A Right internal carotid and **B** vertebral artery injections in lateral view. In a medial frontal arteriovenous malformation (AVM), note the early nonsprouting angiogenesis (*arrowheads* in **B**) around what appears to be remaining AVM, following attempted surgical removal of the lesion. These changes illustrate the early stages of the vascular response to the persistent shunt and to the previous ligations at surgery

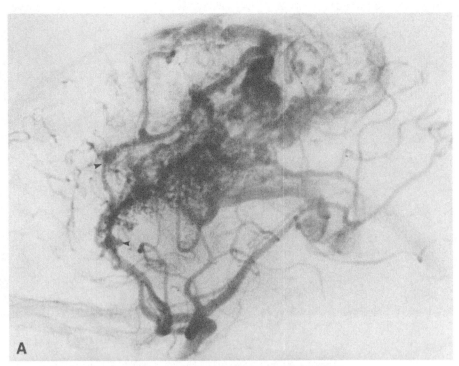

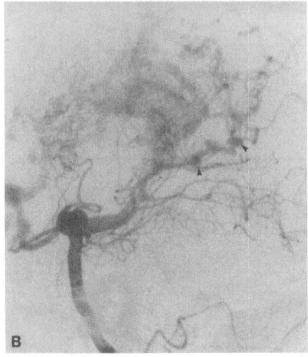

Fig. 1.34. A Right internal carotid and **B** left vertebral artery injections in lateral view of a cortico-callosal arteriovenous malformation similar to that shown in Fig. 1.33. The high-flow angiopathy has modified the aspect of the lesion, with multiple arterial stenoses and ectasias (*arrowheads*). The nonsprouting angiogenesis makes the limits of the nidus difficult to recognize. This stage is considered as a "pre"-Moyamoya situation

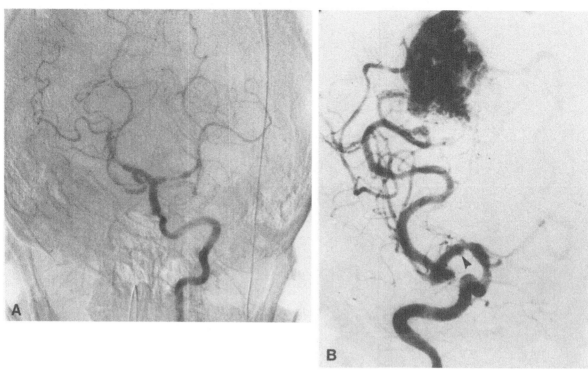

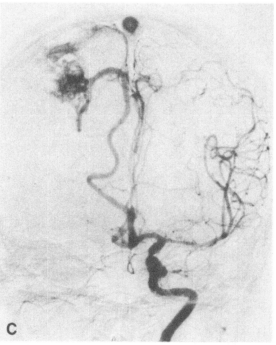

Fig. 1.35. **A** Left vertebral artery injection and **B** right and **C** left internal carotid artery injections in frontal view. Frontal arteriovenous malformation with an associated flow-related aneurysm (*arrowhead* in **B**). Note the arterial vasospasm demonstrated in both P1 segments. This study was performed after subarachnoid hemorrhage

Vasospasm

Vasospasm is very rare following hemorrhage of a BAVM. Parkinson and Bachers (1980), for example, reported only a 1% incidence of vasospasm following hemorrhage from BAVMs. This is reasonable, as it is believed that all CNS AVMs are located subpially. This is the compartment into which hemorrhage will most often occur, and subpial hemorrhage would not be expected to produce the same effect as aneurysm rupture into the subarach-

Fig. 1.36. A Right internal carotid artery in midarterial phase and **B** ipsilateral middle meningeal artery injections in lateral projection. Temporal pole arteriovenous malformation in which the transdural supply opacifies the entire nidus and all the draining venous system

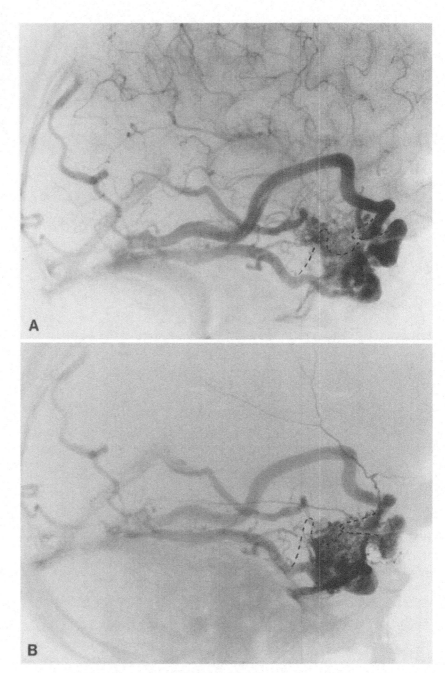

noid space. When present, therefore, vasospasm should raise the suspicion of an associated ruptured aneurysm (Fig. 1.35).

The development of localized spasm following hemorrhage has been implicated in the posthemorrhagic architectural changes of an AVM (London and Enzemann 1981) and was also suggested to be involved in progressive AVM occlusion (Lakke 1970).

Dural Supply

Dural supply to cerebral arteriovenous shunts can further express the hemodynamic and angiogenetic effects of the lesion. Two aspects of dural supply

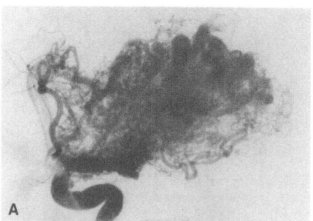

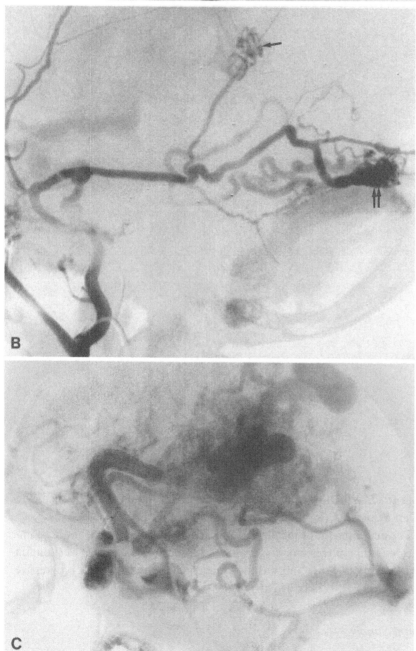

Fig. 1.37. **A** Left internal carotid and **B** internal maxillary artery injections in lateral view. Large temporal arteriovenous malformation. Note the transdural supply to the lesion (*arrow*) and the associated arteriovenous shunt separate from the pial nidus (*double arrow*). **C** Late venous phase of the internal carotid angiogram confirms the absence of a connection between the dural and the pial nidi

can be described: (1) direct supply to the lesion through dural leptomeningeal anastomosis (Newton 1969) (Fig. 1.36) and (2) direct anastomosis
with normal cortical arteries downstream from the lesion (Russell and
Berenstein 1981, Vol. 1). Dural supply was noted in 27% of Newton's (1969)
series and 32% of our patients (Willinsky 1988).

Both aspects of dural blood vessel involvement can be stimulated after
surgery, when adhesions occur between dural layers. Meningeal supply has
also been noted to develop following partial embolization; probably a result
of ischemia (even if subclinical) stimulating (nonsprouting) angiogenesis. In
rare instances, dural supply involves an associated sinus arteriovenous shunt
(Fig. 1.37). Subarachnoid hemorrhage represents an additional factor that
increases dural supply. Six of the seven patients of Faria and Fleischer
(1980) who presented with dural supply had bled. Although no significant
correlation has been established between dural supply to a lesion and the
clinical history of hemorrhage, one should keep in mind that frequent subclinical bleeding observed during surgery may account for some of this
dural participation. In our experience, there is also a possible correlation
between headaches and dural supply to a BAVM.

b) Arterial Variations

Arterial variations seem more frequent in patients with BAVM (24%, Willinsky 1988) than in patients evaluated for occlusive disease or in autopsy
series. However, the true frequency of arterial variation depends on the
ability of the investigator to recognize them (see Vol. 3, Chap. 4). Variations
at the level of the larger vessels (carotid, vertebral), with persistence of embryonic dispositions (trigeminal, hypoglossal, etc.), seem only moderately
increased in BAVM patients as compared to their slightly increased incidence in patients with aneurysms. Conversely, variation of the posterior and
anterior portions of the circle of Willis are very frequent in the BAVM
group. These variations are noted mainly when the area of shunting is
located at the watershed zone. When the lesion develops within the dominant area of supply, only the distal branching pattern of anastomotic arteries shows anatomical variations. Many of these variations remain remote
from the area of actual arteriovenous shunting and probably represent incidental occurrences. Only VGAM seems to be frequently associated with
a truly archaic disposition, such as the limbic arterial ring (see Vol. 3,
Chap. 4, and this volume Chap. 5), as if the early presence of the shunt
prevented maturation of the vasculature. Correction of the shunt allows this
maturation to occur secondarily with disappearance of the archaic disposition (Fig. 5.10).

The arterial territories of these variants should be known, in order to
predict potential risks of endovascular treatment. These territories include
the artery of the corpus callosum (Fig. 4.24, Vol. 3), accessory middle
cerebral artery (Figs. 4.15 and 4.16, Vol. 3), duplicated posterior communicating artery, etc. In addition, these anatomic arrangements may represent additional vulnerable locations that favor the development of flow-
related aneurysms.

c) Arterial Aneurysms

The reported association between arterial aneurysms and cerebral AVMs
varies from 2.7% (Paterson and McKissock 1956) to 16.7% (Miyasaka et

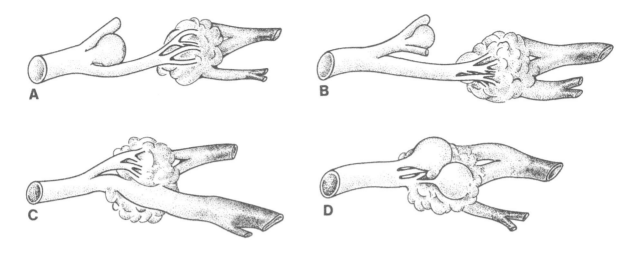

al. 1982). The difficulties in understanding the link between BAVM and arterial aneurysm are due in part to the underestimation of their association. In the series reported by Graf et al. (1983) (191 patients) and Perret and Nishioka (1966) (450 patients), only 6% – 7% of patients presented with aneurysms. These numbers are low compared to reports of series benefitting from complete, high quality, diagnostic angiography.

In our series, the association has been 23%. It reflects our use of high quality pancerebral angiography and may correspond to the true incidence in the overall population of BAVM. The presence of arterial aneurysm constitutes an additional risk factor that needs to be identified and taken into consideration in the treatment strategy. Two types of arterial aneurysms associated with BAVMs can be seen: (1) flow-related aneurysms and (2) dysplastic aneurysms (Fig. 1.38).

Fig. 1.38. Flow-related (**A**) and dysplastic aneurysm (**B**) in brain arteriovenous malformations. Intralesional direct arteriovenous fistulas (**C**) and intralesional arterial ectasias (**D**)

Flow-Related Aneurysms

Flow-related aneurysms develop on the pedicle supplying the BAVM. Two types can be recognized, one group develops near the base of the brain (proximal arterial aneurysms) (Figs. 1.39 – 1.41) while the other is seen close to or at the level of the nidus (distal arterial aneurysms) (Figs. 1.42 – 1.44). From 37% to 82% of arterial aneurysms have been considered to be flow-related (Batjer 1986; Lasjaunias et al. 1988). This includes infundibulae (Fig. 1.41) above 3 mm in size (Hayashi et al. 1981; Miyasaka et al. 1982; Batjer et al. 1986). In our review of 101 patients, the following distribution was observed: (a) 76% were flow-related; of these, 25% were distal (intralesional) and 75% were proximal and (b) 24% of aneurysms were remote to the BAVM and felt to be dysplastic aneurysms.

In the literature, the relationship between the development of arterial aneurysm and the flow of the AVM is mentioned in such diverse ways that a clear-cut approach to the problem cannot be found. However, Okamoto et al. (1984) and Hayashi et al. (1981) demonstrated that patterns of aneurysm distribution in patients with BAVMs were significantly different than in patients without BAVMs. Hayashi's review of 112 aneurysms in 74 patients with BAVMs showed a high incidence of aneurysms in areas where aneurysms usually do not occur, i.e., peripheral, lenticulostriate (Fig. 1.43), anterior choroidal, etc. In AVM patients the great majority of aneurysms

Fig. 1.39. Vertebral artery injection in frontal view demonstrates P1 (*arrow*) and posterior communicating (*double arrows*) flow-related aneurysms in a fronto-parietal AVM

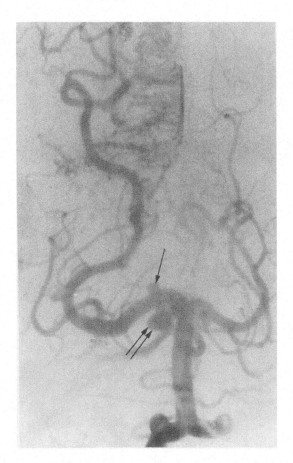

Fig. 1.40. A Right and **B** left internal carotid artery injections in frontal and oblique projections, respectively. Note the multiple aneurysms associated with the arteriovenous malformation (*arrows*)

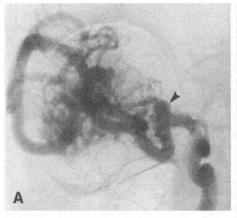
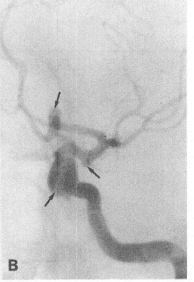

were noted on the feeding arteries of the AVMs, irrespective of the circulation. This finding was confirmed in our analysis (Lasjaunias et al. 1988). It is therefore apparent that the presence of a BAVM predisposes one to the formation of aneurysms on the feeding vessels. The exact pathogenesis of the BAVM and of the aneurysm are, however, probably not related to the same developmental abnormality.

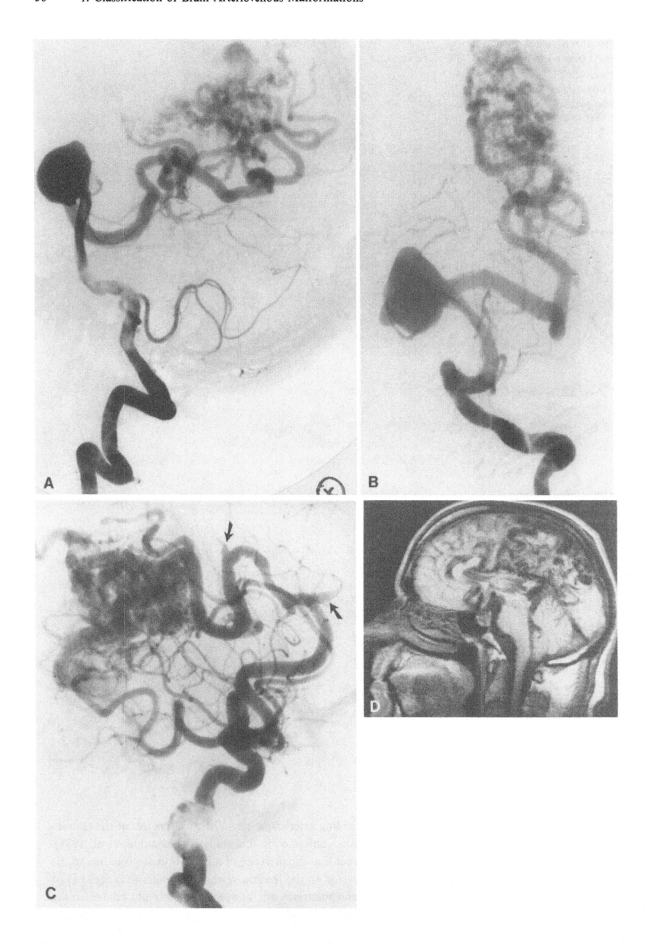

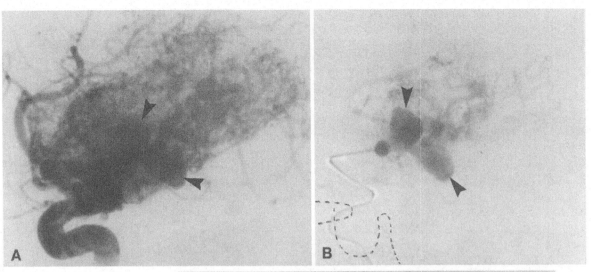

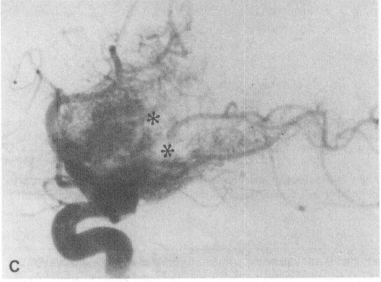

Fig. 1.42. Left internal carotid injection before (**A**), during (**B**) and after (**C**) embolization. Note the large, intralesional, arterial ectasias (*arrowheads* in **A** and *arrows* in **B**). The ectasias were embolized with IBCA at the same deposition as the nidus was occluded and are included in the same cast (*asterisks* in **C**)

◀ **Fig. 1.41. A** Left vertebral artery injection in lateral and **B** frontal views. **C** Right internal carotid injection in lateral view. **D** Sagittal MRI. (Same patient as in Fig. 2.1.) Large medial fronto-parietal lesion associated with a corpus callosum anomaly. Multiple flow-related changes in both the arterial and venous aspect of the architecture are noted. The large basilar tip aneurysm (**A**) cannot be considered as flow-related. Following partial embolization of the posterior cerebral and anterior cerebral arteries, significant reduction of the shunt was obtained as was a decrease in the proximal infundibulum (*arrows* in **C**). A week after the second embolization (3 months after the first), the patient developed a subarachnoid hemorrhage and died. Pathological examination demonstrated a large, hemispheric, hemorrhagic infarction with partial thrombosis of the giant basilar aneurysm and probable dome rupture

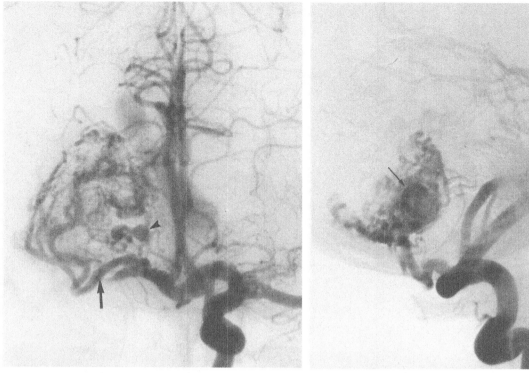

1.43

1.44

Fig. 1.43. Left internal carotid injection in frontal view; caudate nucleus arteriovenous malformation fed by the right recurrent artery of Heubner (*arrow*). Note the proximal arterial aneurysm (*arrowhead*)

Fig. 1.44. Right vertebral artery injection in lateral view. Note the intralesional arterial ectasia (*arrow*) well demonstrated during the early phase of the angiogram

In the rat, aneurysms can be experimentally created by three mechanisms: arterial hypertension produced by ligation of the renal arteries, administration of exogenous estrogen, and unilateral ligation of one internal carotid artery, which increases flow without any other changes in the vascular system. In clinical situations, the augmentation of flow alone, without the addition of estrogens or arterial hypertension, is sufficient to provoke the development of aneurysm (Hashimoto et al. 1980; Alvarez and Roda 1986). For a long time, the link between BAVM-associated aneurysms and increased flow to the malformation has been suspected (Anderson and Blackwood 1959). Arterial aneurysms have been observed to develop: on the internal carotid artery 3–5 years after a surgical occlusion of the contralateral internal carotid artery (Somach and Shenkin 1966); on the superficial temporal artery after a surgical anastomosis of this vessel to a sylvian branch (Lantos et al. 1984); and following spontaneous collateral circulation to the brain (Walsh and King 1942). Rerouting blood in the circle of Willis by proximal ligations for multiple aneurysms in a 12-year-old child was reported to enlarge and rupture a preexisting basilar tip aneurysm 11 days following the ligation (Batjer et al. 1987). Three patients that underwent cervical carotid artery ligation presented 12–15 years later with a basilar aneurysm (Berenstein and Choi 1988) (Vol. 5, Fig. 3.19). Experimentally, in high-flow angiopathy (Pile-Spellman et al. 1988), vessel changes proximal to the shunt

Fig. 1.45. Electron micrograph of normal fusiform ectasias in a cerebral arteriole specimen. (Courtesy of H. Duvernoy)

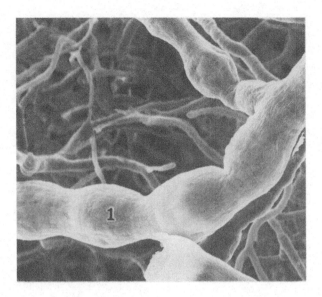

involving the internal elastic lamina have been demonstrated (Table 1.11). These changes may predispose one to the development of an arterial aneurysm. Further evolution of these induced changes could lead to specific clinical manifestations and complications (ischemic symptoms or rupture of an aneurysm). Therefore, when present, an arterial aneurysm worsens the prognosis of the AVM. Nine of 18 patients (50%) treated conservatively and 6 of 16 patients managed surgically, all of whom were in the cooperative aneurysm study (Perret and Nishioka 1966), died. Gamache and Patterson (1985) found that of 42 medically managed patients 38% died, 7% had significant neurological deficit, and only 14% were doing well.

The augmentation of diastolic flow in the ipsilateral or contralateral carotid artery is a feature of considerable interest in cerebral arteriovenous shunts (Pertuiset et al. 1985). In the superficial temporal artery (in which there is normally no diastolic flow) (see Vol. 2, Chap. 1), the aneurysmal and mural changes which occur following surgical anastomosis to the middle cerebral artery suggest specific effects from the diastolic flow that result from the surgery. The chronicity of the increased diastolic fraction could be an important factor in the aneurysmal transformation of the normal ectasias, described by Duvernoy et al. (1981) (Fig. 1.45). Increased diastolic flow may also behave as a trigger factor on the already damaged vessel wall proximal to the shunt (Table 1.11). The problems posed by the endovascular approach to BAVMs associated with arterial aneurysms has only been addressed in a few reports. However, following the occlusion of the AVM, proximal arterial aneurysms have shown partial or even complete regression (Figs. 1.46, 1.47 and 3.14–3.16). Of importance to note is that aneurysms in patients partially embolized with particles showed no change, whereas in a few patients the infundibula decreased in size following embolization (Miyasaka et al. 1982). The problems of arterial aneurysms of the anterior communicating artery (Fig. 1.40) associated with convex AVMs are difficult. However, an augmented diastolic fraction in the internal carotid artery opposite to the shunt will confirm this vessel's actual role in the supply to the AVM and the probable relation to the increased flow accounting for the aneurysm. A regression of the aneurysm after treatment of the

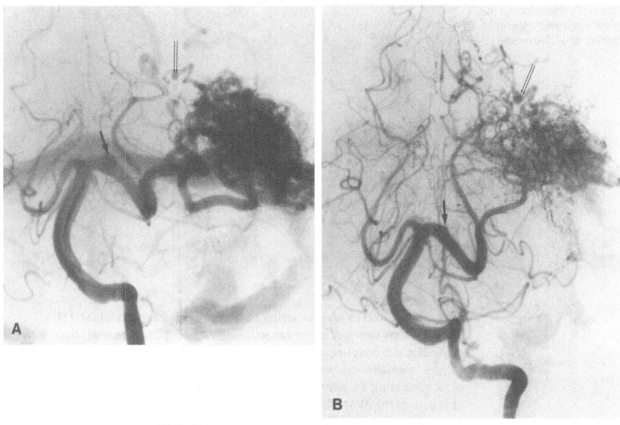

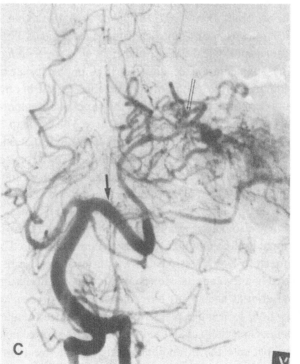

Fig. 1.46. **A** Left vertebral artery injection in frontal view before and **B** during embolization; **C** final control after embolization. Note the different changes observed in the flow-related aneurysm of P1 (*arrow*) and at the level of the leptomeningeal anastomoses (*double arrow*) as the embolization progresses

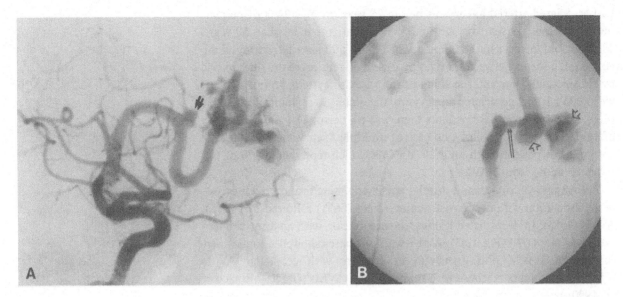

Fig. 1.47. A Right internal carotid injection in lateral view. Medial hemispheric arteriovenous malformation with a proximal flow-related aneurysm (*double arrow*). **B** Superselective injection of the feeding pedicle distal to the aneurysm position for embolization that resulted in complete occlusion of the shunt. Note the venous narrowing (*double arrow*) and ectasias (*open arrows*). Stability of the result is assessed on the 3 month control angiogram (Fig. 3.16B), which demonstrates spontaneous shrinkage of the proximal aneurysm despite the apparent enlargement of arterial collaterals

arteriovenous shunt (by surgical or endovascular means) can be expected (Figs. 1.46, 1.47 and 3.14–3.16). When pressure measurements are made in the feeding vessels to an AVM, either from external pressure measurements, during surgical clipping (Nornes and Grip 1980), or after embolization with particles, the mean arterial pressure immediately rises to equal or approximate the systemic blood pressure. Preocclusion pressure is dampened by the arteriovenous shunt and, although it has not been a problem during acrylic embolization distal to an aneurysm, we recommend blood pressure control during the postocclusion phase (24 h) to avoid the elevation of systolic pressure in the recently occluded feeder with an arterial aneurysm.

Dysplastic Aneurysms

Dysplastic aneurysms develop on an arterial branch independent from the AVM (Batjer et al. 1986; Perret and Nishioka 1966) and are not considered to be flow-related (Figs. 1.40, 1.41).

In most series (Batjer et al. 1986; Miyasaka et al. 1982) there is no overall sex predominance. In our series flow-related arterial aneurysm showed a male predominance of 2:1, whereas a female predominance of 5:1 was seen in the dysplastic aneurysms group. Patients with this association are between 11 and 55 years of age (Batjer et al. 1986); however, flow-related aneurysms are more likely to occur in older patients (Hayashi et al. 1981; Lasjaunias et al. 1988). The association of BAVM and arterial aneurysm in our series showed a distinct increase with age: 8% of the patiens with AVMs had associated arterial aneurysms before 25 years of age, 24% of patients between 25 and 49 years of age, and 37% of patients older than 50 years. The fourfold increase in the frequency of BAVM and associated arterial aneurysm in patients between the ages of 10 and 50 reinforces the roles played by chronic high flow and the aging of the vascular system. In our patients with BAVM and associated aneurysm, the latter were multiple in 44% (Figs. 1.39, 1.40). In these patients there was no personal or family history of vascular disease. Similarly, no case of multiple aneurysms was found in the group of patients with multiple BAVMs, which represented 9% of our series of adults with BAVMs.

With regard to topography, arterial aneurysms were found predominantly in association with corticoventricular AVMs (66%) followed by cortical AVMs (30%). In deep-seated lesions, the association with an arterial aneurysm was rare (4%) (Fig. 1.43). A review of our cases showed a similar percentage of BAVM plus aneurysm in patients with cerebellar AVMs (Fig. 1.44) compared to those with supratentorial AVMs (Garcia-Monaco et al. 1990a).

We consider that the specific presence of flow-related aneurysms is an indicator of which arterial pedicles should be given priority in the sequential planning of an endovascular operation. Considering that in most series 50% of patients (75% in ours) with this association have bled, it is reasonable to believe that certain hemorrhages observed in the natural history of a cerebral AVM may be due to an arterial aneurysm rupture.

d) Nidus Angioarchitecture

The nidus arrangement of BAVMs can be approached in different ways. As previously mentioned, a single-hole fistula represents the simplest aspect of arteriovenous shunting.

In several patients with VGAMs, Dobbelaere et al. (1979) demonstrated an AVF on one side and an AVM on the other side. For them, "the passage from one [AVM] to the other [AVF] is certain;" it expresses the stabilization of the arteriovenous shunting defect "whereas the vein of Galen dilatation is controlled by the straight sinus stenosis." They suggested that all arteriovenous shunts change from one type to the other with evolution or involution. These findings contradict our observations, since the lesions that we have followed have not gone through such a predetermined evolution or involution.

The nidi of AVMs have been classified, primarily for surgical purposes, either by topography, size, or intrinsic morphological or hemodynamic patterns. A description of compartments, as disclosed angiographically, has also been used for classification. AVMs in which a specific and separate venous drainage is seen after each feeder is injected are considered as AVMs with multiple compartments. Those lesions in which a unique or the same venous outlet is opacified after every feeder is injected are considered as AVMs with a unique or converging compartment (Yasargil 1987) (Table 1.12). Most of the multiple compartment lesions are arranged on a radius (cortical and paraventricular nidi in corticoventricular lesions) or a meridian (cerebellar AVMs). Yasargil (1987) made several additional observations on the arrangement of these lesions, pointing to their "compact or diffuse" appearance (Table 1.12).

Table 1.12. Nidus (epicenter)

Single, compact
   Without fistula
   With AVFs
   Only AVFs visible

Multifocal (multicentric or polycentric) compact (subdivided into same types as above)
   Unilateral
   Bilateral
   Supra- and infratentorial
   Orbital and cerebral
   Cutaneous, dural, and cerebral

Diffuse, no visible nidus (scattered pathological arteries and veins without recognizable connections angiographically or at operation)
   Small areas
   Large areas
   Entire hemisphere
   Both hemispheres
   Supra- and infratentorial

From Yasargil 1987.

We observe the same patterns, in which diffuse lesions show less dominant but more numerous feeders. In many cases these more numerous feeders may correspond to the development of secondary arterial stenotic segments, fusiform ectasias, infundibula, "pre"-moyamoya states, and angiogenic activities. The veins draining such diffuse AVMs are surprisingly almost normal in caliber; the transit time in the shunt is often moderate. They are mostly cortico-subcortical lesions and can be seen both supra- and infratentorially. Rarely, a patient with a cervico-spinal cord lesion can present with this aspect (see Vol. 5, Chap. 1).

Most AVMs are composed of several types of arteriovenous communications, including both nidi and fistulas (Fig. 1.5). However we have not encountered both compact and diffuse types within the nidi of genuine AVMs. A diffuse appearance may represent secondarily acquired perilesional an-

Table 1.13. Sizes of AVMs

Cryptic
   Not seen on angiography, not found at surgery, and not demonstrated pathologically

Occult
   Invisible on angiography, invisible at surgery, and may be recognized by histological examination

Micro (0.5 – 1 cm)
   Often invisible to the surgeon; transiently occult at angiography

Small (1 – 2 cm)

Moderate (2 – 4 cm)

Large (4 – 6 cm)

Giant (>6 cm)

AVM, arteriovenous malformation. Modified from Yasargil 1987.

giogenesis, at least in some of the diffuse types of lesions reported by Yasargil. The significance of the size of the nidi lies primarily in their surgical or radiosurgical accessibility (Table 1.13). An exception may be made with microlesions since most lesions with arteriovenous shunting belong to the group of macroarteriovenous shunts since the lesions are at least 1 cm large.

Most authors have grouped BAVMs according to the size of the nidus and considered "small" BAVMs as those less than 2 or 3 cm. It has also been found that smaller BAVMs bleed ten times more often (Crawford et al. 1986; Graf et al. 1983; Parkinson and Bachers 1980; Shi and Chen 1986; Spetzler and Martin 1986; Waltimo 1973b). By contrast, patients with smaller lesions rarely present with seizures, neurological deficits, or headaches (Hashima et al. 1985). In our series, as in that of Crawford, there was no significant difference in the prognostic features (hemorrhage and other complications) of small AVMs as compared to large lesions (vide infra). The former are not more frequent in children, in whom hemorrhage as a presenting symptom is significantly more frequent than in adults. The rebleed rate is the same as that of larger AVMs. The small size probably prevents them from producing seizures or progressive neurological deficits, permitting clinical diagnosis only following a hemorrhagic episode.

Microarteriovenous Malformations

Micro-AVMs and micro-AVFs consist of a small nidus (< 1 cm) or a fistula fed by a "normal" sized artery and draining into a "normal" sized vein (Figs. 1.1, 1.3, 1.7). To explain how obstacles to venous outflow of an arteriovenous shunt can be considered as one significant cause of rupture, one should recall the specific normal disposition of cortical veins (Duvernoy et al. 1981). Small bridging arteries anchor the cortical veins onto the parenchyma and narrow them in the depth of the sulci. These potential anatomical restrictions on increased venous flow may lead to upstream venous hyperpressure and secondary rupture. In fact, when we described a "normal" sized draining vein, the most proximal venous outlet from the micro-AVM actually corresponds to an enlarged subpial cortical vein which is usually not visible angiographically.

Micro-AVMs represent 7% of all AVMs and 21% of the AVMs that were diagnosed following hemorrhagic accident in our series. In the series of Papatheodorou et al. (1961) and in our series (Willinsky et al. 1988), 53% of patients had no history of symptoms prior to the discovery of their lesions; the ages ranged from 8 to 52 years without a sex predominance. All patients presented with intracerebral hematoma with minimal or no subarachnoid blood. Conventional magnification angiography with subtraction demonstrated the micro-AVM in 85% of patients; however, in 18% of these, the AVM could be seen only after resolution of the hematoma, during a second angiographic study 3 months later (Fig. 1.3). In the remaining 15% of patients, the lesions were "angiographically occult" but were seen at surgery during removal of the hematoma.

All of the lesions were "superficial": 77% were cortical supratentorial (Fig. 1.3), 15% were infratentorial (Fig. 1.1), and 3% were at the base of the brain. There was no dural supply and no associated arterial aneurysms. Some 82% of patients were operated upon (13% of patients refused

surgery) and the remaining 5% were referred for radiation therapy. All of
the lesions in patients who were operated upon showed at pathology the
usual aspects of cerebral AVMs. At both angiography and surgery, the intracerebral hematoma helped to localize the lesion, since the micro-AVM
could be seen at the edge of the hematoma. Following surgery there were
no postoperative complications. Control angiograms showed disappearance
of the lesion and no recurrences have been noted. None of the nonoperated
on patients have rebled with 1–5 years follow-ups, but 7% of patients had
previously bled in the same site within 10 years prior to diagnosis and
surgery. Evaluation of the chances of rebled in patients with micro-AVMs
is difficult to assess, since most lesions are surgically removed and most are
operated on at the time of diagnosis. Micro-AVMs have been suspected to
be the cause of many intracerebral hematomas in young healthy individuals
in whom no obvious lesion is found (Krayenbuhl and Siebenmann 1965;
Margolis et al. 1961; Tanaka et al. 1986).

Small vascular malformations have often been included either with the
cryptic or occult vascular malformations (Becker et al. 1979; Bitoh et al.
1978; McCormick and Nofzinger 1966) or with cerebral AVMs.

Systemic (ROW) or nonsystemic multiple AVMs can be associated with
cerebral lesions, including micro-AVMs (Fig. 1.7).

Nontraumatic intracerebral hematoma may be caused by AVMs, aneurysms, blood dyscrasias or a bleeding diasthesis, amyloid angiopathy, drug
abuse, sympathomimetic drugs, or tumors (Lipton et al. 1987). Vascular
malformations have accounted for 10%–40% of lobar hematomas. In
clinical studies no identifiable etiology was found in 25%–41% of patients
with intracerebral hematomas. In autopsy series no etiology was found in
15%.

Nidus Enlargement

Multiple reports have shown conflicting data as to the growth of BAVMs,
with some reporting size increases in cerebral malformations (Hook and
Johanson 1988; Krayenbuhl 1977; Spetzler and Wilson 1975; Stein 1979;
Waltimo 1973b; Minakawa et al. 1989) and others noting decreases in their
size or even complete thrombosis (Eisenmann et al. 1972; Kushner and
Alexander 1970; Levine et al. 1973; Omojola et al. 1985; Sukoff et al. 1972;
Pascual-Castroviejo et al. 1977; Minakawa et al. 1987). In the series of
Minakawa, Hook, Waltimo, and Stein there was a slight discrepancy in the
incidence of decreased, increased, or unchanged malformations. However,
their case material differed significantly, as some of the patients had been
treated conservatively and others had partial surgical intervention. Overall,
a review of 63 vascular malformations with size changes concluded that in
25% there was an increase in size. It is of interest that patients whose AVMs
had enlarged were almost all children at the time of first presentation and
diagnosis. By contrast AVMs which decreased in size or thrombosed without associated hematoma occurred in an older group (vide infra). The issue
of angiogenesis (sprouting or nonsprouting) raises further questions regarding true enlargement of BAVMs.

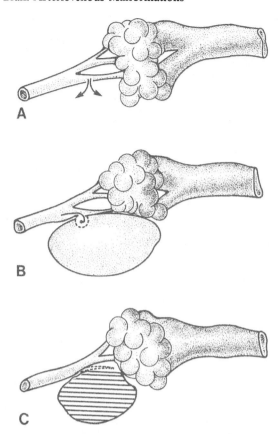

Fig. 1.48 A–C. The mechanisms resulting in an arterial pseudoaneurysm and partial occlusion of the arterial feeder. (See text)

Intralesional Pouches

Ectasia or pouches within the AVM nidus can be either arterial or venous. The former may belong to the group of distal arterial aneurysms or may be very close to the nidus and are difficult to see in global injections. They are thought to be flow-related but represent a weak portion of the nidus. Arterial pseudoaneurysms are usually encountered during the acute stage of an intracerebral hematoma of arterial origin (Fig. 1.48). The aneurysms are usually small in size but may enlarge to produce an early secondary rupture (Figs. 1.49, 1.50).

An enlarging pseudoaneurysm constitutes one of the few indications for emergency treatment. In other instances, venous pseudoaneurysms will evolve favorably with occlusion of the ruptured vessel.

Intralesional venous ectasias are usually opacified after the network of abnormal "capillaries" (Fig. 1.51); ectatic areas can either be open (with an entrance and a distal exit) or closed (where the exit vein is apparently occluded). The open type usually corresponds to ectasia proximal to a mechanical obstacle. However, it may also represent a pseudoaneurysm partially recanalized and annexed to the venous outlet (Fig. 1.52). The latter represents a thrombosed draining vein leaving a proximal stump opacified through the nidus. Acutely following a hemorrhage, closed venous ectasias correspond to pseudoaneurysms of the vein. This feature, when demonstrated, may also represent an indication for emergency treatment. The venous origin of a pseudoaneurysm is difficult to demonstrate. As a sequence of events, however, most of these intralesional pouches do correlate with a recent history of hemorrhage. Such venous pouches are more fre-

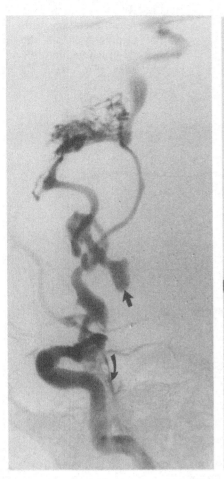
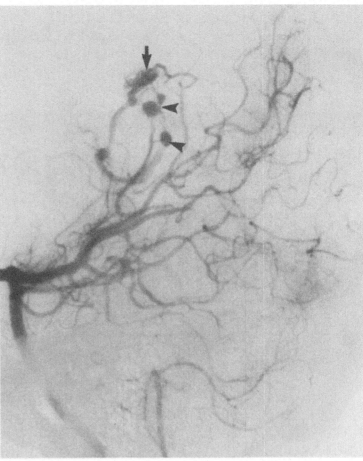

1.50

Fig. 1.49. Left internal carotid angiogram in lateral view. Arterial pseudoaneurysm (*arrow*) in a patient with a frontal arteriovenous malformation with a massive intracerebral hemorrhage. Note the extravasation of contrast material in the subarachnoid space (*curved arrow*). This picture was obtained at the 26th second of a conventional study. Since there was no further flow, brain death had occurred

Fig. 1.50. Left vertebral artery angiogram in lateral view. Multiple small arterial pseudoaneurysms (*arrowheads*) were demonstrated in a microarteriovenous malformation of the singular gyrus (*arrow*). Secondary lethal rupture precluded any therapeutic attempt

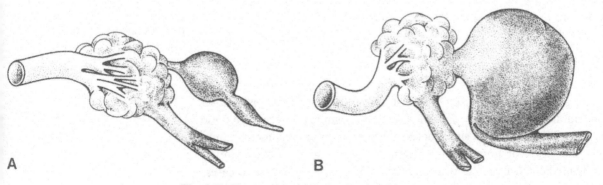

Fig. 1.51. Venous ectasia **A** proximal to a venous thrombosis and **B** proximal to venous kinking. (See text)

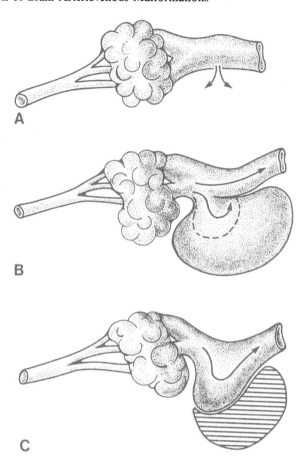

Fig. 1.52 A–C. Evolution of a venous pseudoaneurysm with partial incorporation of the recanalized hematoma into the venous outlet. (See text)

quently encountered in deeply located lesions, in a sulcus infratemporally or within the brain, for example, at the size of a hematoma (Figs. 1.53, 1.54). Their patterns illustrate a common point. Specifically, their acquired nature exemplifies the architectural changes undergone by the lesions.

e) Veins

The venous drainage of AVMs can be very difficult to study due to the vast number of outlets that can be superimposed. Nevertheless, drainage of a shunt should always be analyzed by comparison to or in relation with the venous arrangement of the normal cerebral tissue. In general, the developmental nature of the shunt alters the normal course of the development of the venous system as it does with the arteries.

Venous Variations

Venous variations were noted in 30% of Yasargil's (1987) patients and in 32% of our patients (Willinsky 1988). Variations may involve either cerebral veins, dural sinuses, or both. Careful attention is required to recognize these variations (Figs. 1.2, 1.18), since they may be in the venous channel draining either the lesion or normal brain parenchyma. Drainage of the lesion is usually predictable from the location of the nidus (Fig. 1.15). In some cases, however, thrombosis may hide or reroute the drainage to additional channels which may be ipsilateral, contralateral, or transcerebral (Fig. 1.12).

Fig. 1.53. A Axial noncontrast ▶ CT and **B** left vertebral angiogram in lateral projection at the time of a hemorrhagic episode demonstrate a localized vermis arteriovenous malformation with a venous pseudoaneurysm (*arrowhead* in **B**), corresponding to the larger area of hematoma seen in **A** (*arrowhead*). **C** Noncontrast axial CT and **D** left vertebral angiogram at the time of increased symptomatology with enlargement of the intracerebral hematoma. Note the increased size of the pseudoaneurysm (*arrowhead*) within the vermis

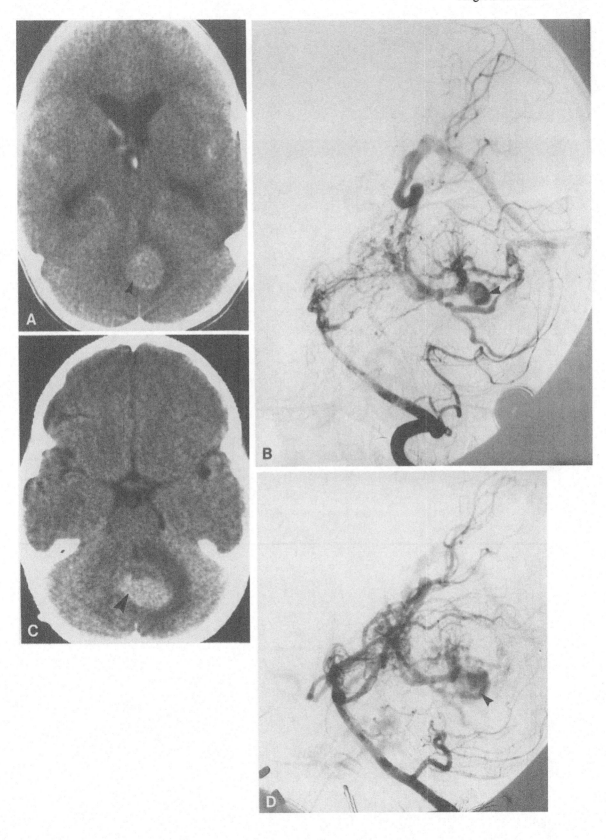

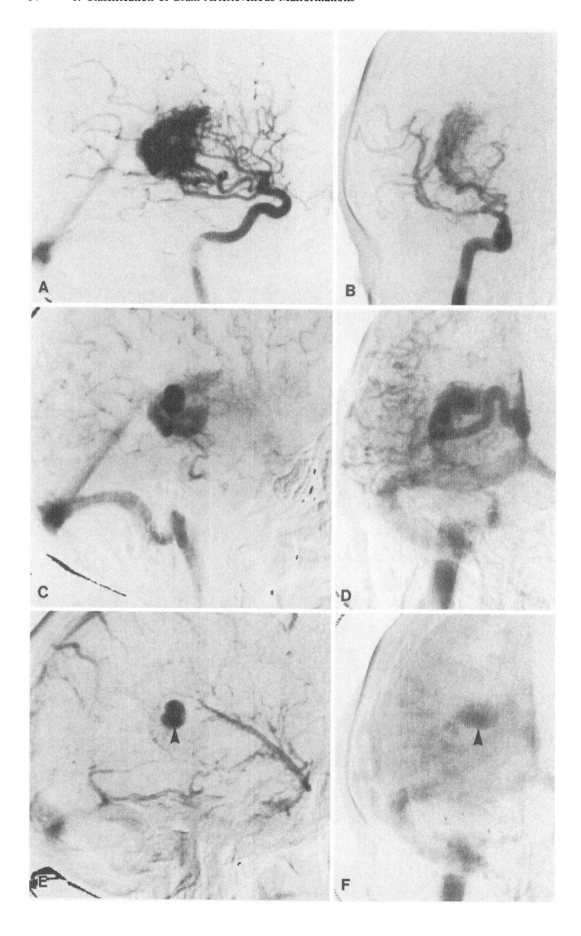

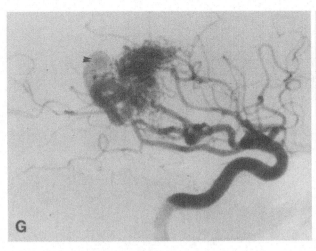
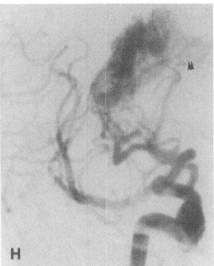

Fig. 1.54 A–H. Cingular gyrus arteriovenous malformation (AVM) supplied by posterior cerebral artery and anterior choroidal artery branches. **A–F** Right internal carotid artery injection in lateral and frontal projections at the time of an intracerebral hemorrhage, the stagnant aspect of venous pseudoaneurysm (*arrowhead*). **G** and **H** Right internal carotid artery injection in lateral and frontal views in the same patient (6 months later) demonstrates the incorporation of the venous pseudoaneurysm into the outlet of the arteriovenous malformation (*double arrowhead*)

These venous variations must be distinguished from collateral circulation that expresses a secondary response to the chronicity of the shunt. Analysis of the connections between both circulations will allow an understanding of some of the symptoms, a prediction of some of the natural history, and will aid in recognition of therapeutic hazards (Laine et al. 1981). Such analysis must include the effects of reflux, due to both venous hyperpressure and collateral circulation. Yasargil (1987) thinks that most hemorrhages occur as a result of venous or vein-nidus junction rupture. Embryonic veins have been described morphologically and histologically to persist in BAVM (Vidyasagar 1979; Deshpande et al. 1980) (Table 1.14).

Venous variations can create specific patterns that constitute an artificial group of lesions; vein of Galen and dural anomalies (see Chap. 5). Schematically:

1. The immediate or developmental venous adaptation tends to compensate for the initial hemodynamic disturbance. It alters the rest of the venous system in an attempt to bypass the higher pressure lesion and is a morphological reaction, creating anatomic variations or permitting persistence of embryonic venous structures.
2. The collateral venous circulation is a secondary adaptation. It tends to preserve the equilibrium of both shunt-related and normal parenchymal drainages. It absorbs into normal channels the increased pressure that exists in the venous outlet of the AVM and represents a pure hemodynamic response. Its failure to compensate will create neurological complications.

Table 1.14. Embryonic veins, in AVMs

Irregular thickness (fibrocollageneous or fibromuscular)
No elastic tissue
No prominent endothelial cells
Fenestrated endothelium

BAVM, brain arteriovenous malformation. From Vidyasagar 1979.

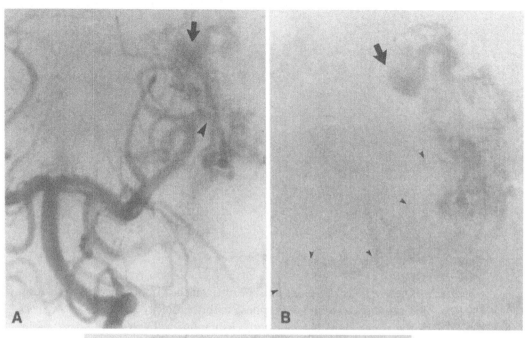

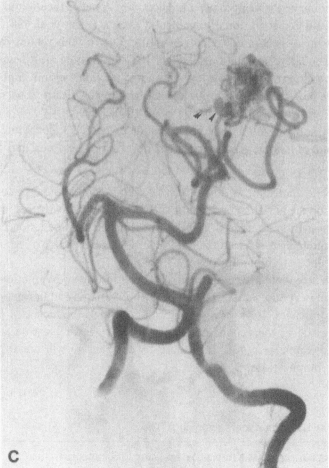

Fig. 1.55. **A** Left vertebral artery injection in frontal view and **B** selective injection of the posterior temporal branch (*arrowheads*) to the arteriovenous malformation. Note the venous ectasia (*arrow*) downstream from the nidus corresponding to secondary thrombosis of one of the venous outlets. **C** Left vertebral artery injection in another patient, demonstrating a small venous ectasia (*arrowhead*) downstream from a malformation and corresponding to secondary thrombosis of the venous outlet (*double arrowhead*). No previous history of hemorrhage could be documented in this patient

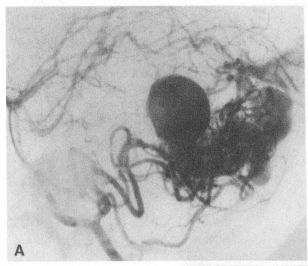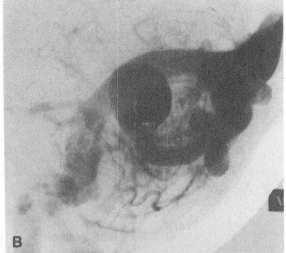

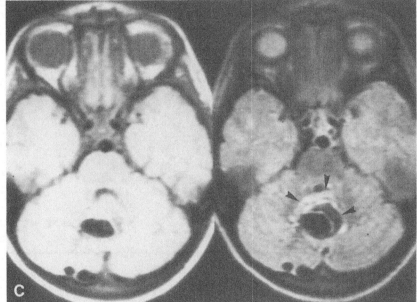

Fig. 1.56 A – C. Inferior vermian arteriovenous malformation. **A** Arterial and **B** venous phases of the left vertebral artery injection in lateral projection show a large, partially thrombosed, venous ectasia as demonstrated in **C** axial MRI studies (*arrowheads*)

Table 1.15. Areas of venous obstacle

Foramen of Monro
Ventricular-choroid fissure junction
Deep sylvian fissure
Tentorial edge
Inferior vermian-dural junction
Vein of Galen-Falco tentorial junction

Venous collateral circulation creates evolving patterns that consistently adapt to the changes created by the evolution of the situation (chronicity of the high-flow conditions, dystrophic changes of the veins, aging of the vascular tree).

Thrombosis and kinking represent some of the obstacles to flow which occur in the venous system draining either the lesion or the brain (Figs. 1.30, 1.51, 1.55, 1.56). Direct venous compression (Table 1.15) by the sphenoid ridge or tentorial edge is frequent and may account for the high incidence of hemorrhagic episodes in lesions developing in the incisura or in the medial temporal lobe (Willinsky 1988) (Fig. 1.57). Some areas of venous narrowing without upstream ectasia can be seen; they may correspond to compression by bridging arteries while in their subpial location (Fig. 1.58). In other instances no venous caliber changes are seen; there is no clinical evidence of previous hemorrhage and yet a thrombosis has occurred producing an unusual venous pattern (Figs. 1.59, 1.60). In these cases, throm-

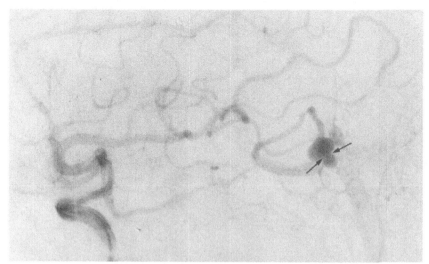

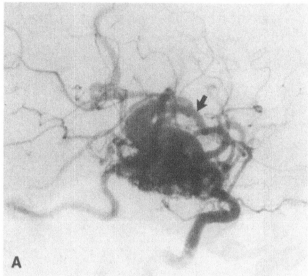

Fig. 1.57. Left internal carotid injection in lateral view demonstrates a venous ectasia above and below the tentorial edge (*arrows*) in a patient with a medial temporal lobe arteriovenous malformation with medial venous drainage

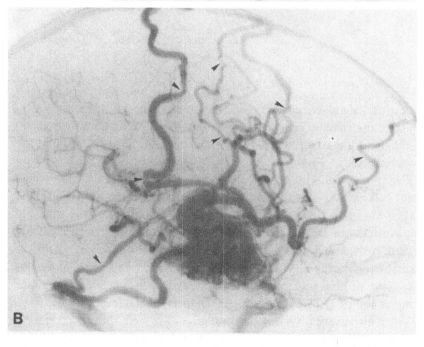

Fig. 1.58. A Early and **B** late phases of the right internal carotid artery injection in lateral view in a temporal arteriovenous malformation draining into a large temporal vein (*arrow*) and then into almost all the cortical venous system (*arrowheads* in **B**)

Fig. 1.59. A Early and **B** late phases of the left internal carotid injection in lateral view. Rolandic arteriovenous malformation in a patient presenting with conjunctival congestion of the left eye. Note the pseudophlebitic aspect of the cortical venous drainage into the ophthalmic vein (*arrow* in **B**) responsible for the ophthalmic symptomatology

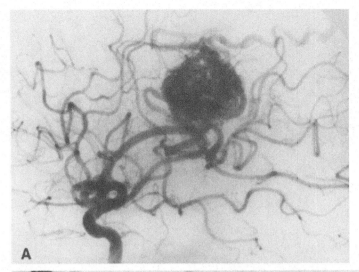

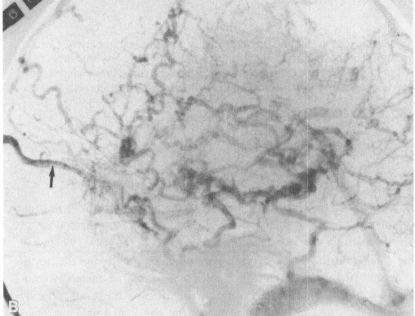

bosis must be differentiated from venous agenesis. The difference of cause refers to the basic distinction between anatomical variation (congenital disposition) and collateral circulation (acquired variation).

Some features may help to distinguish a hereditary vs an acquired variation. For example, hereditary absence of a straight sinus draining a vein of Galen dilatation is often associated with an embryonic sinus persistence (falcine, tentorial). In the acquired absence of the straight sinus, however, the afferents of the basal vein(s) are recruited bilaterally as venous outlets (see Vol. 3, Chap. 7).

Thrombosis of veins can cause hemorrhage; but in some instances, although the vein was patent at the time of the bleed, it thromboses during the immediate evolution of the hemorrhagic episode (London and Enzemann 1981) (Figs. 1.61, 1.62). Complete thrombosis of malformations was reviewed by Nehls and Pittman (1982). In 48% of patients a preceding

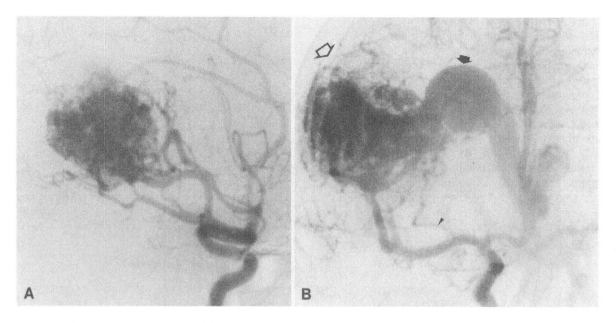

Fig. 1.60. A Lateral and **B** frontal views of the right internal carotid artery. Cortico-ventricular lesion fed by cortical and lenticulostriate arteries (*arrowhead* in **B**). Note the absence of the expected drainage into the cortical vein (*open arrow*) and the prominent deep venous outlet corresponding to a dilated thalamostriate vein (*solid arrow*)

hemorrhagic episode could be documented. The mean age was 39 years and there was no sex difference.

In Einsmann's (1972) review, all spontaneous thromboses occurred following hemorrhage. The compression of a hematoma may thrombose an AVM. Alternatively, it may compress only a portion of the AVM, which will appear smaller during the acute episode and then reexpand after the hematoma has resolved. Even the caliber of some feeders may be altered by compression of the nidus or of draining veins (Fig. 1.63). Repeat angiography is therefore indicated prior to treatment, after the hematoma has reabsorbed.

Additional factors possibly leading to delayed thrombosis have been suggested: thrombosis of abnormal arteries (Svein and McRae 1965), atheromatous lesions of the feeders (Pool and Potts 1965), mechanical compression (hematoma or perilesional edema) (Eisenmann et al. 1972), kinking and stenosis from surrounding gliosis (Lakke 1970), embolism from a proximal aneurysm (Omojola et al. 1982), and partial embolization with IBCA (Vinuela et al. 1983).

The same factors have actually produced increases in the size of AVMs (Peeters 1982). Stein states in his follow-up that one-third of AVMs increased in size and one-third remained stable; this has not been our experience. The limitations in assessing spontaneous thrombosis are illustrated in Becker's review of 18 histologically verified "occult" CVMs (Becker et al. 1979). He reported that 50% were found to be "thrombosed arteriovenous malformations." The criterion he used to call them AVMs was the ability of the small arterial structures within the malformation to be stained using elastic van Gieson preparation. This criterion, however, fails

Fig. 1.61. A Early and **B** venous phases of the right internal carotid injection in lateral view. Posterior temporal arteriovenous malformation draining into a large temporo-parietal vein joining the superior sagittal sinus without opening into it (*solid arrow* in **A**). Note the reflux into a parieto-frontal venous system leading to congestion of the entire hemisphere (*open arrows* in **B**)

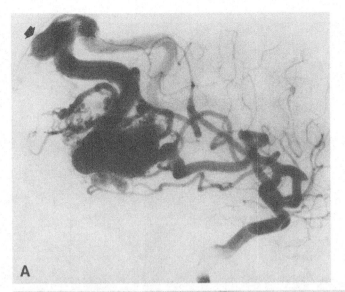

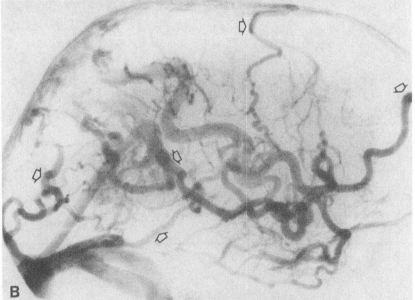

to differentiate AVM from cavernoma. There was a significant female predominance in his series.

Lobato and coworkers (1988), in their review of 21 histologically verified vascular malformations, found 44% to be AVMs, 31% to be cavernous angiomas, and 10% to be venous angiomas. In 4% of patients, a capillary telangiectasia was diagnosed and in 11% the lesions were called mixed or unclassified. The analysis confirmed that there was no essential difference in the patterns of clinical presentation. The diagnosis of thrombosed AVM does not seem to have any prognostic significance. It is felt that, if surgically accessible, the lesion should be removed to decrease the propensity for rebleed and seizures, although clear evidence to support this is lacking. Most "thrombosed AVMs" probably represent cavernomas. Pseudoaneurysms can sometimes be seen in the process of thrombosis, prior to shrinking of the artery (Leo et al. 1979) (Fig. 1.62).

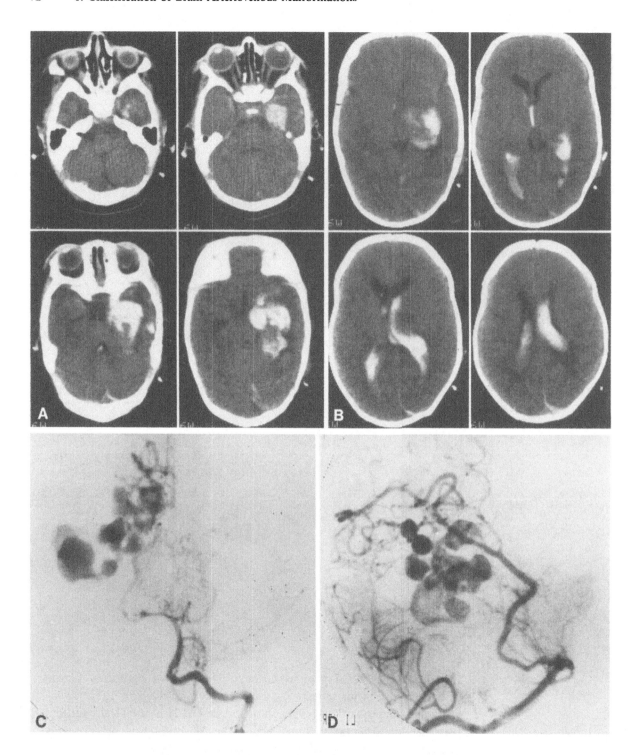

Fig. 1.62. **A** and **B** Nonenhanced axial CT cuts in an infant presenting with an intracerebral hemorrhage with ventricular extension. **C** Frontal and **D** lateral views of the left vertebral artery at the time of the hemorrhagic episode. Note the multiple venous (possible) pseudoaneurysms visualized. Opacification of the lesion is also obtained with injection of the ipsilateral internal carotid artery. **E** Frontal and **F** lateral views of the left vertebral angiogram 3 months following the hemorrhagic episode and after satisfactory clinical recovery. A spontaneous closure of the supply from the right posterior cerebral artery is demonstrated. Note the caliber changes

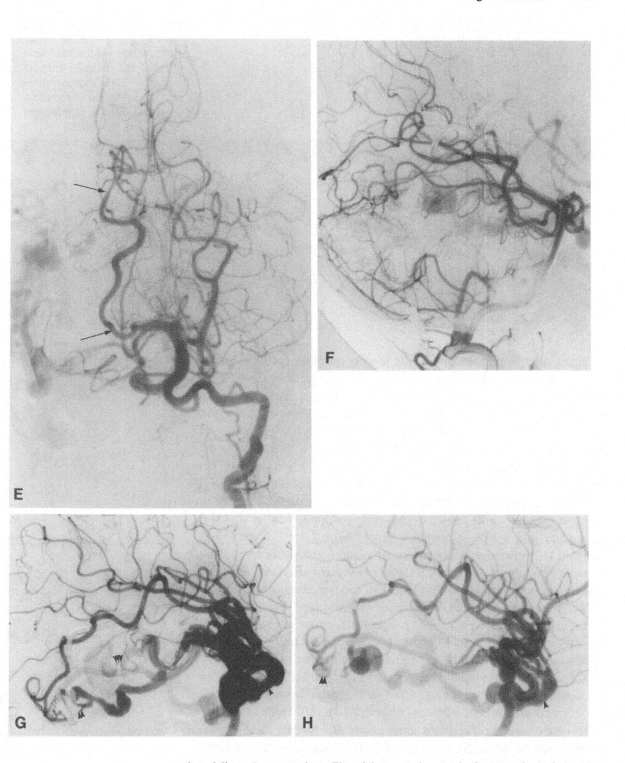

that follow the regression. The right posterior cerebral anatomic variation is unrelated to the arteriovenous malformation. **G** Right internal carotid artery control at the same time demonstrates three areas of shunting: posterior temporal (*double arrowhead*), medial temporal (*triple arrowhead*), and temporo-polar (*arrowhead*). In view of the early thrombotic changes observed, additional thrombosis was anticipated and no treatment was administered. **H** Right internal carotid artery injection 6 months after shows the spontaneous closure of the medial temporal shunt and the decrease in size of the venous outlet of the other two

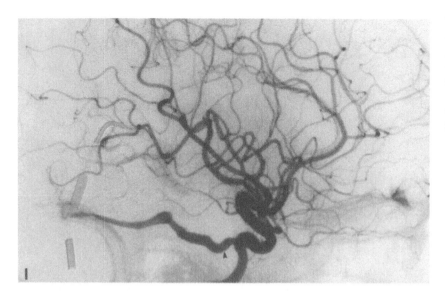

Fig. 1.62. I Right internal carotid artery control 1 year later shows additional occlusion of the posterior temporal shunt. The temporo-polar fistula is the only remaining one. The child is growing normally with no deficits

Finally, the spontaneous thrombotic process that may occur in BAVMs seems more active in children than in adults (as evidenced by the 9.6% incidence of spontaneously thrombosed VGAM in our series) and may be more prominent in adult females than in males. Of interest is the fact that 25.8% of BAVMs in children are multiple, whereas only 6.8% in adults are. Do most of the associated AVMs in children thrombose before being discerned in adulthood? Spontaneous occlusion of AVMs is often symptomatic (Fig. 1.64), whereas occlusion that follows embolization seldom is.

One can question the effect of chronic activation of the coagulation system in a lesion that is known to trap platelets (Sutherland et al. 1988). Association with a true or dominant coagulation (C or S protein, antithrombin III) deficiency can be suspected in some patients (Dusser 1988). A peculiar pattern of anti-factor VIII secretion has been noted in the endothelium of some venous malformations of the face (Berenstein and Choi 1988) and in a few with Von Willebrandt's disease (see Vol. 2, Chap. 6).

Venous ectasias correspond to the progressive response of the venous wall to compromised outflow and/or "turbulence". The aneurysmal dilatation of the vein of Galen illustrates this situation in an extreme fashion. Venous ectasias or pouches are usually encountered where the tortuosity of the enlarged vein meets an obstacle that narrows it or creates kinking (Table 1.15). The venous dilatation results from a failure to find an efficient exit to relieve the increased pressure. Therefore, most converging systems (deep venous, posterior portion of the basal vein, and deep sylvian vein) carry a higher risk of developing ectasias than diverging or highly anastomotic venous systems (cortical veins). The effects of the high pressure in the intracranial venous system will depend on the anatomical variant. Ideally, separation of both venous circulations protects the brain from retrograde venous hypertension; efficient outlets include transosseous, transorbital, and contralateral drainage (Fig. 1.65). Incomplete treatment may further alter this outflow collateralization. In most cases, the closer the lesion to the dural sinus that drains its venous outflow, the less the chance of interfering and impairing the parenchymatous venous drainage. The farther from the sinus,

Fig. 1.63. A Axial CT demonstrates an intracerebral hematoma. **B** Left internal carotid artery injection at the time of the hemorrhagic episode failed to demonstrate the full nidus and shows the mass effect (*arrowheads*) on the venous aspect of the lesion. **C** Following resorption of the hematoma, the nidus is now well demonstrated as is its drainage into transcallosal and subependymal veins

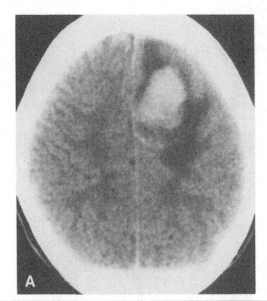

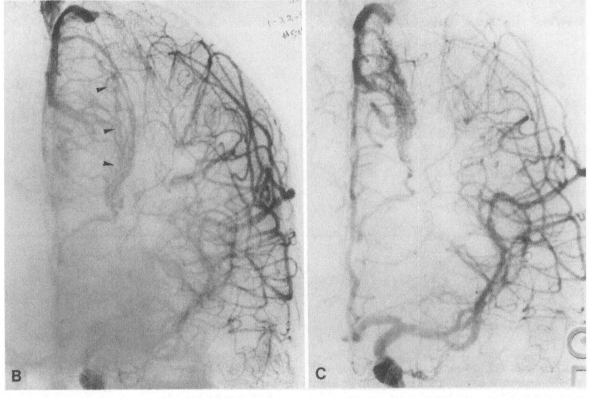

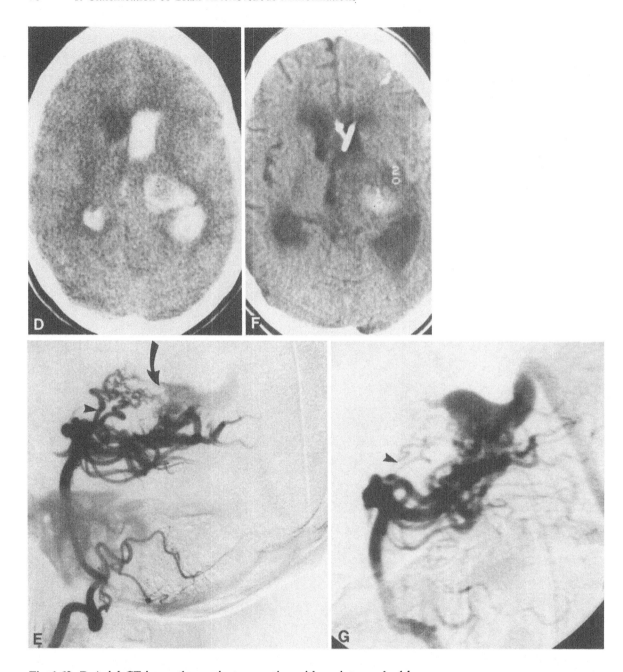

Fig. 1.63. D Axial CT in another patient presenting with an intracerebral hemorrhage with ventricular extension. **E** Left vertebral artery injection in lateral projection at the time of the bleed demonstrates a thalamic arteriovenous malformation,
and its venous drainage, compressed by the hematoma (*curved arrow*). Note the size
of the thalamo-perforators (*arrowhead*). **F** Noncontrast CT and **G** left vertebral
angiogram in lateral view. Following ventricular shunting and resorption of the
hematoma, there is better opacification of the malformation and its venous
drainage. Note the compensatory decreased caliber of the thalamo-perforator
feeders (*arrowhead*)

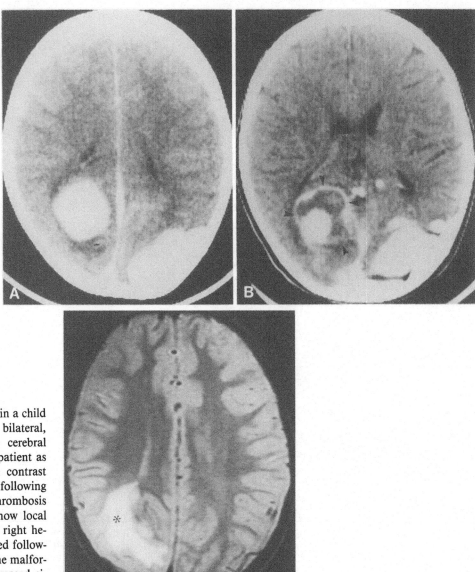

Fig. 1.64. A Axial CT in a child presenting with a bilateral, high-flow, posterior cerebral artery fistula. (Same patient as in Fig. 1.6.). **B** Axial contrast CT and **C** T-2 MRI following partial spontaneous thrombosis of the right fistula show local changes that led to a right hemianopia that regressed following embolization of the malformation. Note the increased signal (*asterisk*) in the white matter of the occipital pole

the higher the chance for the increased flow to reflux into cerebral veins and create retrograde congestive complications (seizures, decreased tissue perfusion) (Fig. 1.66; see Chap. 2).

f) CSF Changes

Alterations in CSF circulation may result from high flow or from thrombosis within the superior sagittal sinus. Reflux into the superior sagittal sinus and stagnation in its posterior segment may in some arteriovenous lesions induce segmental thrombosis that finally separates the shunt drainage from that of normal parenchyma (see Chap. 5). The presence of transosseous and orbitofacial venous collateral circulation will betray this abnormal drainage, but, if efficient, such drainage may allow the abnormal venous reflux to remain neurologically subclinical. Bone hypertrophy (as in

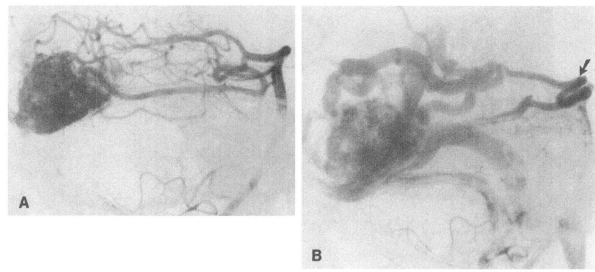

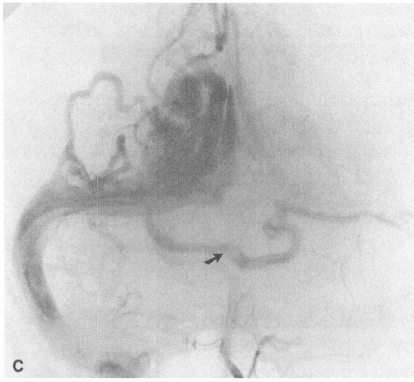

Fig. 1.65. A Early and **B** late phases of the left vertebral artery angiogram in lateral and **C** frontal views. Occipital pole arteriovenous malformation fed by the posterior temporal branch of the right posterior cerebral artery. Note the congested venous drainage that crosses the midline to open into the opposite medial, temporal venous system via the posterior communicating vein (*arrow*)

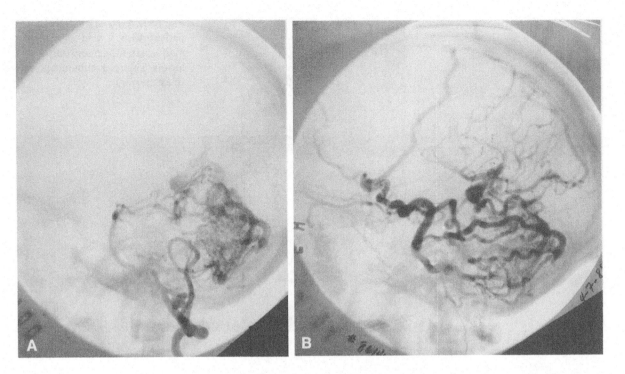

Fig. 1.66. A Early and **B** late phase of the left vertebral artery injection in lateral view. Posterior fossa arteriovenous malformation revealed by temporal seizures. Note on the late phase (**B**) the congested supratentorial venous system, opacified through the lateromesencephalic venous connections

Sturge-Weber syndrome, see Vol. 2, Chap. 10), acts as a constraint applied to the venous drainage of the skull. In addition, CSF alterations which may be purely hemodynamic (dural high flow), functional (multiple subarachnoid hemorrhages), mechanically related (direct destruction to CSF circulation due to intraventricular veins or compression of the mesencephalic aqueduct), or a combination of factors may be seen, particularly in VGAM. Arachnoid "cyst" or enlarged localized subarachnoid spaces can be encountered in association with BAVM but such findings are rare (Fig. 1.67). Many CSF disorders associated with AVM remain unexplained; however, transcerebral vein dysfunction and lack of cerebral compliance represent only two examples of mechanisms which may result in significant modification of the extravascular intracerebral water compartment (see Chap. 5) (Zerah et al. 1992).

g) Calcifications

Calcifications seen in BAVMs are usually located in the venous walls. In children, calcifications may occur at a distance from the shunt, in "normal" veins, probably secondary to hypoxia at the venous watershed zones [medullary venule (Fig. 1.68)] or at the sulpial cortical venous level (Sturge 1879; Weber 1922) (Fig. 1.69). They can appear with age and when present do not disappear. Calcification are rarely parenchymatous but, if so, usually correspond to calcified cerebral hematomas. Sutherland et al. (1988), in two patients with calcified BAVMs, was able to demonstrate platelet aggregation within the malformation (see also Chap. 5).

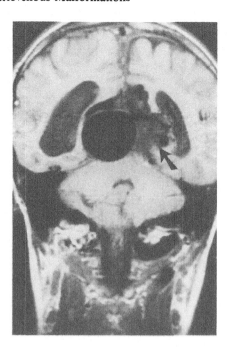

Fig. 1.67. Axial MRI study in a patient with a vein of Galen malformation, demonstrating a locally enlarged subarachnoid space (*arrow*)

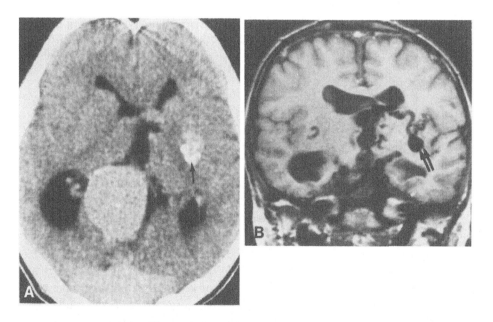

Fig. 1.68. A Axial CT in a patient with a vein of Galen arteriovenous dilatation demonstrates a calcified structure (*arrow*). B Coronal MRI shows that this calcification is on a transcerebral venous ectasia (*double arrow*)

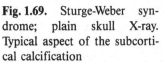

Fig. 1.69. Sturge-Weber syndrome; plain skull X-ray. Typical aspect of the subcortical calcification

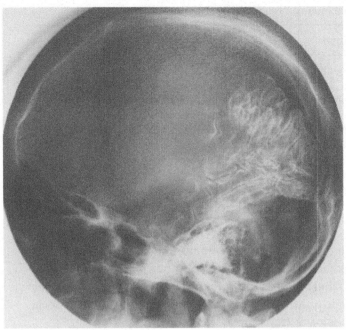

IV. Venous Lesions

Over the years venous lesions of the CNS have generated a large number of publications (Nishizaki et al. 1986; Koussa et al. 1985; Tagle et al. 1986). Among the most controversial venous lesions are the so-called cavernomatous type, which were called venous "angiomas" or cavernous "hemangiomas". Unfortunately the prolific literature contributions have not led to any clear classification. Many of these lesions have been regrouped under the generic name of venous hamartomas (Crawford and Russel 1956). "Hamartomas", however, are simple spontaneous proliferations made up of elements derived from the local tissue in which they develop (Rubinstein 1972, 1981). This proliferation and growth produces a large number of cells that eventually reach maturation and become self-limiting. The resulting mass appears as an "exaggeration" of a physiologic process. In fact, although these lesions present some tumor-like characteristics, they are often erroneously considered as malformations. While capillary hemangiomas of infants correspond to this definition, none of the cerebral venous anomalies or abnormalities can be accurately described as hamartomas (Table 1.16).

1. Developmental Venous Anomalies (DVAs)

Saito and Kobayashi (1981) were the first to consider DVAs (venous angiomas) as anomalies and not as malformations, as claimed by Rigamonti et al. (1990). Subsequently, we have expressed doubts (Lasjaunias et al. 1989c; Jimenez 1989) (Vol. 3, Chap. 7) regarding the role of these lesions in most of the clinical events in which they were demonstrated, thus question-

Table 1.16. Denomination of "venous lesions"

Classical denomination	Proposed denomination
Cerebral venous angiomas	Developmental venous anomaly (anatomical variation)
Cavernous hemangiomas Intraneural (cerebral)	Cavernous malformation (cavernomatous malformation)
Cavernous hemangiomas Dural or epidural (cranial or spinal)	Cavernous hemangiomas (tumor)

From P. Lasjaunias et al. 1988.

ing the need for therapeutic intervention. DVAs represent extreme variations of hemispheric white matter and tectal venous drainage. They are not encountered elsewhere in the CNS, as opposed to other vascular malformations. Secondary failure to efficiently drain cerebral tissue would explain their role in ischemic or hemorrhagic events, independent of their association with true pathologies (cavernoma, AVM, etc.).

2. Cavernous Hemangiomas and Cavernous Malformations

In vitro studies presently allow us to differentiate a proliferative lesion (tumor) from a nonproliferative one (malformation). The clinical and therapeutic consequences of this distinction are obviously very important. Confusion results from the fact that both lesions have always been presented under the same name. Thus, reports discussing the clinical presentation and surgical results of patients with "cavernous hemangiomas", which collect and mix patients with various extradural and cerebral lesions (and sometimes even DVAs), are unusable.

a) Cavernous Hemangiomas

Cavernous hemangiomas are typical tumors. They can be encountered in the intracranial or intraspinal extradural space (Simard et al. 1986; Buonaguidi 1984) and only occasionally occur in the CNS itself. They may also develop in the peripheral nervous system (Fehlings and Tucker 1988). Angiography usually shows a faint homogeneous capillary stain leading to the preoperative diagnosis of meningioma (Numaguchi 1979). If angiography is properly performed, cavernous hemangiomas are seldom angiographically occult. Cavernous hemangiomas are more frequent in females in whom a progressive mass effect may expand the lesion acutely during menstruation or pregnancy (Kobayashi 1984).

These tumors are mostly treated surgically (Padovani et al. 1982), but many authors suggest radiation therapy (Yamasaki et al. 1984), which has not proven to be consistently efficient and may be associated with significant morbidity. These lesions seldom bleed and are absent from autopsy series. They are nosologically close to the lingual or orbital hemangiomas (Harris and Jzkobiec 1979). Thus, they differ completely from the cavernous malformations of the CNS.

Fig. 1.70. A Coronal and **B** sagittal MRI studies in a patient presenting with a mesencephalic cavernous malformation

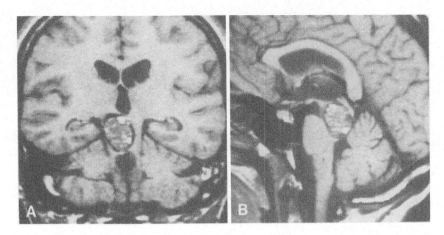

Many authors describe cavernous hemangiomas as tumors, but because of their CNS homonyms (vide infra) they are still improperly called malformations. These lesions, however, are the only ones that deserve the name cavernous hemangioma and represent a separate entity from cavernomas.

b) Cerebral and Medullary Cavernous Malformations

Cavernous malformations (cavernomas) represent the only true venous malformation of the CNS (Fig. 1.70, Table 1.17) (Stein 1985). Their incidence is 0.5% (Otten et al. 1989) and they can be encountered anywhere in the cerebral or spinal cord tissue (Fontaine et al. 1988; Cosgrove et al. 1988;

Table 1.17. Classification of cerebromedullary venous malformations

---

Venous malformation
  Single venous malformations
    Cavernoma (cavernomatous malformation)
    Troncular dysplasia (varix)
  Multiple venous malformations
    Multifocal (familial or nonfamilial)
    Systemic: Sturge-Weber
              Cobb and Klippel-Trenaunay
              Blue rubber bled nevi

Associated forms
  Other vascular malformations
  Telangiectasia
  Arteriovenous malformations
  Venous or venolymphatic extracranial malformations
  Developmental venous anomalies (dural or cerebral)

Secondary vascular changes
  Venous thrombosis
  Collateral circulation
  Angiogenesis
  Ectasias

Secondary morphological changes
  Cortical atrophy
  Calcification
  Cysts

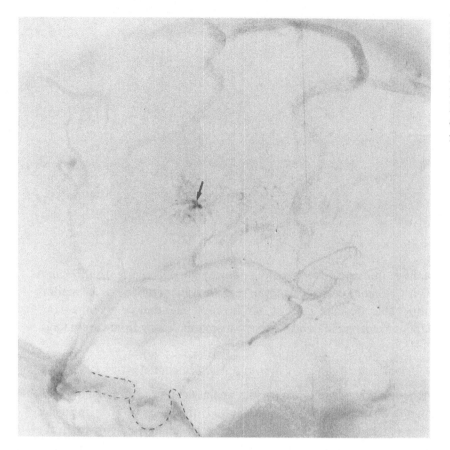

Fig. 1.71. Late phase of the left internal carotid artery injection in lateral view in a patient with a ruptured cavernous malformation at the time of the hemorrhagic episode. Note the late venous puddling at the level of the hematoma and cavernous malformation (*arrow*)

Iplikceoglu et al. 1986; Wang 1988; Lejeune et al. 1989). Cavernous malformations are angiographically occult with the rare exception of partial venous filling encountered at the time of a hemorrhagic episode (Fig. 1.71). Their association with DVAs or confusion with true cavernous hemangiomas (see above) accounts for most of the reports of so-called positive angiography (Simard et al. 1986). Only 4.5% of cavernous malformations are symptomatic (Otten et al. 1989; Steiger et al. 1989).

Fundamentally stable, these lesions can "grow" by confluence of the vascular spaces and further achieve cystic forms through secondary confluence of intralesional spontaneous hematomas (Belloti et al. 1985). There is no cerebral tissue interspaced between the vascular lumens and no evidence of cellular proliferation, capsule formation, or a relationship between the age of the patient and the size of the lesion (Steiger et al. 1989). Numerous cavernous malformations have been reported in newborns or children (El Gohary et al. 1987; Yamasaki et al. 1984; Iwasa et al. 1983; Hubert et al. 1989; Mazza et al. 1989).

These cavernomas, although mostly isolated, often show at pathology adjacent satellite cavernomatous micromalformations. They therefore are often locally multiple and sometimes multifocal (Steiger et al. 1987).

Familial cavernous malformations are not rare; an anomaly of endothelial cell growth factor has been identified in some hereditary forms of vascular lesions (Rutka et al. 1988). In familial disease (Bicknell et al. 1978; Clark 1970; Giombini and Morello 1978; Hayman et al. 1982), intracranial (cerebral) and intraspinal (medullary) cavernous malformations can be present

Table 1.18. Possible causes of angiographically occult vascular malformations

---

Destruction or compression of a vascular malformation (hemorrhage ± edema)

Intraluminal thrombosis
   Stagnant or turbulent flow
   Embolization

Blood vessel changes
   Fibrosis
   Spasm
   Arteriosclerosis
   Plications
   Endoluminal proliferation
   Dysplastic changes

Poor angiographic examination or analysis

Modified from El Gohary 1987.

in the same individual. The transmission, like all inherited CVMs, is autosomal dominant. Even though intralesional hemorrhage is consistently found at pathology, few of these hemorrhages are clinically apparent. Rarely, patients with cavernous malformations present with subarachnoid hemorrhage, including those in spinal cord locations (Ueda et al. 1987). Most of the time they will have a slowly progressive clinical presentation. Some cavernomas, for example, result in seizures. Calcifications and calcified forms are frequent (Occhiogrosso 1983; Shimoji et al. 1984; Tyndel et al. 1985) and may represent the spontaneous and favorable evolution of the lesion (cavernoma calcificans) following intralesional hemorrhage or spontaneous thrombosis. The calcifications could represent homologues or phleboliths which are frequently described in venous malformations of the face (Vol. 2, Chap. 10).

Cavernomas represent most of the angiographically occult vascular malformations and can be associated with telangiectasias (Izukawa et al. 1987; Waybright et al. 1978). Such lesions may undergo an angiogenic reaction following a local hematoma rather than a transitional malformation of the capillary-venous type. In the face of a negative angiogram following an intracerebral hematoma, an MRI study should be performed to identify the underlying cause. MRI has revealed many previously occult malformations and represents the method of choice for diagnosis and follow-up, since it is quite specific except for exclusion of hemorrhagic metastasis.

3. Occult and Cryptic Malformations

Angiographically occult lesions refer to a multifactorial situation in which the quality of the examinations performed is important (Table 1.18). At present no single imaging modality has the ability to diagnose all of the so-called occult vascular lesions. A lesion that would be occult to all modalities including pathology is cryptic. By definition cryptic lesions are mysterious and hidden, whereas occult lesions are difficult to diagnose. This does not mean that occult lesions are invisible to all modalities since their existence is not questioned (Table 1.19). When Crawford introduced the concept of

Table 1.19. Occult CVMs

Permanently angiographically occult
Cavernous malformations
Telangiectasia
Thrombosed arteriovenous malformation
Transiently occult
Microarteriovenous malformations
Small compressed arteriovenous malformations

cryptic AVM in 1956 (Crawford and Russel 1956), examples of intracerebral hemorrhages with AVMs were cited. These cryptic lesions were "encountered" in 4.5% of patients with intracerebral hemorrhage (Russel 1954). Following multiple additional publications, the term "cryptic" has been accepted but has been applied to a heterogeneous group of malformations.

Intralesional thrombosis or compression of an AVM by an intracerebral hematoma may account for the nonvisualization of an otherwise visible lesion at angiography. Only cavernomas and telangiectasias are truly angiographically occult. The former are not occult at MRI; the latter are not occult at pathology.

Cryptic lesions represent neither a specific clinical nor anatomical entity. They correspond to the "remaining" causes for hemorrhagic episodes when other lesions have been excluded. Their incidence reflects our lack of understanding and knowledge; it has no epidemiological value since it corresponds to a postulated disease or group of diseases.

Occult lesions represent our failure to demonstrate with a given imaging tool a heterogeneous group of pathologies. Similar to cryptic lesions but for different reasons, the incidence of occult malformations has no epidemiological value but is mainly of technological interest.

4. Sturge-Weber Syndrome

Two types of Sturge-Weber syndrome can be distinguished angiographically, depending on the patency of the deep venous system and its capacity to collect the drainage of the hemispheres (Bentson et al. 1971) (Figs. 1.69, 1.72).

Although traditionally a pial vascular malformation is described, it does not correspond to our interpretation of the clinical and radiological picture of these patients. The developmental defect (malformation) is probably only manifested by the venular, lymphatic, or mixed malformation seen on the face. The relationship of the facial lesion to the trigeminal nerve root topography is only of historical interest. Any port wine stain of the face will, by definition, involve some or all of the trigeminal root territory without causative relationship. Its topography does not allow any reliable prediction concerning the status of cerebral involvement.

The cortical lesion may arise from an early (in utero) thrombosis of the medullary veins on either side of their opening (deep or superficial), leading to the unusual venous pattern described in the disease. Secondary post-ischemic (venous) atrophy and, eventually, calcification create the traditional reported aspect. The thrombosis could be related to an unknown (or

Fig. 1.72. A Late phase of a right carotid angiogram in lateral view in a patient with Sturge-Weber syndrome. The only draining vein to the hemisphere is a deep-seated vein that connects the superior striate to the inferior striate system (*arrow*). **B** Sagittal MRI confirms this venous anastomosis. No cortical vein is demonstrated in the parieto-temporo-occipital region

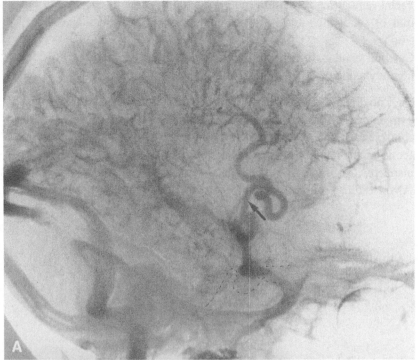

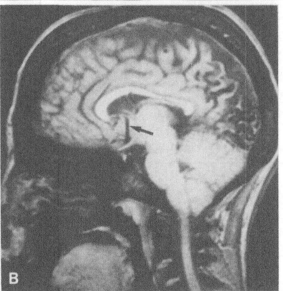

undetected) coagulation problem associated with the venular malformation or to the response of the coagulation system to the presence of anti-factor VIII, as encountered in some venous malformations. Therefore, cerebral anomalies without facial port wine stain (Ambrosetto et al. 1983), enlargement of the choroid plexus (Stimac et al. 1986), evolvement of the disease (Probst 1980; Garcia et al. 1981), localization of the calcifications and atrophy in the hemisphere opposite the port wine stain (Chaudary 1987; Cersoli et al. 1989), and posterior fossa locations (Vol. 2, Chap. 10) characterize the heterogeneity of the disease. Thus, Sturge-Weber syndrome can be summarized as follows:

1. Facial venular malformation (port wine stain), sometimes capillary venular or venolymphatic, with facial bone (maxillary and malar) hypertrophy.
2. Cerebral venular thrombosis due to an associated coagulopathy or local hemodynamic disorder (but eventually isolated).

There is no direct relationship between the facial and cerebral topographies. The trigeminal partition is fortuitous and the port wine stain is stable. The cerebral venular disease is active as long as triggering factors produce ischemia in the venules leading to focal decreased flow into the cerebral hemisphere. Calcification results from this phenomenon (as it does in VGAM), leading to a deficit in cortical functions, atrophy, and seizures.

CHAPTER 2

Clinico-Angioarchitectural Correlations

I. Introduction

"The lobes of the brain involved in the arteriovenous malformation did not influence the mode of presentation" (Crawford et al. 1986).

Patients with cerebral vascular malformations present challenging and difficult problems. The natural history of brain arteriovenous malformations (BAVMs) has been related to every conceivable facet of the lesions, including the size or topography (Shi and Chen 1986; Spetzler and Martin 1986), the age and sex of the patients, the location of the lesion (Crawford et al. 1986; Forster et al. 1972; Jomin et al. 1985), the presence and type of venous obstruction (Laine et al. 1981; Lasjaunias et al. 1986a), and associated arterial aneurysms (Miyasaka et al. 1982; Batjer et al. 1986; Lasjaunias et al. 1988). Most studies have been done in a retrospective manner, the best available prospective study being that of Crawford et al. (1986). A prospective correlation between the angioarchitecture of the AVM and its clinical implications has, however, not yet been done.

Different medical and surgical specialities analyze the morphological patterns using different tools and for different purposes. Picard et al. (1984), for example, looked at angioarchitecture with an eye toward the possibility of embolization.

As we have seen in the previous chapter, analysis of the architecture of BAVMs may permit detection of potential weaknesses in the vascular system and permit identification of some stigmata of previous events. In addition, understanding clinical symptoms as related to a specific angioarchitectural arrangement may lead to more specific treatment options, including partial treatment, to favorably affect both symptoms and the natural history of a specific lesion. The link between AVM architecture and some systemic phenomena (failure to thrive, cardiac overload, hemorrhage, and CSF disorders in children) will be discussed in the section on vein of Galen aneurysmal malformations (VGAMs) and cerebral arteriovenous fistulas (see Chap. 5). This analysis will allow us to individualize the evolution of a given AVM and to assess its risk factors and possible prognosis in a specific patient. Elementary features of the angioarchitecture have already been presented; their link with the clinical symptomatology will now be discussed.

Table 2.1. Equilibrium and symptoms

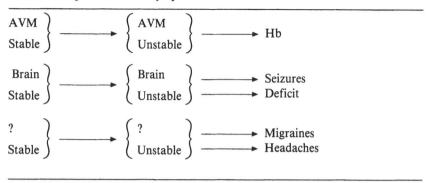

II. Hemorrhage and Angioarchitecture

Hemorrhage in a patient with a BAVM represents a significant change in the compliance of the vascular system; similarly the onset of seizures or neurological deficits in an AVM patient represents an imbalance in the "compliance" of brain function in relation to the AVM (Table 2.1).

One can live normally with an AVM throughout life. However, some angioarchitectures and some acute events may tilt the fragile congenital equilibrium into an unstable situation. From our experience, some features are reversible and make us believe that some specific unstable situations can be reversed and compensated for. Hemorrhage is probably the only event that must lead to complete correction of the congenital defect (i.e., complete obliteration and/or removal of the AVM), since partial surgical treatment does not seem to decrease significantly the risk of future hemorrhage. However, partial treatment with embolization, if properly targeted and achieved, may alter an otherwise dangerous situation and bring favorable results. It has been postulated that sudden headaches, with or without seizures, and other acute symptoms (often transient) can be considered as minor expressions of local hemorrhages. Such small hemorrhages have been noted at surgery (Yamada 1982). If the correlation is true, these minor bleeding events increase the true incidence of hemorrhage in BAVMs; by the same token, they also decrease the real morbidity and mortality risks of an initial or subsequent hemorrhage.

There is evidence that bleeding can result from rupture of the AVM nidus, arterial aneurysm rupture, or from venous rupture, which may occur close to or remote from the lesion. In addition several observations have been made during surgery as to previous subclinical hemorrhages within or in the vicinity of the nidus (McKenzie 1953; Moody 1970; Stein and Wolpert 1980). At surgery, one-third of BAVMs show evidence of previous hemorrhage (Stein and Wolpert 1980). Bleeding in AVMs has a high incidence of resultant hematoma and intraventricular hemorrhage. Vasospasm following bleeding from an AVM is, however, a rare occurrence (1 patient in 500 in Yasargil's series, 1% in Parkinson's series, and 2 patients in the 900 we have seen) (Figs. 1.35 and 3.31). In a surgical series of BAVM patients, Yamada (1982) pointed out the venous topography associated with 16 out of 18 hematomas. He also emphasized the probable hemorrhagic significance of acute, intermittent, severe headaches. Hematomas resulting from brain

Table 2.2. Cerebral AVM: Hemorrhage and type in adults

Type of AVM	Incidence of each presenting with hemorrhagic episode (%)
Cortical and subcortical	
Micro-AVM	100
Macro-AVM	13
Cortico-ventricular	40
Deep	75
Posterior fossa	64
Total	44

AVM, arteriovenous malformation. From Willinsky 1988.

AVM rupture seem to be better tolerated than those from other causes, although no real comparative study exists comparing the outcome of hematomas of the same size resulting from different etiologies (Mohr 1984; Ruscalleda 1986).

There are two different pathophysiologic mechanisms that produce hemorrhage in BAVM: (1) the arterial or anterograde pressure-related rupture and (2) the venous or retrograde pressure-related rupture. Both are linked and can provoke a rupture at the weak point of the lesion either separately or together. Possible hemorrhage secondary to ischemic infarction will not be considered here but may occur.

In Morello's series (Morello and Borghi 1973) of over 154 patients, 86% of small AVMs bled, while 75% of mixed sized and 46% of large AVMs bled. These numbers illustrate the more frequent presentation of small AVMs as hemorrhagic episodes (Tables 2.2, 2.3). Patients with small AVMs do not usually present with seizures or progressive neurological deficits. Crawford et al. (1986) found that recurrence of bleeding episodes was not linked to AVM size. Associated arterial aneurysms (75%) and venous stenosis (52%) were the most common angioarchitectural features associated with hemorrhage (Willinsky 1988) (Tables 2.4, 2.5). Analysis of Crawford's patients who bled reveals that venous stenosis (52%) (Table 2.6) and arterial aneurysms (41%) were significantly more frequent in the hemorrhage group

Table 2.3. Hemispheric cerebral AVM[a]: Hemorrhage and topography in adults

Topography	Patients who bled (%)
Frontal	6
Parietal	11
Occipital	8
Temporal	44
Insular	66
Corpus callosum	66
Total	28

AVM, arteriovenous malformation. From Willinsky 1988.
[a] Only cortico-subcortical and corticoventricular macro-AVMs included.

Table 2.4. Clinical hemorrhagic episodes and arterial angioarchitecture in adults

	Incidence in all AVMs (%)	Incidence in AVM with hemorrhage (%)
Arterial aneurysm	21	41
Arterial infundibulum	14	11
Arterial stenosis	17	11
Arterial variation	24	27
Arteriovenous fistula (isolated or within AVM)	4	5
Micro-AVMs	9	21

AVM, arteriovenous malformation. From Willinsky 1988.

Table 2.5. Incidence of BAVM with and without arterial aneurysm by topography and by symptoms

	BAVM with aneurysm (%)	BAVM without aneurysm (%)
Topography		
Cortical	30	41
Corticoventricular	66	34
Deep-seated	4	13
Posterior fossa	0[a]	12
Total	100	100

BAVM, brain arteriovenous malformation. From Lasjaunias et al. 1988.
[a] At present we have seen flow-related aneurysms of both the proximal and distal type in posterior fossa AVMs.

Table 2.6. Hemorrhagic episodes and venous angioarchitecture in adults

	Incidence in all AVMs (%)	Incidence in AVM with hemorrhage (%)
Venous stenosis	38	52
Venous ectasias	43	47
Venous variation	32	32
Transcerebral venous drainage	10	9

AVM, arteriovenous malformation. From Willinsky 1988.

than in the overall population of those with AVMs. Some 73% of the patients who bled showed either a venous stenosis or an arterial aneurysm.

When comparing the incidence of the various features present in the entire population with those present in patients that bleed, only arterial aneurysms and venous stenosis have a clearly increased frequency in the hemorrhagic group. In the group that bled, two-thirds of the venous stenoses were encountered in females and two-thirds of the arterial aneurysms were encountered in males. Despite the almost equal number of males and females in the hemorrhagic group, we found that in the third decade of life there is a female predominance, whereas in the fifth decade there is a male predominance. The increased chances (89%) of rebleed in an AVM patient

Table 2.7. Brain AVM prognostic factors[a]

	Overall risk (%)	Risk factors			
		Increased	(%)	Decreased	(%)
Hemorrhage	42	Previous Hb	51	No Hb	33
		Temporal	67	No Hb and no epilepsy	8
		Age > 60	89	Incidental	0
				Parietal	32
Handicap	27	–		–	
Epilepsy	18	Previous Hb	22	No Hb	0
		Age 10 – 19	44	Age > 30	6
		Temporal	37	–	
Death	31	Previous Hb	32	Epilepsy	21
				Parietal	25
				Incidental	27
				No Hb	28

AVM, arteriovenous malformation. Modified from Crawford et al. 1986.
[a] 217 patients; data collected over 20 years.

diagnosed after the age of 60 (Crawford et al. 1986) (Table 2.7) may testify to the acquired rigidity of the vascular system with aging and its vulnerability to the presence of the AVM.

Some 89% of patients harboring both venous stenosis and arterial aneurysm have had a hemorrhagic episode (Willinsky 1988). Yasargil (1987) questioned the fact that, if the AVM is the determining factor for the occurence of the arterial aneurysm, why are aneurysms so infrequent an accompanyment of AVM? At least the higher flow lesions and direct fistulas should be associated with a higher incidence of associated aneurysm. He observed that in giant and small AVMs there was a 10.5% – 13.1% association with arterial aneurysm, respectively, but no aneurysms were present in patients with VGAMs or in those with arteriovenous fistulas (AVFs). We agree with these comments and confirm from our experience the range of numbers given (see Chap. 5). We believe, however, that some weakness of the angioarchitecture are only revealed with time. VGAMs and AVFs, the highest flow lesions, are diagnosed at an early age therefore flow-related arterial aneurysms (time related) have not developed. In addition, each individual reacts differently to disease. Consequently although acquired features are linked to the AVM, they also express the host's capacity to compensate for the presence of an AVM and his overall resistance and flexibility. It is of interest to note that all of the patients harboring arterial aneurysms with their AVM had more symptoms than those without aneurysms, except for headaches, which were half as frequent in the population with aneurysms (Lasjaunias et al. 1988). These observations may indicate that the unstable state that exists in patients with associated aneurysms can express itself in various clinical manifestations.

In our series, temporal, insular, and callosal AVMs were as likely to bleed as deep-seated or posterior fossa lesions (Garcia-Monaco et al. 1990a). Crawford et al. (1986) also noted an increased risk of hemorrhage in temporal AVMs (Table 2.7) but found that neither deep-seated nor posterior fossa AVMs produced a higher incidence of rebleeding. It should also be

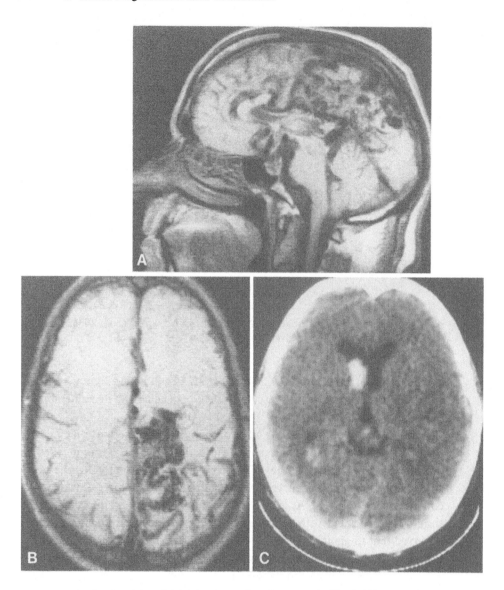

Fig. 2.1. A Sagittal and **B** axial MRI of a patient (same as in Fig. 1.41) presenting with a medial parietal and singular arteriovenous malformation associated with a corpus callosum abnormality. **C** Note on axial CT, the topography of a hemorrhagic accident that involves drainage of the malformation into the thalamostriate and internal cerebral veins. This hemorrhage cannot be linked either to the arterial feeders and their secondary anomalies or to the nidus that is more posteriorly located

noted that patients with AVMs in the temporal region have the highest incidence of seizures (37%). The only specific anatomoarchitectural characteristics of the temporal lobe are its cortical nature (with increased incidence of arterial aneurysms) and its deeply located venous drainage (basal vein), with its natural tendency to loop and kink at the tentorial edge (Willinsky 1988). Both characteristics lead to possible explanations as to the higher incidence of hemorrhage and seizures in patients with temporal AVMs. One can postulate that hemispheric lesions have a higher incidence of bleeding from their associated aneurysms, whereas deep and posterior fossa AVMs tend to bleed as a result of venous obstruction. Both risk factors are encountered in temporal lesions. In the literature 41% – 50% of BAVM pa-

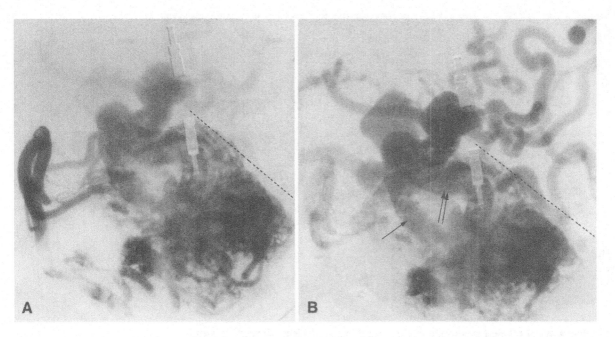

Fig. 2.2. A Early and **B** venous phase of the left vertebral artery injection in lateral view in a 30 year old male who presented with four hemorrhages that required a ventricular shunt. Large cerebellar arteriovenous malformation without brainstem involvement. Note the huge precentral (*arrow*) and superior vermian (*double arrow*) veins that reach the vein of Galen confluence. Enlargement proximal to a thrombosed straight sinus leads to additional congestion of all the afferents of the great cerebral vein. Falco-tentorial junction (*interrupted line*)

tients with aneurysms presented with hemorrhage and 78% of these events were thought to result from the aneurysm rupture (Batjer et al. 1986; Miyasaka et al. 1982), although documentation was not always conclusive.

It is also relevant that the incidence of both associated aneurysms and hemorrhage increases with age. Therefore, it becomes evident that, in a given AVM patient, the overall 2% – 3% risk of hemorrhage per year may not apply. The chance of developing an arterial aneurysm and bleeding from it increases fourfold between 10 and 50 years of age (Lasjaunias et al. 1988).

Venous causes for hemorrhage are more difficult to document. Laine et al. (1981) and Dobbelaere et al. (1979) have pointed out the importance of the venous outlets in the maintenance of hemodynamic equilibrium within the AVM. Luessenhop and Rosa (1984), quoting Kaplan (1961), supported the pivotal role played by the venous structures in determining the course of "embryologically mature AVMs" (those that develop from the cortical mantle).

Hemorrhages located at a distance from the nidus are usually related to venous bleeding (Fig. 2.1). Yasargil (1987) found the venous pressure in ruptured AVMs to be higher than in nonruptured ones (as measured during open surgery). Viñuela et al. (1985), in their review, pointed out the high frequency of venous abnormalities in deep-seated lesions, but did not separate the population into groups with and without anomalies or assess the relationship of anomalous venous drainage to symptoms. Thrombosis and hemorrhagic infarctions are probably part of venous group of com-

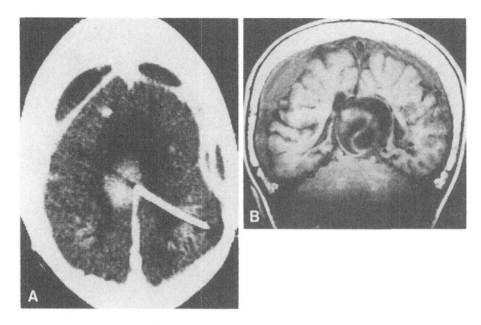

Fig. 2.3. A Axial CT and **B** coronal MRI in two different patients presenting with vein of Galen vascular malformations. Note the sequelae of bilateral subdural hematomas that followed surgical ventricular shunting

plication (Fig. 2.2). In large AVMs, hemorrhage is a rare event, and such lesions usually do not present significant venous obstacles. Most commonly, the obstacles include kinking of dolicho veins and mechanical compression within a sulcus, the tent, or the choroidal fissure. As long as the vein can enlarge, however, or more proximal venous outlets can be recruited, no hemorrhage occurs. This point is well illustrated in our series; stenotic veins have a significantly increased incidence in patients with lesions that have bled, whereas venous ectasias do not. When interference with drainage is present, chronic venous congestion may produce "referred" hemorrhagic accident within the ischemic zones. Conversely, deep-seated lesions draining into the vein of Galen confluence, regardless of their size, present a higher risk of bleeding. Thrombosis of the straight sinus, often observed in this location, forces the venous collateral circulation to open additional channels. In addition, the converging nature of this system constitutes an obstacle that may well end by producing vessel rupture (Fig. 2.2).

Interaction and interference between the venous changes and CSF circulation as a cause of hemorrhage is of importance, but is difficult to assess. Operative observations of these phenomena are difficult to reproduce during endovascular approaches since CSF counterpressure on the veins is preserved. In one of his patients Dobbelaere (1979) noted a threefold increase in a vein of Galen ectasia within months after ventricular shunting, pointing to the importance of CSF vascular pressure equilibrium. Similar observations have been made several times in our series since this report (see Chap. 5). Other reports in the literature refer to the changes in lesion angioarchitecture following ventricular shunting. Several extracerebral effusions have been noted in patients in our series, some of them leading to seizures or major cerebral damage following subdural drainage and secondary intracerebral hemorrhage recurrence (Fig. 2.3).

Table 2.8. Algorithmic representation of symptoms and angioarchitecture

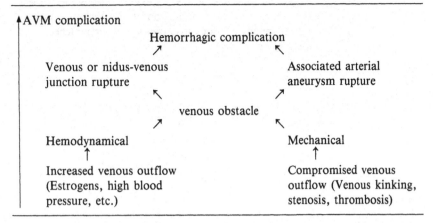

Ventureyra's (1984) patient bled twice and died within 1 month following ventricular shunting. The patient was 14 years old, had a pineal region BAVM, and presented with gaze problems, precocious puberty, and hydrocephalus. We have seen a patient with a pineal region AVM and hydrocephalus who bled within 3 days after shunting. Transient increased intracranial pressure (ICP) as a cause of thrombosis and consequent hemorrhage is possible. Pre- and postoperative bleeding have been observed following clipping of the venous outlets. However, interruption of the vein proximal to the first "normal" afferent vein (draining normal brain) prevents transfer of abnormally elevated pressures to the normal venous system and may lead to thrombosis and cure of the AVM. Hemodynamic and morphological changes that follow partial thrombosis can result in regional increased blood volume and pressure. These changes may enhance the hemodynamic significance of a minor area of venous narrowing and transform it into a significant obstacle (Table 2.8).

Although increases in regional blood flow have been documented during physical activity, there is no relationship to hemorrhage (Pelletieri 1980). Regional blood flow changes occurring with cerebral function may, however, change the hemodynamic conditions of the equilibrium between the AVM and the brain.

A 65 year old female presented with grand mal seizure with a musical aura. She recognized it as being the introductory tune for her radio-broadcasted English lesson which she had heard every week for two years prior to the onset of the first symptoms. CT and angiography revealed a left temporal mid-size AVM located in the region of Heschl's gyrus. Had "function" created flow changes in the AVM?

Brown et al. (1988) demonstrated that, in 166 patients with unruptured AVMs, 5.4% were hypertensive at the time of presentation, while 16% of 31 patients that subsequently bled were hypertensive. This suggests that systemic hypertension increased the risk of hemorrhage in this group of patients. Heavy lifting, sexual intercourse, or emotional stress are associated with hemorrhage in less than 25% of patients with a bleed. Some 36% of hemorrhagic complications occurred during sleep (Perret and Nishioka 1966). Thus, there is no definitive relationship between hemorrhage and physical exertion (Pelletieri 1980) or mild trauma.

Table 2.9. Neurological deficit and seizures in BAVMs

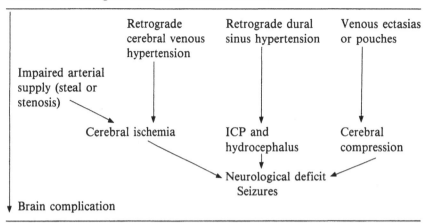

In conclusion, a hemorrhagic episode accounts for the failure of the host vascular system to compensate for the morphological alterations created by the AVM. Arterial aneurysm, venous stenosis, and kinking express the weakening process of the vascular tree and often presage its ultimate failure.

III. Cerebral Function and Angioarchitecture of BAVMs

The interaction between cerebral AVMs and brain function represents the most challenging aspect of analysis of these lesions. Clinical experience in managing BAVMs shows that, beside the regional blood flow interaction, two gross types of interference with brain function exist which are reflected in identifiable pathology: (1) "scar" formation, with perilesional gliosis and tissue destruction, and (2) an ischemic territory remote from the nidus.

The goal of analysis of lesion angioarchitecture is to appreciate specific patterns that have or will create symptoms. Such analysis must, of necessity, be mostly retrospective, but the deductions from it, as they relate to the natural history, will help us to outline the vascular arrangements responsible for further clinical problems.

Schematically, neurological deficits and seizures can be linked to two broad categories of interference with function (Table 2.9); (1) ischemia, either arterial or venous, and (2) direct or indirect mechanical compression.

Clinical symptomatology may often result from more than one type of interference. No clear distinction between the two categories may be present. We can, however, separate the various underlying causes artificially into arterial and venous.

Arterial ischemia may arise from two types of mechanisms: a "steal" phenomenon and occlusive changes. In our experience, evidence of the steal phenomenon has never been demonstrated, except by angiographic studies.

Since the recognition of preferential blood flow towards the low resistance area of an AVM, significant controversy has existed as to the hemodynamic steal in vascular malformations of the brain. The first suggestion of such phenomena occurred following both the recognition, during cerebral angiography, of preferential blood flow towards the AVM (Bergstrandt et al. 1936) and the various blood flow studies (Shenkin et al. 1948).

Norle (1949) described the significant dilatation of arteries leading to an AVM which would take up to 3 weeks to return to normal size following excision of the AVM. He suggested an elevated blood flow via the dilated arteries to the lesion. In 1971, Feindel reported steal in the cerebral micro-circulation as a syndrome and based this conclusion on evidence from fluorescine angiography and microregional blood flow using radioisotopes during excision of a BAVM. There was a diminished microcirculation in the brain surrounding the AVM prior to excision or ligation of the feeding arteries which returned to a more normal appearance after the operation.

Cerebral blood flow studies undertaken with xenon-131 have been disappointing even after cerebral stimulation (visual or speech). Deutsch (1983) showed that visual activity could steal blood from the AVM towards the occipital cortex. The concept of steal in angiography is based on the non-visualization of vessels in a normal area of the cerebrum. However, careful angiographic evaluation always visualizes the "missing" branches through leptomeningeal anastomoses, thus expressing the real adaptive capability of the brain circulation. Most of the "stolen territories" are not symptomatic, even if the flow within the AVM was important enough to steal the contrast material from the ipsilateral hemisphere. Although we have doubts with regard to the symptomatic aspect of this feature, the finding itself cannot be rejected. Thus, the phenomenon of steal remains a possible mechanism. Improvement in flow, noted following partial correction of the steal either by hypotension (autoregulation test by Ancri and Pertuiset 1985; Pertuiset et al. 1985), embolization, or surgery (Mohr 1984; Luessenhop and Rose 1984), does not support this concept. Several authors have expressed doubts with regard to the significance of steal (Yasargil 1987). Empiric experience contradicts the steal theory, leaving a hypothesis which requires further investigation.

Gliosis, presumably postischemic, has been found at some distance from an AVM by Constantino and Vitners (1986). Description of the arterial supply of the lesion was, however, not presented nor was the venous drainage of the AVM and of the normal brain noted. The gliotic transformation of tissue surrounding the nidus region can be attributed to: (a) venular dysfunction (secondary to venous hyperpressure) with resultant decreased tissue perfusion, (b) mechanical pulsation of the enlarged vascular channels, or (c) a combination of both mechanisms (Fig. 2.4). Dystrophic calcifications at a distance from high-flow lesions suggest that venous hyperpressure is an important factor in decreased tissue perfusion and ischemia.

The steal phenomenon is, however, considered by some authors as the only satisfactory hypothesis for explaining these remote gliotic changes. One of the first quantitative demonstrations of arterial steal was obtained in a territory distal to the AVM following intracarotid injection of contrast material. No study was performed in the posterior circulation (which frequently provides the compensatory flow) (Prosenz et al. 1971). The steal areas found by Homan (1986) were variably located ipsi- or contralaterally: "distal to the main arterial supply of the AVM in areas supplied by arteries not directly involved in the AVM." Again, venous congestion was not analyzed, and the study demonstrated quantitatively the absence of steal phenomena in the arterial tree that supplied the lesion. Hypoxia, originating arterially in a vascular territory which functions with apparently normal

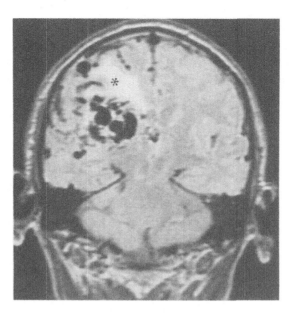

Fig. 2.4. Coronal MRI study (same patient as in Fig. 1.30). Note the abnormal increased signal (*asterisk*) of the white matter posterior and superior to the nidus of the arteriovenous malformation

arterial hemodynamics, was suggested. Although the territory is subject to impaired drainage secondary to venous constraints from the adjacent AVM, this possibility was not discussed.

Experimental or traumatic AVFs (CCF or others) reroute an already functioning system and shift a previously established equilibrium of the vascular supply. In such cases, clinical steal is not observed. Cerebral ischemia is only seen when an incompetent circle of Willis exists. The congenital nature of AVMs, with the resulting morphological adaptation, favors the venous hypothesis for ischemia.

Arterial stenosis and occlusion may range from a single narrowing to a moyamoya pattern but always express acquired failure of the remaining arterial tree (see Chap. 1). Such changes are, however, usually slowly progressive, allowing stepwise compensation and probably accounting for their clinically silent development. Patients with occlusive changes may be more symptomatic (neurological deficits, headaches) and have less hemorrhagic complications than those patients without such changes.

Displacement of watershed zones and the changes in them after embolization, as seen during follow-up angiography, testify to their role and importance in compensation. Often, changes in arteries providing collateral circulation are considered more likely responsible for arterial ischemia than are the occlusive changes (high-flow angiopathies) that develop on the branches of the AVM. The various types of watershed zones changes represent the possible evolution of the lesion over the years (Figs. 1.24, 1.26–1.29). Congenital vs acquired watershed transfer can be assessed from careful analysis; additionally, postischemic angiogenic features can often be identified. For example, chronic hypoxemia may increase the capillary density by up to 50%.

The concept of venous ischemia is accepted by most authors involved in the management of cerebral arteriovenous lesions but is never recognized as the dominant one. Laine et al. (1981) pointed out the key role played by the venous patterns in understanding the symptoms presented in dural and brain AVMs. The absence of arterial steal or even of any contribution of pial arteries to the supply of dural AVMs, in the face of often identical neurological manifestations in brain BAVMs, points to the predominant role played by the venous drainage in this type of anomaly. Spetzler and Selman (1984), commenting on Nornes and Grip (1980) work, emphasized the role played by the locally increased venous pressure, but only as a secondary (additional) factor in decreasing tissue perfusion. Like most other authors, they related ischemic symptoms mainly to the arterial steal. Even when discussing the "sump effect" after resection of the AVM, only the capillary bed was considered, and its loss of autoregulation was proposed to explain the breakthrough perfusion theory. Nornes (1984), in his attempt to demonstrate the quantitative aspects of the sump effect, was successful only when he took into consideration the venous consequences of AVM resection. One should remember that 60% – 80% of the cerebral blood volume is located in the cerebral venules. These present all the cytologic characteristics of active exchange with the surrounding tissue, testifying to their role in nutrient exchange. Flow in venules is bidirectional in the white matter, allowing them to fulfill their nutrient role even in a retrograde fashion. Most of these nutrient functions involve catabolic reabsorption (Auer and McKenzie 1984).

Conversely, the congestion of the system that occurs either hemodynamically or by stasis, due to stenosis or thrombosis, will produce ischemic phenomena of venous origin and accumulation of catabolic substances in the parenchyma. Abnormal signals obtained on MRI are often encountered around veins draining AVMs (Fig. 2.4). The same observation is made in dural AVMs draining into cerebral veins and spinal dural AVFs draining into the cord. At some point the white matter can no longer tolerate the venous congestion. The acquired nature of the congestion makes it become quickly (as soon as it occurs) symptomatic, since no anatomical compensation has occurred embryologically.

The venular changes associated with aging may account for the delay observed in the development of these deficits. The progressive nature of the deficits and their fluctuation in severity reflect the attempts of the collateral circulation to overcome the increased pressure in the venous outlet of the shunt.

Decreased tissue perfusion secondary to venous ischemia may produce virtually any type of neurological symptom (motor or sensory deficits, neuropsychological alteration, seizures, etc.). Noteworthy is the fact that complete failure of the venous system (retrograde congestion and secondary thrombosis) has led, in some of our patients, to dementia without focal neurological deficits (Figs. 3.1, 3.2). Involuntary movements are rare in patients with BAVMs (Tamaoka et al. 1987; Lobo-Antunes 1974). A few reports can be found in the literature: ten such patients were described by Tamaoka et al. (1987).

A link between the nidus topography and symptoms may sometimes be constructed. Analysis of the drainage pattern ipsilaterally and contralaterally will, in most cases, explain the remote character of symptoms (Fig. 2.5).

Brain atrophy that is observed in the vicinity of the lesion probably also has a venous origin. As Yasargil pointed out, the atrophic changes do not correlate with the areas of arterial steal and most venous diseases of the cor-

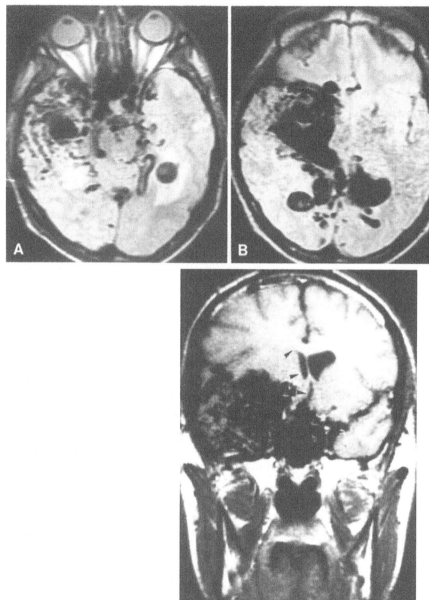

Fig. 2.5. A and **B** Axial and **C** coronal MRI studies in a patient presenting with a large temporal arteriovenous malformation on the right side and several venous ectasias related to obstruction of the venous outlet to the deep venous system. (Same patient as in Fig. 1.12.) This patient presented with a bilateral corticospinal tract syndrome with generalized seizures. Note the mass effect (*arrowheads*) at the level of the nidus and the large ectasias clearly demonstrated on the angiogram shown in Fig. 1.12

tex produce atrophy (Sturge-Weber syndrome). In our series, we have been unable to correlate atrophy with the intensity of the flow or the topography of the angiographic steal.

The longer the venous channel from the shunt site to its emptying into a dural sinus, the higher its chances of interfering with the normal brain circulation. This simple observation has not been made in the discussion of the "normal perfusion pressure breakthrough" (NPPB) (Nornes 1984), although it was recognized that the length of the arterial feeders correlated with an increased chance of a perfusion abnormality developing during or shortly after resection. It is of importance to mention that in BAVM pressure in the jugular vein is usually normal. This emphasizes the ability of the venous system to absorb the abnormal pressure from the arteriovenous shunt. It also illustrates its potential role as a valve, fulfilled by the transdural portion of the cerebral veins.

IV. Seizures and Angioarchitecture of the BAVM

Seizure is the second most frequent presenting symptom in all BAVM patients, present in over 50% at one time or another. The most frequent AVM locations associated with seizure production are the motor-sensory strip and the temporal areas, representing close to 70% of patients with seizures (Crawford et al. 1986).

In patients without an obvious hematoma or subarachnoid hemorrhage, the cause of seizures has been controversial. It has been said that this symptom is frequently associated with small hemorrhages, discovered only at the time of surgery (Stein 1985). However, only 6.5% of Yasargil's operated on patients who presented with a seizure had evidence of bleeding at the time of surgery. Some of the discoloration noted at this time may have represented old areas of previously thrombosed malformation or veins. The onset of seizures in a previously healthy individual must reflect an acute or abrupt change in hemodynamics, which may be due to rerouting of drainage from the malformation through a vein that previously drained normal brain. The increase in pressure produces secondary neurological dysfunction and seizures. A patient with a posterior fossa vascular malformation had venous drainage that was rerouted into the temporal lobe prior to presenting with temporal lobe seizure (Fig. 1.66). Patients with lesions in the basal ganglionic area and posterior fossa do not present with seizures unless there has been some venous thrombosis.

Mass effect has been observed for a long time (Terbrugge et al. 1977) from 17.5% to almost 40% of patients with AVMs as determined by CT. However, mass effect was seen in almost half of the patients in whom previous hemorrhage has occurred. In unruptured AVMs the size of the venous component is the dominant factor responsible for mass effect (Fig. 2.5).

Remote causes of increased ICP include CSF obstruction and associated subarachnoid cysts. Unilateral occlusion of the foramen of Monroe by an enlarged thalamostriate vein may lead to ipsilateral ventricular enlargement (Pribil et al. 1983; Sang 1983). Oversecretion of CSF by a choroid plexus AVM has been suggested; however, in our experience it has never represented a satisfactory explanation for any form of hydrocephalus. Papilledema without evidence of hydrocephalus has also been reported (Schiffer et al. 1984). As mentioned previously, venous thrombosis, secondary ectasias, and hemorrhage may create secondary ICP changes and unilateral or bilateral hydrocephalus. ICP changes are seen more frequently in patients with high-flow lesions (cerebral or dural) with rapid sinus drainage. Most of these lesions are encountered in BAVMs (Gibson et al. 1959) or dural high-flow lesions (Young 1979; Sroobandt 1986; Cronqvist et al. 1972). Hydrocephalus can be seen in children without mass effect when venous hypertension and reflux into the superior sagittal sinus compromise CSF reabsorption (Berenstein 1981; Seidenwurm et al. 1989). Transcerebral venous disorders and extravascular intracerebral water compartment dysfunction have also been shown to be responsible for ICP changes in children with BAVMs (Zerah et al. 1992) (see Chap. 5).

V. Systemic and Remote Effects

Most of the systemic manifestations secondary to a BAVM will be address-ed in the Chap. 5, in the section devoted to vein of Galen aneurysmal malformations. Others include: *Cardiac overload with failure to thrive* and *consumption of coagulation factors.* Ross et al. (1986) reported on a large, intracranial, dural lesion in a newborn, which was partially thrombosed and was associated with anemia and thrombocytopenia. Hydrocephalus, brain atrophy, and cardiac insufficiency were also noted. The baby subsequently died.

Endocrine manifestations with precocious puberty (Ventureyra and Baj-dedo 1984) and associated VGAM and galactorrhea remain anecdotal.

Facial veins enlargement or pseudovenous malformation can be seen when the transosseous venous system drains the normal brain (see Chap. 5).

Finally, children with VGAMs often develop seizures following intraven-tricular shunting (see Chap. 5).

VI. Headaches and Angioarchitecture of BAVMs

Headaches are subjective and difficult to quantify and therefore to study. In patients with BAVMs, headaches can be divided into those that accom-pany the episode of a subarachnoid hemorrhage or intracerebral hemor-rhage and those that are more subacute and chronic in nature.

Constant headaches or episodes of throbbing ("migraine-like") head-aches can occur in the same patient. The headaches seem to remain on the same side as the AVM. Headache is the first symptom in approximately 60% of patients and is present in over 20%–30% of our patients.

The acute headaches associated with hemorrhage are those typically re-lated to an acute event, presenting abruptly and usually severe in nature, as-sociated with photophobia, nausea, vomiting, convulsion, and loss of con-sciousness. The patient may deteriorate acutely with generalized cerebral dysfunction and may progress to respiratory and/or cardiac arrest.

Subacute and chronic headache may be related to the vascular distribu-tion of the malformation or to partial thrombosis, edema, mass effect, or hydrocephalus.

The headaches associated with various vascular distributions are those that relate specifically to the dural supply and/or external carotid participa-tion in a vascular malformation or to an adjacent territory. These types of headaches may have a precise distribution. They are usually throbbing in nature and often are associated with some eye symptoms.

Patients with stenotic lesions in association with an AVM appear to have chronic headaches which occur more frequently and which are less respon-sive to treatment.

Patients with significant or predominant posterior cerebral supply to a purely pial vascular malformation may have associated headaches, most often localized to the same side as the malformation. These may also be as-sociated with various types of visual prodromes and/or intermittent epi-sodes of field defects or other ophthalmic symptoms.

Patients having AVMs in the distribution of the middle cerebral artery also complain of headaches, although less frequently and most often if their venous drainage is to superficial veins. However, any patient with a vascular malformation, regardless of the primary blood supply, may complain of headaches.

Headaches associated with BAVMs tend to be periodic and may be disabling on some occasions. Headaches were present in 37% of our patients; 14% referred to them as "disabling". Concerning migraine headaches and vascular malformation, no true relationship exists. Lees (1962) failed to find any evidence of vascular malformation while investigating 300 migraine patients, including 23 in whom angiography was performed. None had a vascular malformation.

The management of headaches will vary depending on the cause. Embolization, in general, may relieve headaches of vascular nature. When the meningeal participation to an AVM is properly embolized, associated headaches usually resolve or diminish. On occasion, the visual prodrome (tearing, etc.) may persist, but the headaches will not appear. In patients with lesions with posterior cerebral artery participation, the headaches may actually be exacerbated for a short period of time, usually days, after embolization and then improve or disappear. Conversely, in patients with middle or anterior cerebral artery contribution, in addition to posterior cerebral artery supply, the headaches may increase after embolization of the former and will respond to embolization of the latter, a pattern suggesting an initial increase in posterior cerebral artery flow and its inversion.

Conservative management of nonhemorrhagic headaches in patients with AVMs or those that do not respond to embolization may include the use of hypotensive medications (see Chap. 3).

VII. AVM and Pregnancy

Although there appears to be an increased rate of presenting symptoms at the time of pregnancy, much controversy has existed as to the increased risk factor of neurological complications, primarily hemorrhage, during pregnancy. In neither our experience nor that of Yasargil was there any increased bleeding rate during pregnancy. Controversy also exists as to the increased risk of hemorrhage during delivery. Although there appears to be an increased venous pressure during Valsalva maneuvers with delivery and some patients with AVMs have had acute symptoms or aggravation of preexisting symptoms during the third trimester of pregnancy or during delivery, a significant number of patients have gone through multiple pregnancies and deliveries without manifestations of their disease (Dias 1990; Horton 1988). It therefore appears prudent that, if a vaginal delivery is contemplated, the procedure should be done with an epidural block and no nausea-producing drugs (also see Chap. 3).

CHAPTER 3

Indications and Objectives in the Treatment of Brain Arteriovenous Malformations

I. Introduction

Decisions regarding endovascular treatment of brain arteriovenous malformations (BAVMs) require complete information concerning the clinical setting and demonstration of the angioarchitecture of the lesion and remaining brain. From these factors a clinico-morphological analysis can be made to formulate the best plan for therapy. The hemodynamics of the condition are therefore of significant importance in determining both the approach to the lesion and the expected chances of reaching the therapeutic goal. Treatment modalities represent an evolving part of this strategy and may change with time, whereas the original objective, as determined by clinical and angioarchitectural features, remains the same.

II. Hemodynamic Basis of BAVMs

Blood flow through cerebral vessels has a parabolic velocity profile, with its maximum in the center. In such so-called laminar flow patterns, all "particles" move parallel to the vessel axis (Hassler 1986). At bifurcations, flow variations occur at different areas, slower flow patterns at the bifurcation itself. Depending on the angle of a bifurcation, the pressure will be different.

The blood flow through feeding vessels to malformations shows high velocity, and laminar flow may be transformed into "turbulent" flow, especially where an arteriovenous fistula (AVF) exists (Nornes and Grip 1980). Particularly, at the level of the shunt, significant turbulence is encountered, with blood flow in the first several centimeters of a major draining vein often being very turbulent.

There is a significant difference in the distensibility of arteries and veins. On average, a vein is six to ten times more distensible than an artery; a vein holds three times the blood volume of a comparable artery and therefore its compliance or capacity tends to be 18 – 30 times as great (Yasargil 1987). Hassler, in studying experimentally produced AVFs, noted that enlargement was much more pronounced in draining veins (up to 250%) than in feeding arteries (average 23%). In venous structures, the intercellular spaces of the tunica media widens; fibrous elements proliferate; and dysplastic collagen, matrix vesicles, and muscle cells of the N-type occur (Fischer 1979). Similar changes are seen in varicose veins. Large volumes of blood are needed to raise the pressure in the venous sinuses. To offset each increase of 1 mmHg, approximately 100 ml of blood are needed (Yasargil 1987).

The phenomenon of delayed compliance describes how acute pressure changes in blood vessels are followed by slow adaptation towards normal.

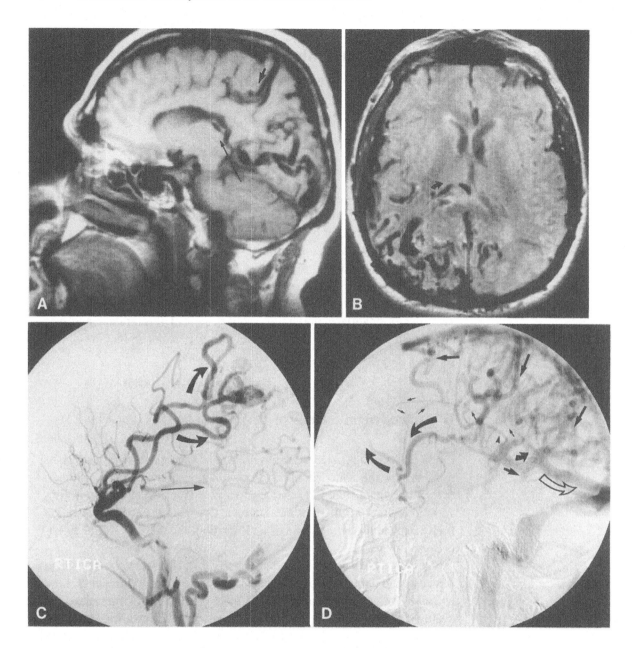

Fig. 3.1 A–L. Venous hypertension. **A** 78 year old male, previously asymptomatic, presents with progressive mental deterioration over 6 months and more abrupt deterioration over the last week to a semistuporous state prior to embolization. **A** Sagittal and **B** coronal MRI examination (T1-weighted images) 3 months prior to admission demonstrates an arteriovenous malformation in the parietal occipital region with venous drainage through the superficial venous system in a reverse manner (*arrow*) and to the deep venous system (*long arrow*). Note prominence of the transcerebral venous system on the right (*curved arrow* in **B**). **C** Early phase of the common carotid artery injection on the right in lateral projection demonstrates two main middle cerebral artery branches supplying the parietal portion of the malformation (*curved arrows*). There is filling of the posterior cerebral artery (*long arrow*), which contributes small distal branches to the malformation in the parietal occipital region. **D** Late venous phase of the same injection. Lateral digital subtraction angiography (DSA) demonstrates the significant venous drainage of the malformation congesting the superficial venous system (*arrows*). Note filling of the internal cerebral vein (*arrowhead*) and the inferior sagittal sinus (*small arrows*) fill-

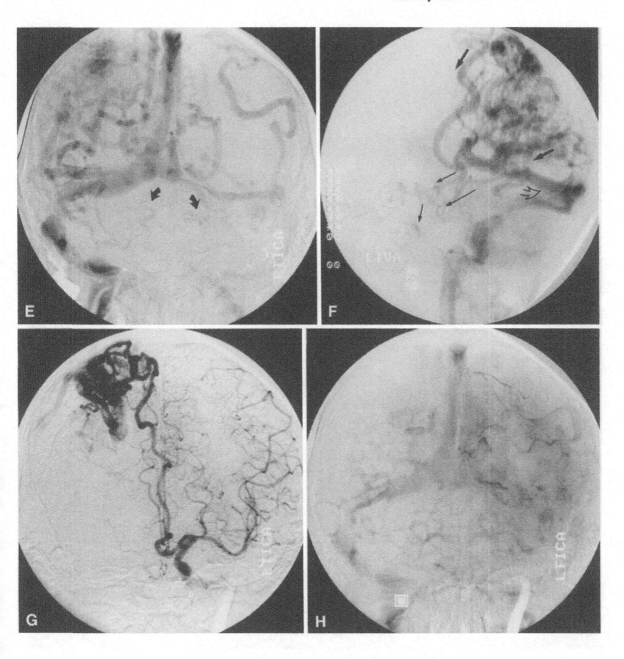

ing in a retrograde manner. There is additional reflux into the vein of Galen (*curved arrow*) and towards the straight sinus (*curved open arrow*). Note also filling of the posterior portion of the basal vein of Rosenthal (*arrow*) and transcerebral venous drainage into the middle cerebral veins which drain towards the superior sagittal sinus (*long curved arrows*). **E** Late phase of the right internal carotid injection in frontal projection demonstrates the significant venous congestion on the right hemisphere, basal veins bilaterally (*curved arrows*), and venous drainage towards the contralateral hemisphere. **F** Lateral DSA, late phase, of the left vertebral artery injection which demonstrates the significant retrograde venous cortical drainage (*broad arrows*). Note retrograde filling of the lateral mesencephalic veins draining into the anterior pontomesencephalic venous system (*long arrows*). There is also reflux towards the straight sinus (*curved open arrow*). **G** Frontal view of the opposite (left) internal carotid injection demonstrates the contribution of the anterior cerebral artery to the malformation. **H** Late phase of the left internal carotid artery injection demonstrates congestion of the venous system on the left hemisphere and the remaining drainage of the malformation on the right

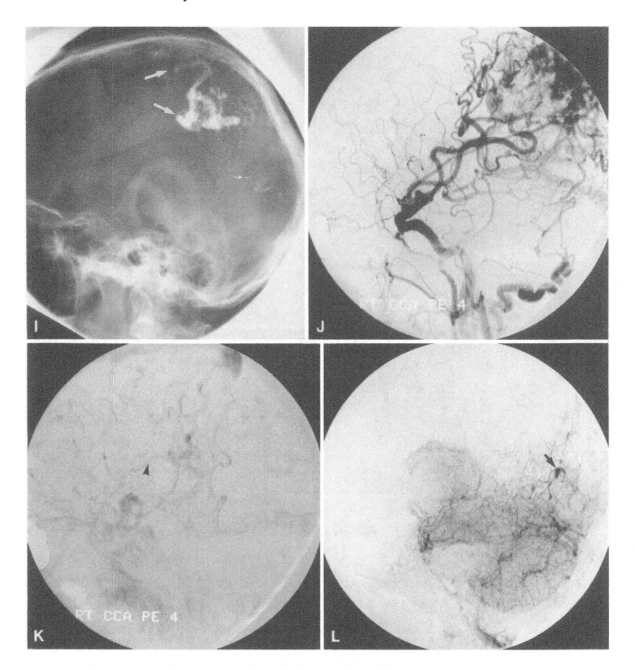

Fig. 3.1. I Lateral plain film of the skull demonstrates the cast obtained of the middle cerebral artery (*large arrows*) and posterior cerebral artery (*small arrow*). **J** Mid-phase control angiogram of the right common carotid artery after embolization of the middle, posterior cerebral, and external carotid supply demonstrates significant slowing of the shunt. **K** Late phase; there is better opacification of the remaining cortical venous drainage and internal cerebral vein (*arrowhead*). **L** Late phase of the left vertebral artery injection demonstrates significantly better opacification of the posterior fossa and parietal venous drainage and stagnation in the distal posterior cerebral artery (*arrow*). Rapid improvement followed treatment with nearly complete recovery at 1 month

This is explained as follows: after maximal stretching of the muscular and/ or fibrous wall (in smooth muscle this is called stress relaxation), vessels that have undergone enlargement are no longer able to constrict appropriately in response to rises in blood pressure or vasodilate in response to lower blood pressure, therefore losing autoregulation for some time (Yasargil 1987).

Pertuiset et al. (1982) used technetium-99 to measure the blood volume in the brains of normal individuals and in patients with AVMs during normotension and hypotension. He demonstrated that patients with AVMs continued to have autoregulation in normal brain; however, perfusion of the AVM was dependent only on the systemic blood pressure. Yamada and Cojocaru (1987), using intravenous injections of xenon-133, showed a prominent decrease in regional cerebral blood flow in areas adjacent to the AVM. However, this phenomenon occurred in other more remote brain areas and could also be seen during postoperative recovery in regional cerebral blood flow. Malis (1982b) suggested that "steal" in occlusive disease is actually a steal from one system of circulation to the other. In an open system with a shunt, as in AVMs, the hydrodynamic steal is not present. The angiographic steal shown during fluorescein studies by Feindel (1979) did not consider venous hyperpressure as part of the mechanism leading to decreased tissue perfusion.

Yamada and Cojocaru (1987) have demonstrated that there is a decrease in the number of mitochondria in areas surrounding the AVM. This decrease may represent either chronic hypoxia, with a decreased capacity to produce energy, or decreased energy consumption, so that the balance between supply and demand remains constant. Accordingly, behavioral disorders, mental slowness, and progressive dementia in patients with AVMs may be compensatory changes rather than a reflection of primary dysfunction. Such compensatory changes may be reversible if local perfusion is improved by ameliorating the venous hyperpressure (Fig. 3.1) (see Chap. 5, Vein of Galen Aneurysmal Malformation). In contrast, patients with significant, generalized, cerebral dysfunction resulting from venous thrombosis and/or irreversible tissue damage from venous hypertension may not improve even after complete AVM exclusion (Fig. 3.2) (similar to the irreversible venous hypoxia in some advanced, long-standing, spinal dural AVMs, see Vol. 5, Chap. 1, Spinal Dural Arteriovenous Fistulas and Vol. 2, Chap. 3). This syndrome of generalized cerebral dysfunction based on venous hypertension is more frequently seen in older patients or in very young patients.

As noted above, flow through vascular malformations is dependent primarily upon the systemic blood pressure (Nornes and Grip 1980) and therefore may decrease during hypotension or increase in hypertensive states. Measuring hemodynamics in AVMs using intraoperative ultrasonography, Nornes et al. (1979a) noted that in one of his patients there were marked variations in the systemic blood pressure with parallel changes in the flow of the AVM feeders. Similar findings have been noted in patients in whom hypotension is induced prior to the excision of the AVM, the pressure within the AVM paralleling the systemic blood pressure. These findings confirmed the absence of vasomotor control within the AVM (Nornes and Grip 1980; Pertuiset et al. 1982, 1985).

The surrounding brain, however, still maintains autoregulation, as demonstrated by ultrasonography (Nornes and Grip 1980; Hassler 1986, 1987),

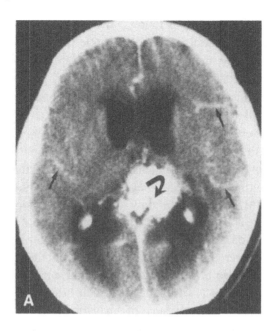

Fig. 3.2 A−F. Irreversible mental deterioration secondary to venous hypertension. **A** Axial CT scan after intravenous contrast administration demonstrates ventricular enlargement with periventricular lucency, enhancement of the malformation and its deep venous drainage (*bent arrow*), and prominent venous cortical enhancement bilaterally (*arrows*). **B** Lateral view in intermediate phase of the left internal carotid artery injection demonstrates a relatively slow flow vascular malformation of the midline (*bent arrow*) draining towards a congested deep venous system and towards the basal vein and transcerebral venous system. There is no filling of the internal cerebral vein or vein of Galen systems. **C** Later phase of the same injection; significant delay in brain drainage, with cortical venous drainage and no opacification of the internal cerebral vein or vein of Galen complex. **D** Frontal view of the left internal carotid artery after embolization in midarteral phase; the radiopaque cast of the filled nidus has been subtracted (*arrowheads*). **E** Laterial views in midarterial and **F** late venous phase of the left internal carotid artery after embolization demonstrate no filling of the malformation and good cortical venous drainage. Note the better opacification of the venous system towards the cavernous sinus (*curved arrow*) and stagnation in the veins that drained the malformation (*open arrow*). Despite successful treatment, the patient continued to deteriorate and eventually died

PCO_2 reactivity during hypocapnia, single photon emission tomography, and direct cortical blood flow measurements (Takeuchi et al. 1987; Barnett et al. 1987; Lindergard et al. 1985).

Deutsch's (1983) study of changes in blood flow during behavioral activation in patients with cerebral AVMs demonstrated that there are focal regulatory mechanisms in the normal brain. During periods of nonvisual attention-demanding activities, the flow decreased from more than 170 ml to less than 100 ml per 100 g/min in the region of the malformation. It is interesting to note that the AVM stood out as a region of high blood flow during the relaxed state, since it approached normal flow levels when there were attentional demands. We believe that these findings are compatible with a simple passive reflection of substantial redistribution of blood flow in other parts of the normal brain.

Pressure recordings from the feeding arteries at the entrance of the AVM were significantly below systemic arterial blood pressure, with a mean pressure ranging between 15 and 56 mmHg (Nornes and Grip 1980). On tem-

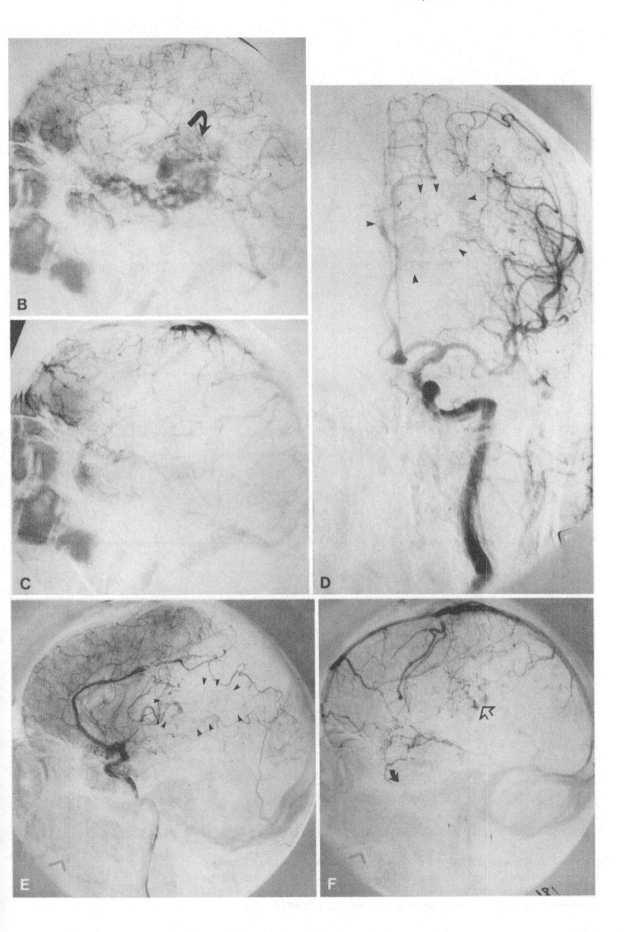

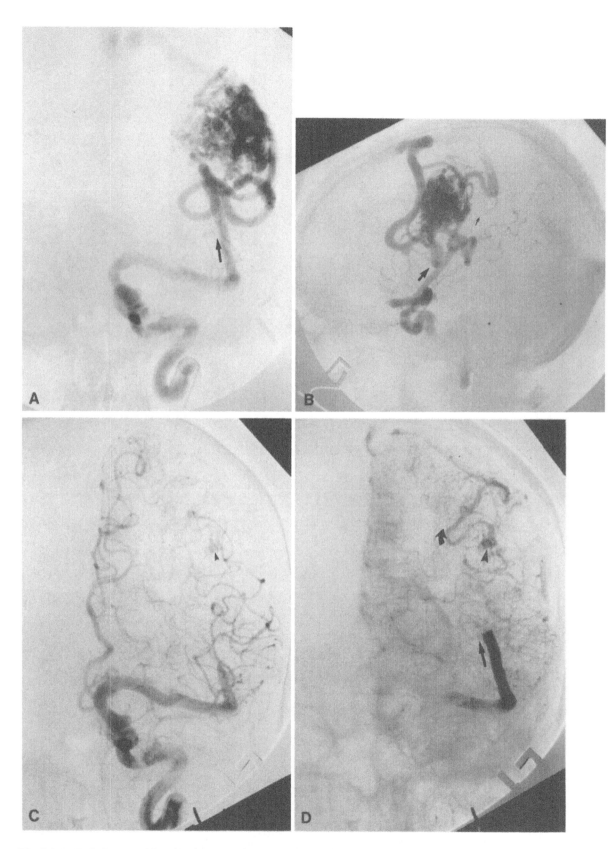

Fig. 3.3 A – F. A 60 year old male with a transient aphasia and hemiparesis immediately after 90% obliteration. **A** Frontal and **B** lateral views of the internal carotid artery injection demonstrate an arteriovenous malformation of the parietal region supplied by a main trunk of the middle cerebral artery trifurcation (*arrow*). **C** Fron-

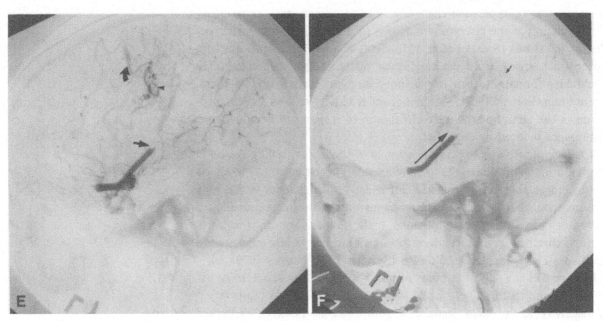

tal angiogram in midarterial phase after embolization and **D** in later arterial phase demonstrate almost complete obliteration of the malformation with only a small remaining nidus (*arrowhead*) and one draining vein (*curved arrow* in **D**). Note the stagnation in the middle cerebral artery main trunk that supplied the malformation (*arrow*). **E** Later midarterial phase and **F** late film of the series following embolization demonstrate the small remaining nidus (*arrowhead*) and draining vein (*curved arrow*) and the filling defect in the stagnant middle cerebral artery trunk (*arrow in* **E**). Note lack of filling of the normal artery shown in **B** (*small arrow* in **B**). The same parietal branch is filling in a retrograde manner (*small arrow* in **E**). The patient had a transient aphasia and hemiparesis

porary occlusion, the stump pressure rapidly rose to a mean pressure of 76 mmHg, resulting in a concomitant rapid increase in cortical artery perfusion pressure (Barnett et al. 1987). Similar findings have been confirmed by intravascular pressure measurements (Duckwiller 1989; Jungreis and Horton 1989).

The pressure in the draining vein(s) is also elevated, with a mean pressure of 50 mmHg prior to treatment. After excision of the malformation the venous pressure decreases to 0–2 mmHg. The drop in venous hyperpressure contributes further to the increase in normal tissue perfusion after embolization and/or resection of the AVM. This synergistic combination of factors has been postulated to produce progressively first a relative hypertensive state in the adjacent normal microcirculation, followed by cerebral edema, and finally by "circulatory breakthrough" (Nornes et al. 1979 a, b), "proximal hyperemia" (Mullan et al. 1979 a), or "normal perfusion pressure breakthrough" (NPPB) (Spetzler et al. 1978). In rat models of AVFs, blood-brain barrier disruption, as measured by Evans blue dye technique, occurred only in hypertensive rats but not under normal tension or in control animals with AVFs (Morgan et al. 1987).

Scott et al. (1978) and Spetzler et al. (1978) studied the vascular dynamics of experimental arteriovenous shunts in a primate and in carotid jugular fistulas in cats, respectively. Both authors suggested that an AVF that enlarges will produce secondary abnormal autoregulation of cerebral vessels in response to both pressure changes and PCO_2 variations. The return of autoregulation in the cerebrovascular bed to normal may occur after occluding the fistula (Spetzler et al. 1978; Scott et al. 1978). Significant controversy has arisen as to the validity of this reported phenomenon. In cerebral malformations there may be poor vascular reactivity to CO_2 in adjacent brain (Barnett 1987). Such abnormal reactivity reflects a decompensation in the ability of the microcirculation to respond to hemodynamic disturbance induced by the shunt.

The lack of response to pressure changes of the major feeding vessels to the malformation is due to the stress relaxation phenomena, i.e., the vessels are no longer able to vasoconstrict sufficiently with changes in pressure. This may contribute to some of the problems with hemorrhage encountered during surgery of cerebral vascular malformations or in the early postoperative period. The length of the arterial feeders is also suggested to relate to a higher incidence of NPPB (Spetzler 1978; Nornes 1979a, b).

Muraszko et al. (1990), in a study of reactivity in feeding vessels to AVMs in vitro, found that in 20 out of 24 lesions studied there was preservation of reactivity in the AVM feeders. In four patients, however, there was neither reactivity to various vasodilators nor spontaneous contractility. Those four patients had significant complications postoperatively.

In patients following embolization, one can frequently see persistence of the vascular dilatation with stagnation of contrast material in the occluded feeders. These features are also seen in postoperative angiograms. Usually no clinical manifestations are present. However, a transient aphasia and hemiparesis occurred in a 60 year old male with these angiographic findings following 90% occlusion of a left temporal AVM (Fig. 3.3).

In patients with distal AVMs, the venous drainage and its proximity to the superior sagittal sinus may play a role in the genesis of generalized postoperative edema. A sudden decrease in the sinus pressure following acute occlusion of the shunt may result in retrograde venous stagnation and generalized cerebral edema. However, in the great majority of patients, there is a natural protective system at the venous-sinus junction (see Vol. 3, Chap. 7). In most BAVM patients pressure in the jugular veins is within normal limits.

Hassler (1986) showed that, in surgically created cervical AVFs in cats (utilizing an H-fistula model), the blood flow rates across the fistula can increase up to tenfold. This increase is limited by: (a) output volume, (b) diameter of the fistula vessels, (c) cross-sectional area, and (d) systemic blood pressure. In this AVF model, cortical microcirculation was reduced by 25%. Spetzler's model only slightly affects microcirculation. In neither Hassler's nor Morgan's AVF models was there any evidence of disturbance of autoregulation following acute occlusion of chronic fistulas. The blood-brain barrier remained intact and, as in the rat model (Morgan 1987), only blood pressure increases above the upper limits of vascular autoregulation (hypertensive rats) resulted in Evans blue extravasation.

Following removal of AVMs, as monitored by Doppler sonography and angiography, Hassler and Steinmetz (1987) assessed the various hemodynamics described above. They showed that the flow velocities in former AVM feeders are considerably reduced, with often undetectable diastolic values. This would indicate a sharp increase in arteriolar resistance ("stagnating" arteries). Intraoperative measurements in these vessels showed an increase of 53% in intravascular mean pressure (Nornes and Grip 1980). However, in no instance was there evidence of hyperperfusion, hyperemia, or petechial edema. CO_2-dependent vasoreactivity was normal following AVM removal. This data therefore fails to support the NPPB theory. Rosenblum (1987a, b), using SPECT scanning with ^{123}I-labeled *n*-isopropyl *p*-iodoamphetamine (IMP), showed normal perfusion in the region surrounding the malformation both before and after surgical removal of AVMs, suggesting that there is autoregulation around the AVMs but not supporting the concept of "steal".

Batjer et al. (1988a, b), using xenon-133 SPECT, showed pressure vaso-reactivity to acetazolamide (CO_2 reactivity) to produce even greater vasodilatation. He proposed a "paradoxical" dissociation between the vaso-constrictive and vasodilatory capacities of neighboring areas. However, if the microcirculation is maximally dilated (NPPB theory), acetazolamide vasodilatation should not occur.

These experiments were undertaken in parallel with the neurosurgical experiences. Predictably the same controversies and contradictions are seen in the neurosurgical literature. A number of factors have been incorporated into the NPPB theory, including size of the malformation, the caliber of the feeding vessels, their length, the rapidity of filling, evidence of "angiographic steal," and watershed shifts; however, the theory remains unproven. It is at least conceivable that some technical difficulties, such as leaving a portion of the malformation (Yasargil 1987), occluding venous outflow to normal areas, or compromising feeding arteries to normal brain, contribute to the "unexplained and delayed postoperative massive swelling of the brain." Such swelling is thought to occur in large malformations with very high flow but has also been observed in small ones (Barnett, case 5).

Yasargil (1987) reported that none of his six patients with high-flow fistulas of the brain in which the fistula was abruptly occluded showed any evidence of perfusion pressure breakthrough. Similarly in all the high-flow fistulas that we have closed acutely by embolization, no evidence of perfusion pressure breakthrough has been observed (Fig. 3.4). Patients with extreme high-flow fistulas, such as carotid cavernous fistulas (acute or chronic), in whom the fistula is abruptly occluded with preservation of the carotid artery do not develop this syndrome.

There are, however, some reports of patients with high-flow fistulas in whom occlusion produces neurological deficits which may either be reversible following deflation of the balloon (Halbach et al. 1987) or may be fatal. Both situations have been explained by NPPB (Kondor et al. 1988). Progressive occlusion was better tolerated than acute occlusion in Halbach's patients.

The NPPB theory has also been invoked in reperfusion following carotid endarterectomy (Sundt et al. 1981; Powers and Smith 1989), but this is most likely due to reperfusion of irreversible ischemic territory (Pomposelli et al. 1988; Heros and Korosue 1989). It is therefore difficult to accept this theories to explain certain cases, when several hundred similar situations in which NPPB should have happened were complication free. Closed skull surgery vs open craniotomy may account for the lack of NPPB seen following embolization.

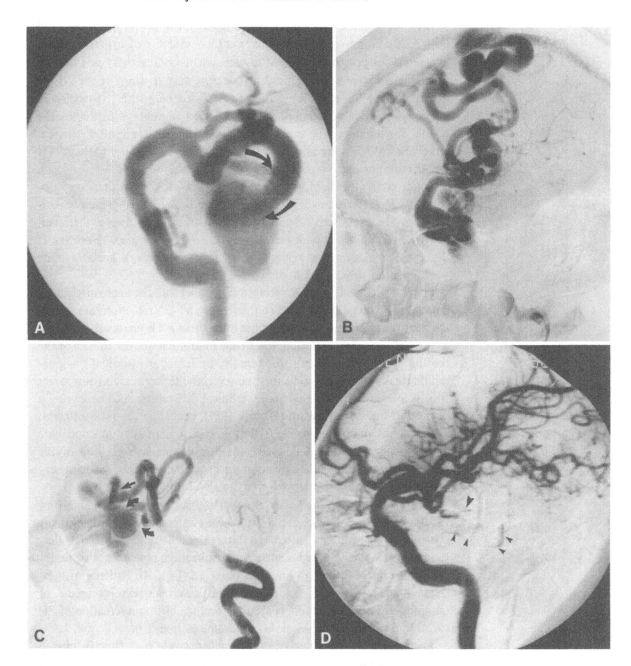

Fig. 3.4A–G. Asymptomatic abrupt closure of multiple high-flow arteriovenous fistulas. **A** Digital subtraction angiography (DSA) in frontal projection of the left internal carotid artery in early phase demonstrates marked hypertrophy of the middle cerebral artery in its anterior temporal branch (*curved arrows*) supplying multiple fistulas of the anterior temporal region. **B** Later phase in lateral projection demonstrates the prominent venous drainage, with a rapid transit time and draining towards the superior sagittal sinus. **C** Lateral view of the left vertebral artery injection demonstrates the hypertrophy of the posterior communicating artery (*arrow*) and a lateral fistula from the lateral temporal branch of the posterior cerebral artery (*curved arrows*) entering the venous sac at a different point than the middle cerebral artery. **D** Immediate postembolization control angiogram of the left internal carotid artery in oblique projection demonstrates the balloon (*large arrowhead*) closing the largest fistula. There was no clinical consequences of this acute occlusion. **E** Frontal view of the left internal carotid artery 6 months after embolization. **F** and **G** Lateral projections of the same injection in arterial and venous phases show complete disappearance of the malformation. Note the regression in the size of the internal carotid and middle cerebral arteries

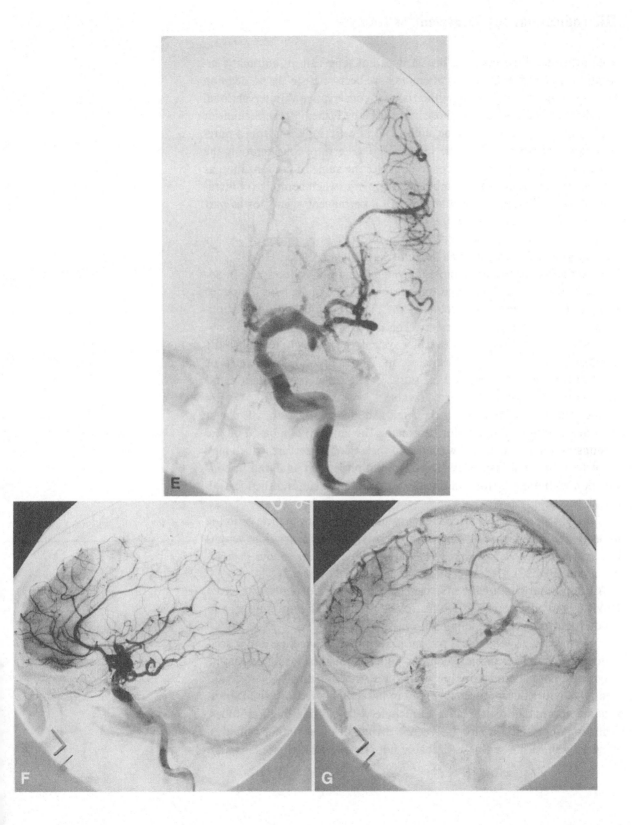

III. Indications for Treatment of BAVMs

The incidental discovery of a BAVM does not represent an automatic indication for treatment. Various attempts have been made to devise decision analysis programs to determine the risks of conservative vs interventional treatment of BAVMs, such as those introduced by Fisher (1989), Steinmeier et al. (1989). All are based on the ability to deal with the lesion from a purely surgical viewpoint. All fail, however, to take into consideration the angioarchitecture of the lesion or to consider the value of embolization as a preoperative adjunct, a sole mode of treatment (when complete obliteration of the malformation is obtained with a permanent agent), or as part of a combination of treatments.

None of the patients analyzed by Crawford (1986) in whom the AVMs were diagnosed incidentally had a hemorrhage 20 years later. However, for more complete conclusions a more thorough evaluation is necessary. In addition to the original computed tomography (CT) or magnetic resonance imaging (MRI) study that discovered the malformation and its location, pancerebral angiography is necessary. This is performed with the aim of obtaining a complete study of the vascular system: the supply to the AVM, the angioarchitecture of the malformation, its venous drainage, associated or additional vascular lesions, and the status of the collateral circulation and the venous drainage of the normal brain.

The information obtained by the angiographic investigation will play a key role in deciding the need for treatment. The latter will be based on the demonstration of evidence of weakness in the angioarchitecture, which may point to a potential instability. This information is then analyzed in conjunction with other factors such as the age of the patient and the location of the lesion.

If there is an associated arterial aneurysm in the feeding pedicle or in the nidus (Fig. 3.5), evidence of venous thrombosis, outflow restriction, venous hyperpressure, venous pouches or dilatations (Fig. 3.6), or venous pseudo-aneurysm (Fig. 3.7), treatment is recommended (see Chap. 2).

An important part of the management of such incidentally discovered BAVMs is to educate the patient as to the problem, its implications, and what is known about the long-term outcome.

If no significant weakness is present in the angioarchitecture and a decision is made not to treat the lesion, the patient should be reassured that he may lead a normal productive life with no restrictions. Some suggested caution in activities that produce increases in intracranial and/or venous pressure are appropriate. Such activities include weight lifting, high altitudes, flying in nonpressurized airplanes, scuba diving, or other similar activities. Pregnancy in such a setting is probably not contraindicated (see Chap. 2).

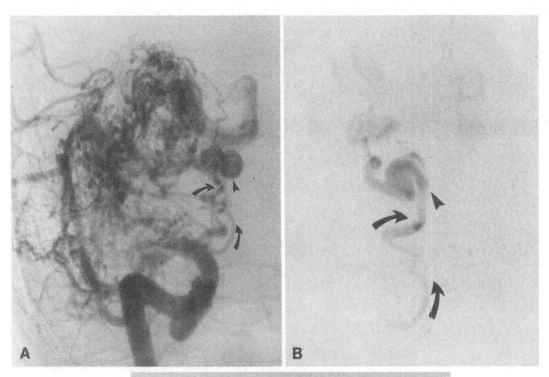

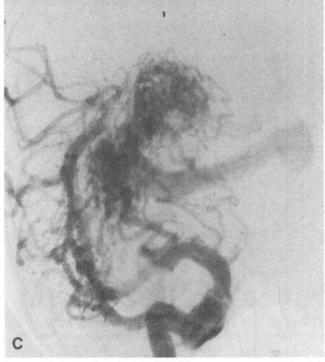

Fig. 3.5 A–C. Thalamic malformation with an intralesional aneurysm. **A** Frontal view of the right internal carotid artery demonstrates a basal ganglionic malformation supplied by the lenticulostriate arteries. Note the intralesional aneurysm (*arrowhead*) from a prominent lenticulostriate artery (*curved arrows*). **B** Superselective catheterization of the lenticulostriate artery (*curved arrows*) demonstrating partial filling of the dysplastic aneurysm (*arrowhead*). **C** Potembolization angiogram of the right internal carotid artery in the frontal projection. The lesional aneurysm does not fill

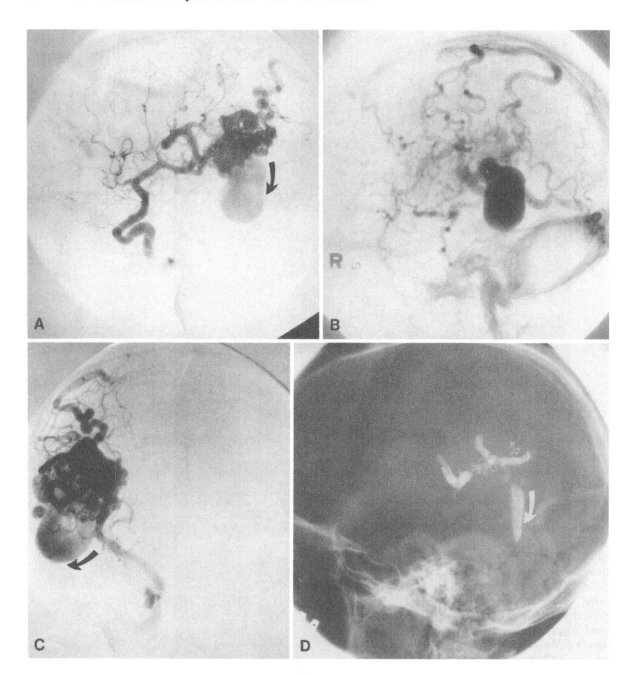

Fig. 3.6 A–J. Large venous pouch; preoperative embolization. **A** Lateral view of the right internal carotid artery in midarterial phase demonstrates a posterior temporal vascular malformation draining into a large aneurysmal pouch (*curved arrow*). **B** Later phase of the same injection demonstrates the giant aneurysmal sac and the venous drainage of the malformation. **C** Frontal view of the right internal carotid artery prior to treatment. **D** Plain film of the skull after two major pedicles have been embolized. Note stagnation in the venous pouch with a fluid-fluid level (*curved arrow*). **E** Lateral midarterial phase and **F** late venous phase after embolization demonstrate almost complete obliteration of the malformation, with stagnation in

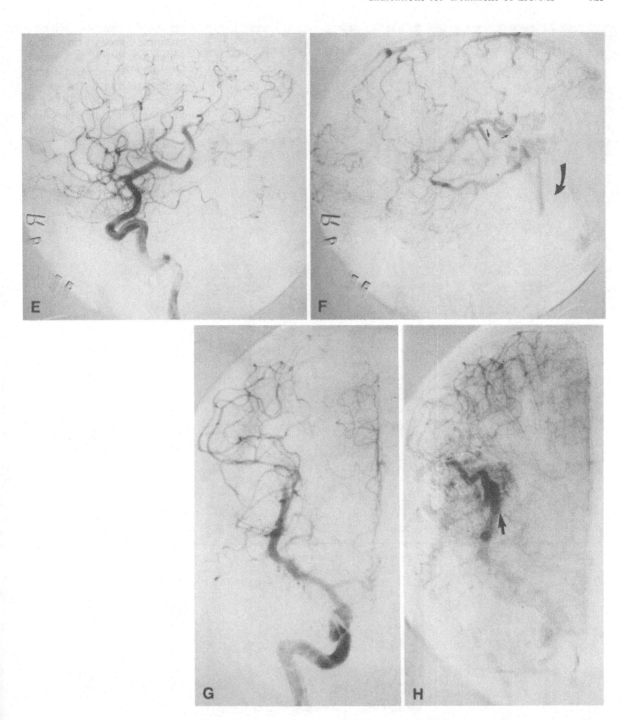

the venous pouch that is partially subtracted from previous stagnant contrast material (*curved arrow*) and stagnation proximally in the embolized feeding pedicles of the middle cerebral artery (*small arrows*). **G** Frontal view of the same injection in early arterial and **H** later phase after embolization in the main middle cerebral artery trunk (*arrow*). The venous pouch was thrombosed at the time of the surgical removal of the AVM

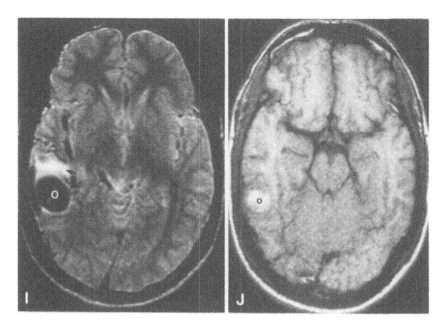

Fig. 3.6. I Axial MRI prior to treatment shows the large venous pouch (*O*) as a signal void and the increased signal changes anterior to the venous dilatation (*arrow*). J MRI after embolization. Note the complete thrombosis of the venous pouch (*O*)

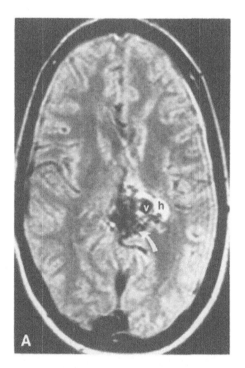

Fig. 3.7 A–G. Venous pseudoaneurysm. **A** Axial MRI, T1-weighted image, shows a midline malformation (*curved arrow*). There is a signal void (*v*) adjacent to an area of hemorrhage (*h*). **B** Lateral view of the left vertebral artery injection in late venous phase demonstrates a pseudoaneurysm of the venous type (*arrowhead*) corresponding to the signal void (*v*) in **A**. **C** Late phase of the internal carotid artery injection also fills the same pseudoaneurysm (*arrowhead*). **D** Lateral digital subtraction angiography of the posterior cerebral artery on the left side shows the choroidal supply to the malformation, the venous pseudoaneurysm (*arrowhead*), and the deep venous drainage. **E** Postembolization of the left vertebral artery in midarterial phase demonstrates thalamoperforator supply to the malformation (*arrows*), with shunting into the deep venous system. **F** Late venous phase of the vertebral artery injection and **G** late venous phase of the left internal carotid artery injection show no filling of the venous pseudoaneurysm

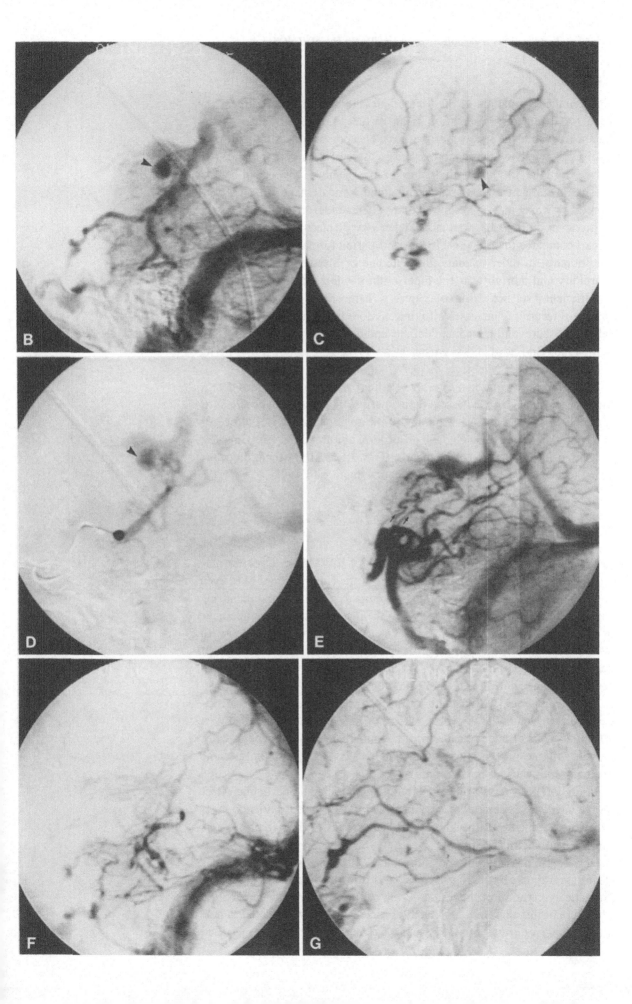

1. Age

The younger the patient at the time of presentation, the more urgent the need for treatment. Presentation at an early age represents an early imbalance between the lesion and the host. Newborns presenting with congestive heart failure are the most severe example of such an imbalance (see Chap. 5). In the fifth and sixth decades of life, the high incidence of hemorrhage and subsequent poor patient outcome mandate aggressive intervention. Crawford et al. (1986) showed that patients older than 60 years of age at presentation (Fig. 3.8) were at a higher risk of bleeding, up to 89% by 9 years compared to a 15% risk in the same period for patients aged 20–29. Additionally, in older patients, the outcome of bleeding has a very high morbidity and mortality, as the older brain has less plasticity to recover.

Sufficient evidence exists that once a hemorrhage has occurred the chance of recurrence increases with time, as does the probability of both developing seizures and permanent deficits and death (Ondra 1990; Crawford et al. 1986; Graf et al. 1983; Forster et al. 1972; Luessenhop 1984; Perret and Nishioka 1966; Michelsen 1979; Wilkins 1985).

Over time, the condition may evolve, with progressive neurological deterioration secondary to decreased tissue perfusion (venous hyperpressure, thrombosis, stenotic changes from high-flow angiopathy, etc.). Hydrocephalus may also occur following CSF absorption abnormalities (see Chap. 5). Decreased mental status and dementia (Figs. 3.1, 3.2) are therefore more prone to occur the earlier the malformation manifests itself.

2. Sex

In the general discussion of the management of BAVMs, sex does not play a major role, with the exception of females in the childbearing age or even younger women in whom symptoms are already present prior to having children. There is some controversy as to the increased risk of hemorrhage or other symptoms during pregnancy. It is not infrequent that women with BAVMs have had one or more normal pregnancies and deliveries without being aware of the malformation, whereas other women present with an acute syndrome related to the malformation for the first time during pregnancy. In his series, Crawford found no statistical difference in the incidence of affected males vs females; however, one in four women between 20 and 29 years of age presented with a hemorrhage while pregnant, comparable with the one out of four women in the same age group that became pregnant and who did not have an AVM.

Yasargil's (1987) results suggested that pregnancy had no particular effect on the incidence or severity of bleeding from AVMs. In our patients, pregnancy did not increase either the risk of hemorrhage or the risk of progression of neurological symptoms.

However, in patients with maxillofacial AVMs, there is a group that has clear aggravation of symptoms several days prior to their menstruation or dramatic aggravation of the lesion during or immediately after pregnancy. The cause of this aggravation in maxillofacial lesions may be related to hormonal changes during both menstrual cycles and pregnancy, the increased

Fig. 3.8 A–D. A 67 year old male originally presenting with a grand mal seizure (**A**) and 6 months later hemorrhage (**B**). **A** Frontal view of the right common carotid artery injection at the time of the original seizure demonstrates an arteriovenous malformation on the parietal region supplied by the middle cerebral artery. **B** 6 months later the patient has had an intracerebral hemorrhage. At this time angiography examination demonstrates an intralesional aneurysm (*arrowhead*) not present before. **C** and **D** Postembolization control angiogram of the right common carotid artery demonstrates remaining malformation but no filling of the intralesional aneurysm (*curved open arrow*). The remaining malformation was treated with radiosurgery

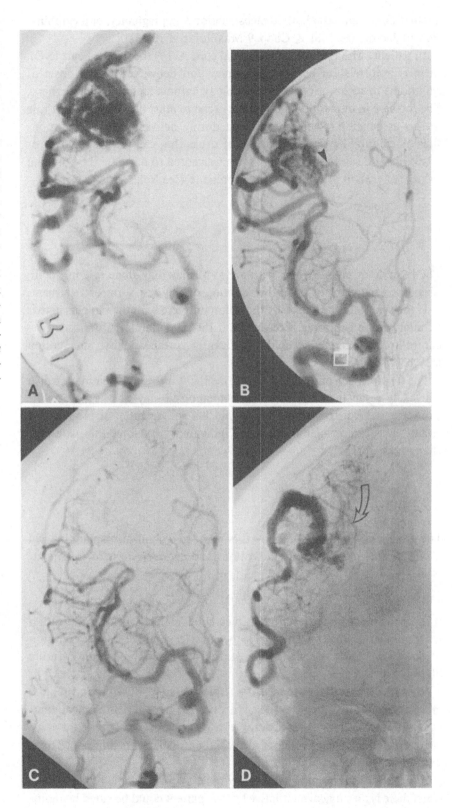

circulating volume seen both in menstruation and pregnancy, or a combination of factors (see Vol. 2, Chap. 9 Maxillofacial AVMs).

In patients with thoracolumbar spinal cord AVMs (below the heart level), there is a correlation between pregnancy and delivery with the onset of symptoms or aggravation of preexisting symptoms including hemorrhage. The increase in intraabdominal venous pressure must play a significant role in this association. Therefore, at least during delivery, some precautions such as epidural block, minimal use of drugs that can produce nausea or vomiting, and careful monitoring seem warranted to decrease the potential risks of increased arterial or venous pressure (see Vol. 5, Chap. 1).

3. Lifestyle

The lifestyle of an individual with a BAVM may play some role in the indications for treatment or in the selection of the best form of treatment.

If the symptoms produced by the lesion interfere with the patients activity, intervention is favored. Conversely, if the potential deficit that may occur following treatment would significantly curtail activity, intervention may be discouraged.

For example, in a pilot with a medial occipital AVM, any treatment which will likely result in a homonymous hemianopsia may not be acceptable. Conversely, the discovery of a lesion that has the potential of producing a seizure or a hemorrhage in the same individual may force the patient to change his work.

4. Presenting Symptoms

The presenting symptoms and how they relate to embolization planning will play a significant role in the indications and aggressiveness of treatment.

a) Hemorrhage

It is for the most part agreed that intracerebral hemorrhage is an indication for treatment of BAVMs. The goal is the complete and permanent exclusion of the lesion from the circulation as the only guarantee against future bleeds.

Repeated hemorrhages represent a more pressing situation and require more aggressive treatment, as the chances of permanent neurological damage and death increase significantly with each recurrence (Crawford et al. 1986; Graf et al. 1983; Forster et al. 1972), particularly in children (Berenstein et al. 1990).

In patients with lesions that are incurable by all available modalities or when there is no surgical alternative but the patient could be cured by radiosurgery or a combination of embolization and radiosurgery, partial embolization appears warranted. The true rebleed rate following partial embolization is not known, as not enough time has elapsed. Evolving strategies and technical advances cannot yet be taken into full account but will be major factors in the long term.

At this early stage and based on limited data, in our analysis of 279 pa-

Table 3.1. Bleeding after embolization[a] (Berenstein 1978–1990)

First hemorrhage	8
Rehemorrhage	19
Total	27 (9.6%)

[a] $n = 279$.

tients treated in the last 12 years, mostly by embolization alone (AB, 1978–1990) (Table 3.1), 27 patients (9.6%) have bled after embolization. The mean follow-up time was 6.5 years. (The present strategy has been used since 1983.) Of these 27 patients, 19 had bled at least once prior to embolization, while in 8 their first hemorrhage occurred after embolization (Table 3.1).

Six patients had embolization of the external carotid artery only (palliation of headaches), 6 had silicone sphere embolization, and 15 had isobutyl-2-cyanoacrylate (IBCA) embolization (Table 3.2). In 10 of the 15 in whom IBCA was used, a suboptimal proximal vessel occlusion resulted (our early experience with IBCA and Kerber's calibrated leak balloon microcatheter described in Vol. 2, Chap. 1). Only 5 of the 27 patients with an apparently "good" embolization with IBCA went on to bleed.

Table 3.2. Bleeding after embolization, by embolic agent (Berenstein 1990)

Agent	Patients treated (n)	Patients who bled (n)
ECA[a] (IBCA and/or PVA)	17	6
SS	36	6
IBCA/NBCA	226	15[b]

$n = 279$; IBCA, isobutyl-2-cyanoacrylate; PVA, polyvinyl alcohol; NBCA, N-butyl-cyanoacrylate; SS, silicone spheres.
[a] ECA, external carotid embolization only.
[b] Ten patients had proximal vessel occlusion and only five (2.2%) with a "good" embolization bled (see text).

Of a total of 36 patients who had silicone sphere embolization, 6 bled afterward. The rebleed rate is therefore 16.6% in this subgroup, making it evident that silicone spheres give no protection against bleeding. In contrast, of the 226 patients treated with IBCA or NBCA only, 5 (2.2%) bled within a mean of 6.5 years (a 0.33% annual rate), suggesting that significant protection is conferred by this therapy. At present, however, insufficient follow-up time has elapsed to reach a significant conclusion (mean follow-up of 6.5 years in the acrylic group).

Ondra (1990) found the rebleed rate of symptomatic BAVM patients treated conservatively (probably mostly inoperable and similar to the referral pattern for embolization) was 4% per year regardless of the form of presentation. The rebleed rate in our series thus appears very favorable, even at this early stage. The serious morbidity in Ondra's untreated patients was 1.7% per year, and the mortality was 1% per year (Ondra 1990).

The decreased life expectancy in Ondra's population is impressive. The mean life expectancy in patients that died from AVM hemorrhage was 44.4 years, and the overall life expectancy of those patients harboring a BAVM who died from other causes was 59.4 years. These figures are highly significant when compared to the general Finnish population without BAVM who had a life expectancy of 73 years.

Table 3.3. Outcome of postembolization bleeding

Outcome	n	(%)
Deaths	14	(51.8)
Severe deficits	1	(3.7)
Mild deficits	2	(7.4)
No residual effect	10	(37.1)

27 out of 279 patients (9.6%); Berenstein 1978–1990

Patients that bled (or rebled) in Ondra's series (1990) had an 85% chance of having a major morbidity or of dying from the recurrent hemorrhage. Of our 27 patients that bled after embolotherapy, 14 (51.8%) died and 1 (3.7%) had a severe deficit, for a combined major morbidity and mortality of 55.5% (Table 3.3).

b) Seizures

In most series, seizures represent the second most common form of presentation. This manifestation is seen primarily in lesions located at or near the primary motor-sensory cortex or temporal or frontal regions. Multiple reports dealing with surgery performed in patients presenting "only" with seizures found evidence of subclinical bleeds. It is also accepted that there is a higher incidence of hemorrhage in patients that have had seizures previously (Crawford et al. 1986; Graf et al. 1983; Forster et al. 1972, etc.) than those who have not had seizures.

In Crawford's study (1986), patients that originally presented with seizures had a lower risk of bleeding (22% in the next 10 years and 30% at 15 years) than patients who had a previous bleed (10 years 26%, 20 years 51%). The clinical presentation of epilepsy should be considered in deciding intervention. The frequent argument that the patient "only" has seizures should not be considered as of minor importance, as it may predict loss of equilibrium.

The hardest decision in the management of a patient with seizures "only" and a malformation in an "eloquent" area of the brain is to decide if treatment should be postponed until the patient has "more" symptoms in order to justify intervention.

Ondra (1990), in a prospective review of 160 symptomatic patients harboring a BAVM and followed for a mean of 23.7 years in the Finish population, found that, irrespective of the mode of presentation, the long-term outcome ("natural history") was poor. This was true for patients presenting with seizures, with a 1% mortality per year (cumulative), and a combined yearly severe morbidity and mortality of 2.7%.

The risk of endovascular intervention, even if incomplete, is low: 1.6% mortality and 1.4% severe morbidity (see below, Results and Complications from Embolization), similar to 1 year risk factor in the natural history of untreated BAVMs (Ondra). Embolotherapy may result in a return to the previous state of balance between the malformation and the host, averting the complications of the disease. Alternatively, it may create a new situation, such as converting a nonsurgical lesion to one that can be cured by surgery or radiosurgery. In patients in whom seizures are difficult to control, embolization can reduce seizure activity (Luessenhop and Rosa 1984; Stein and Wolpert 1980).

New seizures after embolization were noted in eight of our patients, six had prior intracerebral hemorrhage, or silicone sphere embolization. In only two of our patients (out of 279) did a new seizure occur after acrylic embolization (Table 3.4). In both instances the ictus paralleled thrombosis of the lesion, one complete (Fig. 3.9) and one partial. Both patients had only a single seizure episode (both generalized) and both have a normal EEG at present. Therefore, embolization may be considered in patients presenting "only" with seizures, especially if weakness in the angioarchitecture can be identified angiographically.

Luessenhop et al. (1965), Luessenhop and Presper (1975), Wolpert et al. (1981), and others have observed an improvement in seizure control after embolization (with particles). Similarly, there appears to be improved control in patients with difficult or refractory seizures (Table 3.5). However, in at least some of these patients, the changes due to medications, dose adjust-

Table 3.4. New seizures after embolization

ICH	2
Surgery	2
SS	2
IBCA/NBCA[a]	2

279 patients; March 1990; ICH, intracerebral hemorrhage; SS, silicone spheres; IBCA, isobutyl-2-cyanoacrylate; NBCA, N-butyl-cyanoacrylate

[a] Both patients had a single generalized seizure, one associated with complete thrombosis (Fig. 3.9) and one with partial thrombosis.

Table 3.5. Seizure outcome in 257 patients (1989)

Present prior to embolization (*n*)	Seizure-free (*n*)	New seizures (*n*)
134	91	8

ment, and compliance in a controlled (hospital) environment may account for some of these improvements. Patients with "uncontrollable seizures" despite therapeutic levels of medication, in status epilepticus (an infrequent occurrence in BAVMs), or in whom venous thrombosis or venous hyperpressure is noted are the best candidates for improved seizure control after embolization (Fig. 3.10).

c) Headaches

As discussed in the previous chapter, headaches may be those that accompany intracerebral hemorrhage and are treated as discussed for hemorrhage. Nonhemorrhagic headaches may be related to other causes and are usually accompanied by other neurological signs or symptoms. Such headaches could be related to vascular changes, such as posterior cerebral artery contribution to the AVM, meningeal supply, or, less frequently, middle cerebral artery supply.

In our series, some patients developed headaches de novo some weeks or months after embolization. At angiography, these patients frequently demonstrated increased supply to the AVM from the posterior cerebral or meningeal arteries. Other patients with severe "incapacitating" headaches had significant amelioration or even disappearance of their symptoms after embolization of the posterior cerebral artery and/or dural supply. Similarly, Troost and Newton (1975), Troost and Mark (1979), and others have reported the resolution of headaches after the removal of an occipital AVM.

In other patients, embolization of the meningeal contribution to the malformation resulted in dramatic symptomatic relief; recurrence of the headaches correlated with recanalization from incomplete, proximal occlusion, or "new" dural supply.

Patients with large malformations also appear to have headaches more frequently. Despite the above generalizations, headache relief is difficult to predict even after careful review of the angioarchitecture.

One additional cause of nonhemorrhagic headaches in patients with BAVMs (primarily in the posterior fossa) is the development of hydrocephalus, either because of mechanical distortion in the flow of CSF or alteration of CSF reabsorption. In some of these patients, the hydrocephalus may be relieved following embolization without the need of a shunt (see Chap. 5) (Fig. 3.11).

Therefore, embolization may play a role in the palliative treatment of headaches in lesions that otherwise would not be considered for intervention "only" for headaches.

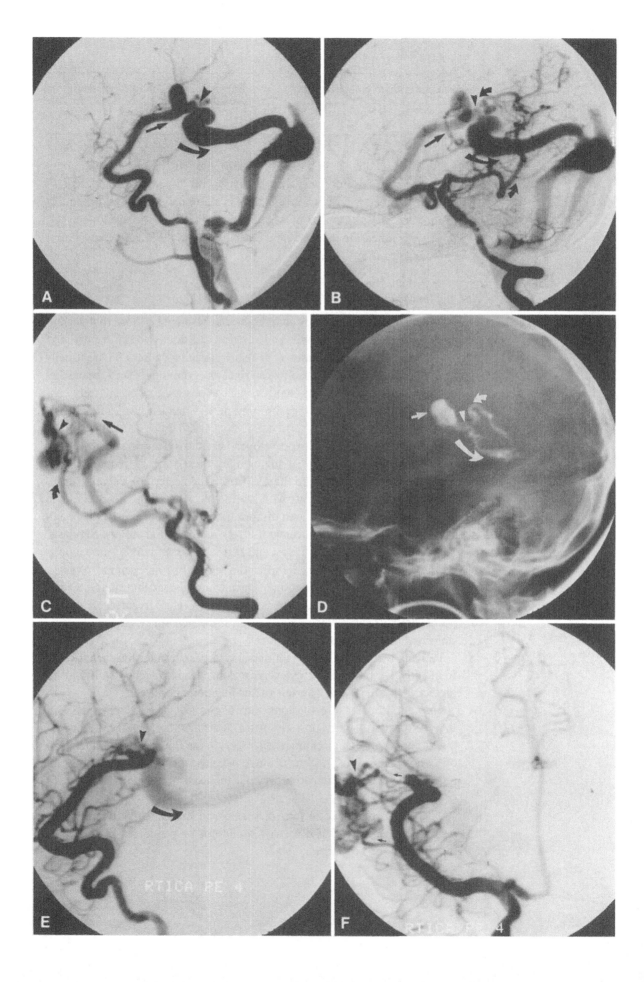

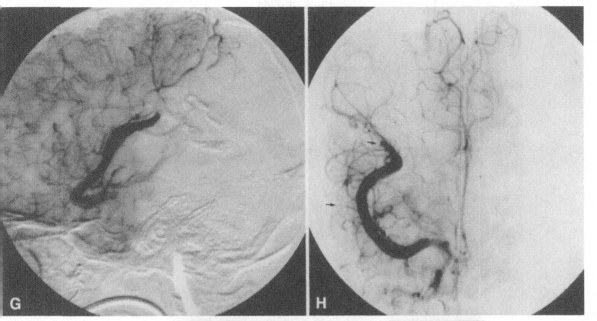

G

H

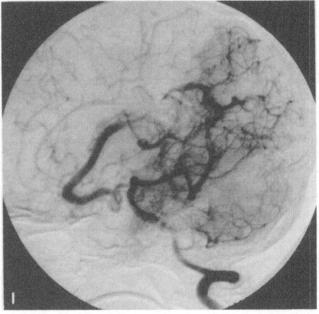

I

Fig. 3.9 A–I. Delayed thrombosis producing a grand mal seizure and Todd's phenomena. **A** Lateral view of the right internal carotid artery demonstrates an arteriovenous fistula from the middle cerebral artery (*arrow*) towards a single-hole fistula (*arrowhead*) draining into a prominent sylvian vein (*curved arrow*). **B** Left vertebral artery study demonstrates additional supply to the fistula via a lateral temporal branch (*curved arrows*). **C** Frontal view of the left vertebral artery injection shows filling of the middle cerebral artery (*arrow*) through the left posterior communicating artery, the temporal branch of the posterior cerebral artery (*curved arrow*), and the fistula site (*arrowhead*). **D** Plain film after embolization. Note the radiopaque cast in the posterior cerebral contribution (*curved arrow*), middle cerebral artery (*arrow*), fistula site (*arrowhead*), and the proximal portion of the draining vein (*curved arrow* in **E**). **E** Lateral and **F** frontal subtraction angiograms immediately after embolization demonstrate some remaining arteriovenous shunting and filling of the fistula (*arrowhead*) and draining vein (*curved arrow* in **E**). Three days later the patient had a single grand mal seizure followed by transient hemiparesis. **G** Lateral and **H** frontal digital subtraction angiography (DSA) 1 week later demonstrates complete thrombosis of the malformation. The middle cerebral artery remains dilated; there has been retrograde thrombosis of one middle cerebral artery branch and regression of a second branch (*small arrows*). **I** Left vertebral artery control angiogram at the same time confirms complete thrombosis of the arteriovenous fistulization. The seizure is probably related to thrombosis of the vein that drained the fistula

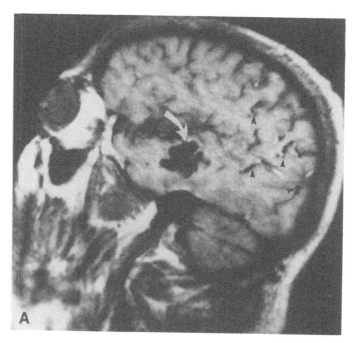

Fig. 3.10 A – G. Venous hypertension producing grand mal seizure which, despite proper levels of anticonvulsants, progressed towards status epilepticus and required general anesthesia for control. **A** MRI scan in sagittal projection demonstrates the relatively small malformation (*curved arrow*) and the prominent cortical venous pattern (*arrowheads*) 3 months prior to status epilepticus. **B** Lateral view of the left internal carotid artery demonstrates a relatively slow-flow BAVM. Note filling of the vein of Labbé (*open curved arrow*). **C** Later arterial phase of the same injection and **D** late venous phase; additional venous drainage superiorly towards the cortical venous system (*curved arrowheads*), towards the medial and lateral aspect of the temporal lobe, and towards the cavernous sinus (*curved arrow*) producing congestion of the main venous outflow of the entire hemisphere. **E** Postembolization angiogram demonstrates a small remaining shunt towards the vein of Labbé (*open curved arrow*). **F** Late phase shows the remaining drainage but significant reduction in the arterial outflow. **G** Normal venous transit time of the same cortical veins draining primarily normal cerebral parenchyma. The patient has been seizure free 3 years on anticonvulsants

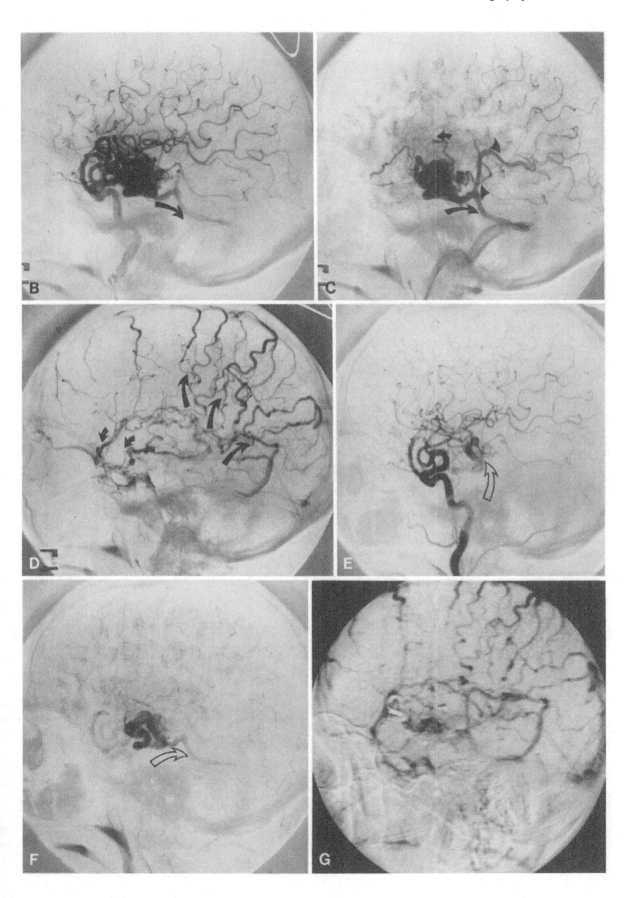

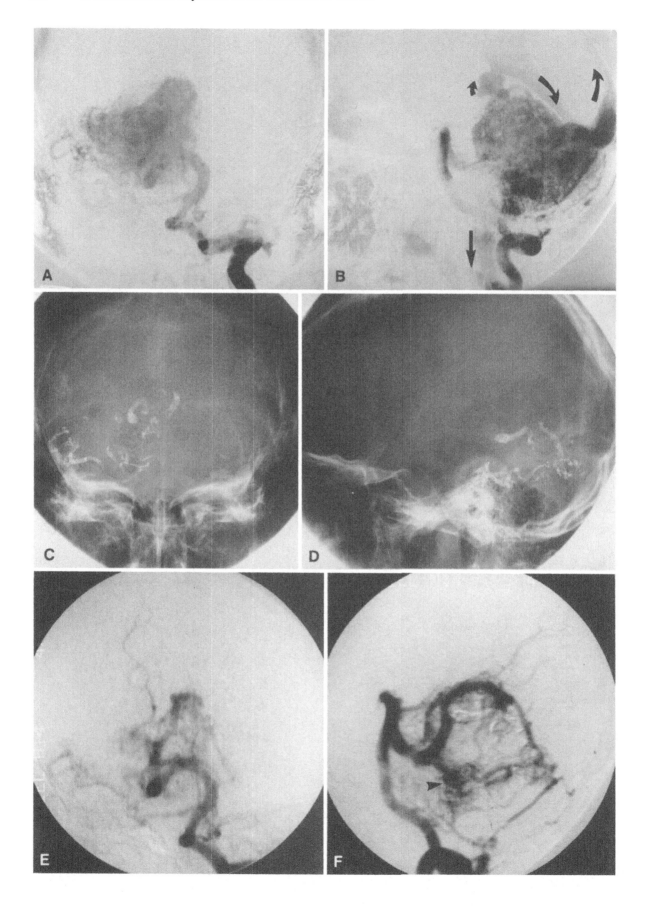

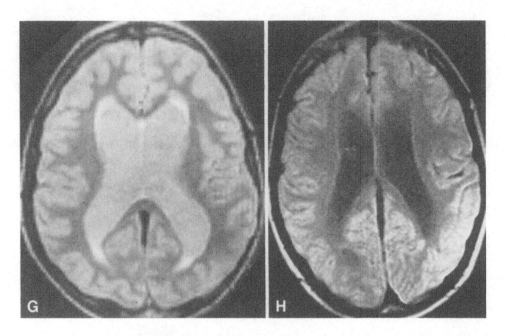

Fig. 3.11 A–H. Posterior fossa malformation in a patient presenting with headaches and ventricular dilatation. **A** Frontal and **B** lateral angiograms of the left vertebral artery in midarterial phase demonstrate an extensive cerebellar vascular malformation draining to the precentral cerebellar vein and towards the vein of Galen (*small curved arrow*) and straight sinus, with reflux into the superior sagittal sinus (*large curved arrows*), and downward towards the jugular vein (*arrow*). **C** Frontal and **D** lateral plain radiograms after partial embolization demonstrate the radiopaque cast. **E** Frontal and **F** lateral digital substraction angiography in midarterial phase after embolization demonstrates significant reduction in the amount of malformation, with the remaining supply coming from the marginal branch of the superior cerebellar artery (*arrowhead* in **F**), and preservation of the normal posterior inferior cerebellar and superior cerebellar arteries, with significant relief in the venous hypertension. **G** Axial MRI, T2-weighted image, prior to treatment. Note the ventricular dilatation. **H** After the partial embolization there was a decrease in the size of the ventricular system and relief of the headaches

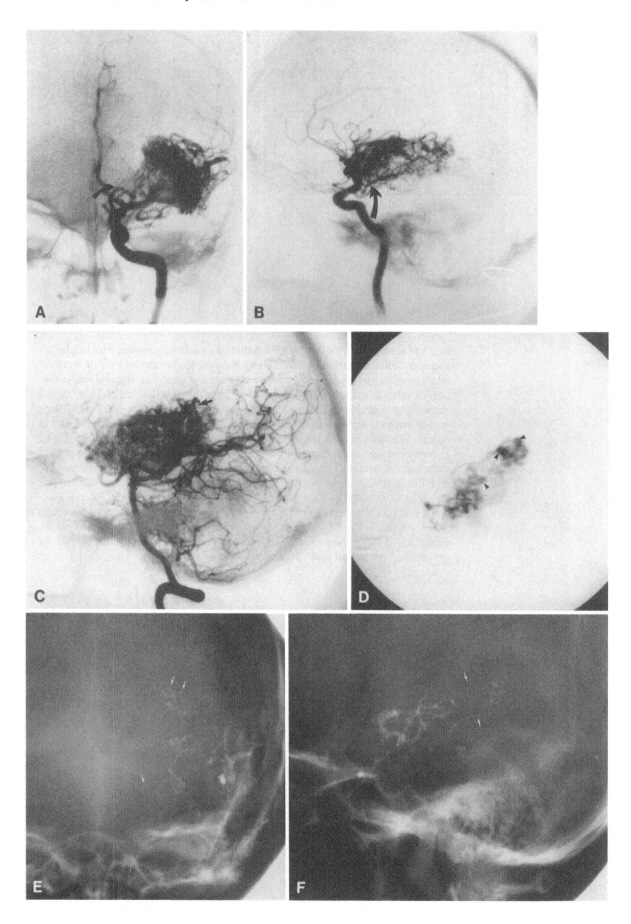

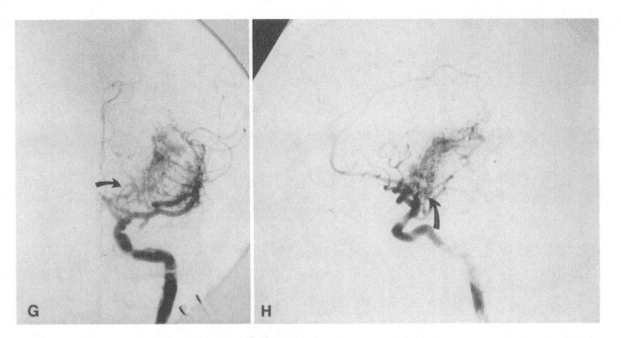

Fig. 3.12 A–H. Dominant hemisphere malformation in a patient presenting with progressive neurological deficit. The patient was embolized 6 years previously with silicone spheres and had a hemorrhage. **A** Frontal and **B** lateral views of the left internal carotid artery demonstrate a vascular malformation involving the left insula. There is an important contribution from the anterior choroidal artery (*curved arrow*). **C** Left vertebral artery injection in lateral projection shows additional supply from the posterior choroidal arteries (*arrow*). Significant reflux through the posterior communicating artery is also seen. **D** Representative film of one of the superselective catheterizations demonstrates the malformation with multiple intralesional aneurysms (*arrowheads*). **E** Frontal and **F** lateral projections of the cast obtained. Note the patient has been previously treated with silicone spheres (*white arrows*) which did not give her protection. **G** Frontal and **H** lateral views of the internal carotid artery after embolization with acrylic demonstrate the significant reduction in the nidus of the malformation with preservation of all normal arteries. The main remaining contribution is from the anterior choroidal artery (*curved arrow*). The posterior cerebral artery supply was also embolized (not shown). Significant improvement in neurological deficit followed the acrylic embolization

d) Neurological Deficits

As discussed in Chaps. 1 and 2, neurological deficits not related to hemorrhage represent decreased tissue perfusion from stenotic lesions on the arterial side, arterial "steal", venous hypertension, or a combination of these factors. Less often they may be secondary to mass effect from dilated venous structures or from hydrocephalus. The risk of hemorrhagic complications in patients presenting with neurological deficit was only 8% over 10 years in Crawford's series (1986), similar to our experience. The final outcome, however, was similar to that of Ondra's (1990) 23.7 year follow-up. Therefore, although complete obliteration and/or resection of AVM would be ideal, patients presenting with nonhemorrhagic neurological deficits more frequently harbor large diffuse lesions and complete eradication may be more difficult. Partial treatment of large lesions in patients presenting with nonhemorrhagic neurological deficits by embolization is probably the first and best method of palliative treatment, as it may stabilize or even result in neurological improvement (Fig. 3.12). Partial embolization may

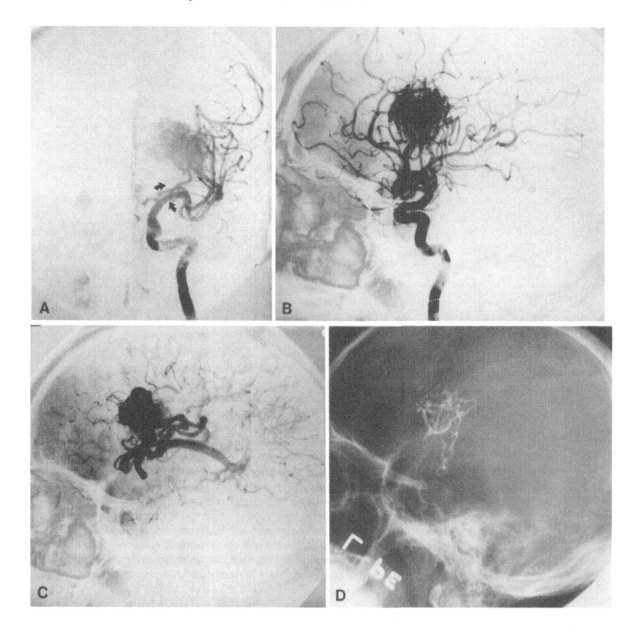

Fig. 3.13 A–H. Basal ganglionic vascular malformation. **A** Frontal subtraction angiogram of the left internal carotid artery demonstrates a basal ganglionic malformation supplied by lenticulostriate arteries (*curved arrows*) and transinsular supply from the middle cerebral artery (*arrow*). **B** Lateral projections in arterial phase and **C** in later phase show the nidus (**B**) and the deep venous drainage (**C**). **D** Lateral and **E** frontal plain radiograms showing the radiopaque cast of the malformation. **F** Frontal and **G** lateral subtraction angiograms after embolization and in midarterial phase show complete obliteration of the malformation. **H** Late venous phase shows normal drainage of the venous system

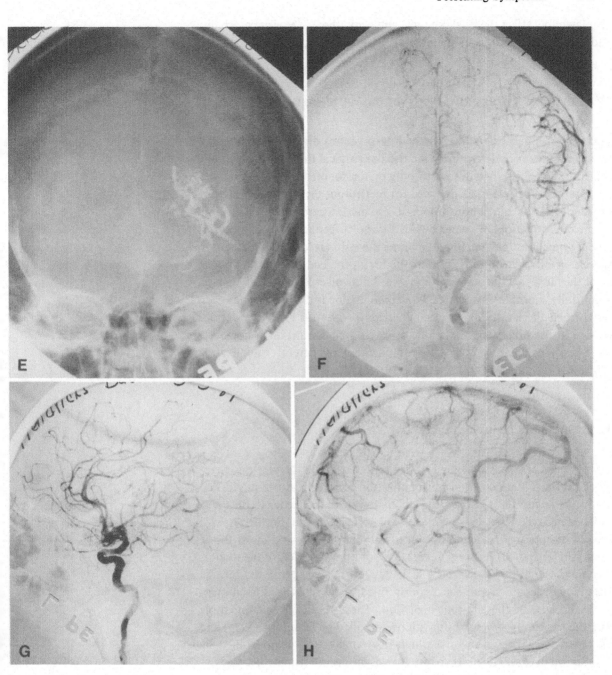

also favorably effect the final outcome and avoid the 2.7% severe morbidity and mortality regardless of presentation (Ondra 1990).

IV. Location, Size, and Deep Venous Drainage

Location of a malformation, size, and deep venous drainage are the most important factors in determining the risks of surgical therapy (Spetzler and Martin 1986). These features are of only minor concern for the endovascular approach to BAVMs, as the need for meticulous technique and sparing of all normal noncontributing arteries is essential, regardless of the location of the malformation. We concur with Yasargil's feelings, that any normal parenchyma has some function; therefore, if a lesion is located in the motor, speech, or other "eloquent" area of the brain, the endovascular approach is for the most part the same as if the location involves "ineloquent" cortex. Technically, morbidity associated with embolization is related to the capacity to reach the lesion and to remain strictly within it; therefore, lesions located in the brainstem, thalamus, or basal ganglia, although obviously more risky to treat, can be safely obliterated by careful embolization (Fig. 3.13).

V. Associated Lesions

The presence of an associated aneurysm, as discussed in the previous chapters, is not a contraindication to embolization or resection of a malformation if the aneurysm is in the same circulation or in the feeder to the AVM (flow-related). Flow-related aneurysms will decrease in size (Figs. 3.14, 3.15) or even disappear after embolization of the high-flow lesion distal to the aneurysm (Fig. 3.16) (TerBrugge et al. 1987) or after resection of the malformation (Yasargil 1987; Rizzoli 1983). A flow-related aneurysm located distally may actually represent a poorly filled vessel that has dilated proximally because of the adjacent high flow. These findings are compatible with the narrowing at vessel bifurcations described by Duvernoy (1981) and the vascular changes seen in the high-flow angiopathy demonstrated by Pile-Spellman et al. (1986). If so, the true situation will usually become apparent after occlusion of the AVM (Fig. 3.17). If the aneurysm clearly is of the developmental type, is not related to the main flow to the AVM, or has increased in size (Fig. 3.18), one may argue that the aneurysm should be treated first. The same holds true if it is clearly demonstrated that the aneurysm has bled (Fig. 3.18).

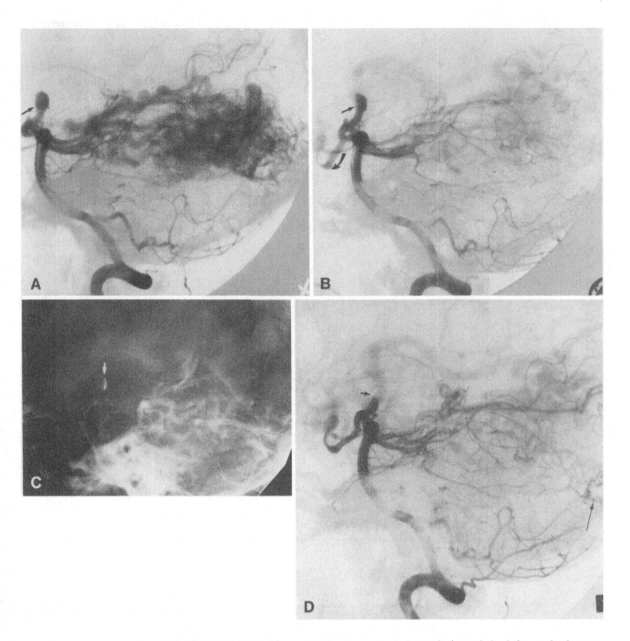

Fig. 3.14A–D. Flow-related aneurysm. **A** Lateral view of the left vertebral artery shows a flow-related basilar aneurysm (*arrow*). Note the dysplastic appearance of this aneurysm. The aneurysm is proximal to a high-flow occipital malformation. **B** Immediate postembolization angiogram of the left vertebral artery in lateral view. There is significant decrease in the supply to the malformation and slight decreased filling of the aneurysm. Note the compensatory filling of the posterior communicating artery (*curved arrow*). **C** Lateral view of the same injection in late venous phase. Note the fluid level stagnation at the dome of the aneurysm (*white arrow*). **D** 3 month follow-up angiogram demonstrates partial thrombosis of the upper dome of the aneurysm (*arrow*). Note also the development of collateral circulation of the nonsprouting type in the occipital region (*arrow*)

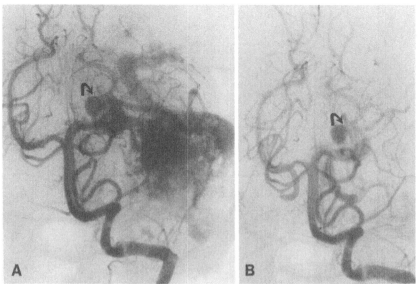

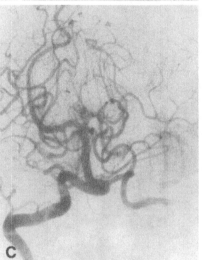

Fig. 3.15 A – C. Flow-related aneurysm. **A** Frontal subtraction angiogram of the left vertebral artery supplying a temporal arteriovenous malformation (AVM) also fills a large aneurysm at the posterior communicating level (*broken arrow*). **B** Immediate postembolization control study shows stagnation in the aneurysm and no filling of the AVM. **C** At 3 month follow-up, no filling of the aneurysm. The distal posterior cerebral artery is filled by the carotid circulation, without filling of the aneurysm (not shown)

Fig. 3.17 A, B.   Flow-related ▶ aneurysm. **A** Frontal view of the left vertebral artery injection demonstrates a vermian malformation. There is what appears as a flow-related aneurysm in the superior cerebellar artery (*arrowhead*). **B** After embolization of the distal superior cerebellar artery, the flow-related dysplasia represents the proximal portion of a vessel which also supplies the malformation (*curved arrow*). Changes of caliber in the proximal portion of a vessel in a high-flow situation are compatible with the microanatomy demonstrated by Duvernoy and the changes of a high-flow angiopathy (see text)

Fig. 3.16 A, B. Flow-related aneurysm at a bifurcation. **A** Lateral view of the internal carotid artery on the left, prior to embolization, shows a flow-related aneurysm at a bifurcation (*arrowhead*) in the feeding pedicle to a frontal malformation (*curved arrow*). **B** 3 months after embolization, regression of the aneurysm (*open arrow*) is noted. Note the enlargement of the natural collateral branch (*single* and *double arrows*)

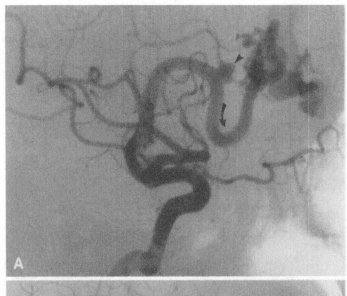

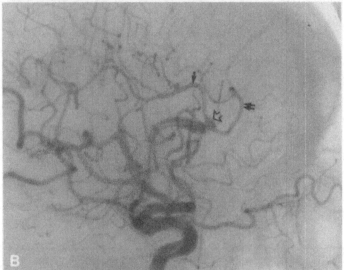

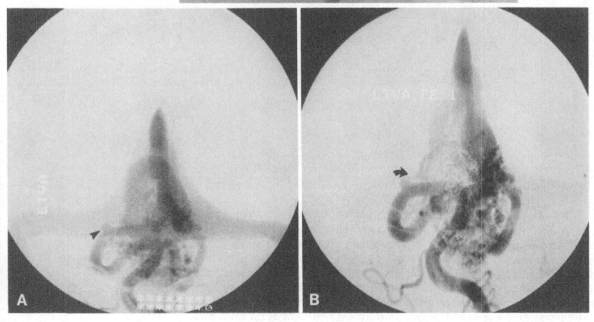

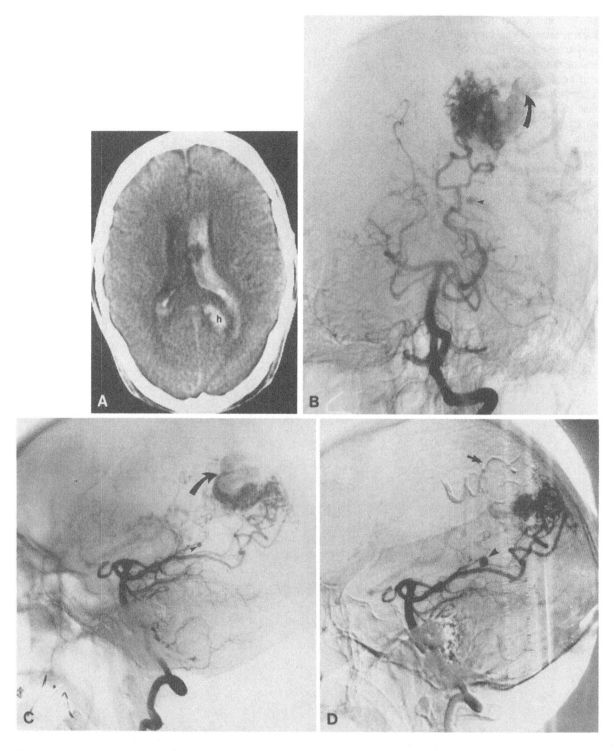

Fig. 3.18 A – D. Pseudoaneurysm of the arterial side. **A** Axial CT scan demonstrates
an intraparenchymal hemorrhage (*h*) with ventricular extension. **B** Frontal and **C**
lateral views of the left vertebral artery injection demonstrate a small arterial
aneurysm (*arrowhead*) from a posterior choroidal artery, corresponding to the location of the hemorrhage. There is a distal malformation in the parietal area with cortical venous drainage (*curved arrow*). **D** Control angiogram of the left vertebral
artery 2 days after middle cerebral artery embolization (*arrow*) shows the aneurysm
to have increased in size (*arrowhead*), with increased flow towards the malformation. The posterior cerebral artery at the level of the choroidal artery was closed at
that time

VI. Therapeutic Modalities

Once the indication for treatment has been established, a decision as how best to treat the patient must be made. In general, the main objective of any treatment of a patient with a BAVM is to completely and permanently exclude the lesion from the circulation. Such exclusion represents the only guarantee of cure.

The indications favoring interventive vs conservative treatment in BAVM patients are determined by comparing the risks of the treatment to the natural history of the individual lesion. Such risks are judged by the clinical picture and the apparent influence of the angioarchitecture of the "natural history" of the individual BAVM.

The decision to treat and the plan to be carried out (in general) is arrived at by a multidisciplinary approach. In such an approach, the various specialists involved (surgical neuroradiologist, vascular neurosurgeons, neurologist, neuro-ophthalmologist, neuropsychologist, etc.), assess the patient and design a plan to accomplish the goals of treatment. As our understanding of the disease is evolving and technical capabilities advance, the ability to properly and safely treat more complex lesions is expanding.

Initially, evaluation of pretreatment angiographic studies is conducted. A preliminary assessment of the technical possibilities and difficulties as well as a formulation of the desired objectives is made. This process, based on consideration of reasonable risks and expectations, results in an initial therapeutic plan. As treatment progresses, adjustments are made based on short-term results.

Various modalities are available which may accomplish a cure. These include surgical excision, complete embolization, radiosurgery, or a combination of treatments.

1. Surgery

Surgery alone should only be recommended when complete excision can be accomplished with a reasonable risk; there is no place for partial surgical intervention. Similarly, there is no place for partial embolization with non-permanent agents. The need for surgical evacuation of a hematoma, ventricular shunting, or other supportive measures is dictated by the clinical situation.

2. Radiation

The use of radiation in the management of BAVMs was considered ineffective until the report of Johnson (1975). He found that 9 out of 20 malformations were obliterated at a 2 year follow-up after therapy with conventional radiation. All nine obliterated AVMs, however, were small deeply placed lesions; 11 larger lesions were unaffected. The term "radiosurgery" was introduced by Leksell (1971), who used a cobalt unit with multiple fixed sources. Kjellberg et al. (1978, 1983), who used a unit that could deliver Bragg peak protons (a heavy particle beam) very accurately to produce focal targeted irradiation, demonstrated similar results in small AVMs and poor results in larger lesions. Steiner (1972, 1984, 1985, 1987) and Steiner et al. (1972, 1979), using the Leksell gamma unit, have reported impressive results in the treatment of small malformations ($20 \times 30 \times 40$ mm or 24 cm^3). Other methods, employing modified linear accelerators, seem to produce similar results in small lesions (Fabbrikant et al. 1984, 1989; Levy et al. 1989; Colombo et al. 1987, 1989; Avanzo et al. 1984). In large lesions the dose must be reduced, with no effect on the majority of lesions irrespective of radiosurgical technique.

To obtain complete occlusion after radiosurgery, a latency period of 14–24 months must elapse. During this period the patient is without protection from symptom progression or hemorrhage (Steiner 1987). Therefore, in our opinion, radiosurgery alone should be reserved for small lesions not accessible to endovascular or conventional surgery and is of no value (or contraindicated) in large AVMs.

3. Curative Embolization

Curative embolization refers to complete anatomical obliteration of the malformation by the endovascular route. If embolization is to be curative, a permanent nonbiodegradable agent must be used to form a cast of the pathological angioarchitecture (see Vol. 2, Chap. 1 and this volume, Chap. 4). We believe that there is no place for particulate or reabsorbable agents in this instance, with the possible exception of direct brain AVFs, in which a detachable balloon(s) or coils may accomplish a cure (Vinuela et al. 1982; Halbach et al. 1989a; Berenstein et al. 1990).

Cure by the endovascular route, as demonstrated by the immediate post-embolization angiogram, must be confirmed by a follow-up at least 6 months later and preferably 1 or 2 years later (Fig. 3.19). Immediate post-embolization studies are not sufficient, as small remnants may not be apparent immediately or the mixture of embolic material (even if radiopaque) with nonopaque autologous blood may recanalize at a later time (see Vol. 2, Chap. 1). Of importance is the potential recruitment of arterial collaterals, probably via a mechanism of nonsprouting angiogenesis if the shunt remains patent. If venous thrombosis is the result of the decreased shunt, however, there is no recruitment of new veins. Delayed thrombosis can occur if the nidus and draining veins are also occluded (Fig. 3.9).

In general, when a good embolization results in complete obliteration of the malformation with no residual opacification of the malformation, no arteriovenous shunting, and without stasis in the nidus, recanalization does not occur (Fig. 3.19). When some stagnation is noted in the immediate post-embolization study, in our experience delayed thrombosis of the malformation does not usually occur (Fig. 3.20) (Vinuela et al. 1983a). Delayed thrombosis can be seen mostly in fistulas if the outflow vein is occluded (Figs. 3.9, 3.32 and Chap. 5).

Complete obliteration of BAVMs by embolization has been reported to be possible in 10% (Debrun, presented at Val D'Isere, France, 1987), 16% (Berenstein, presented at Val D'Isere 1989), and 18% (Picard, Moret presented at Val D'Isere 1989), with the discrepancy related to referral patterns.

From a purely statistical point of view, at present, in only a very limited number of patients can complete cure be obtained by embolization alone.

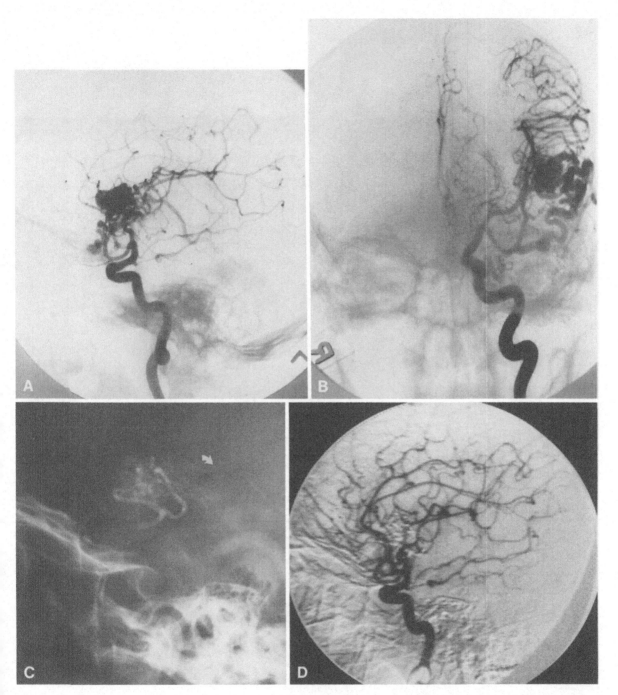

Fig. 3.19 A–G. Complete obliteration. **A** Lateral and **B** frontal subtraction angiograms of the left internal carotid artery demonstrate a vascular malformation in Broca's area, with evidence of mass effect secondary to an intracerebral hematoma. **C** IBCA cast obtained under flow arrest. Note a small amount of acrylic in the venous outflow (*curved arrow*). **D** Immediate postembolization lateral digital subtraction angiogram demonstrates no filling of the malformation. **E** Frontal and **F** lateral views of the internal carotid artery injection 2 years later in arterial phase and **G** venous phase confirm the entire obliteration of the malformation and regression to normal caliber of the middle cerebral artery (*arrow*)

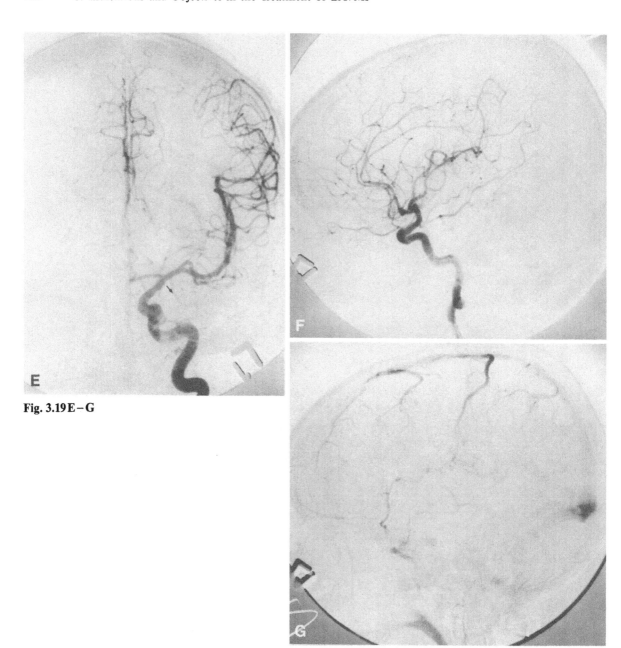

Fig. 3.19 E–G

Fig. 3.20 A–N. Nonthrombosis of a malformation. **A** Right internal carotid artery ►
injection in lateral projection, midarterial phase, shows the malformation supplied
by callosal marginal branches (*arrowhead*). **B** Late phase of the same injection.
Note some drainage of the malformation towards the deep venous system (*curved
arrow*). **C** Frontal subtraction angiograms of the right internal carotid artery in midarterial phase and **D** late phase demonstrate the deep extension of the lesion (*arrowheads*), the cortical venous drainage (*curved arrow*), and the deep venous drainage (*small curved arrow*). **E** Superselective injection of the anterior frontal polar
artery shows the balloon (*arrow*), the feeding pedicle being diluted (*curved arrow*),
and the deep portion of the malformation formed by small vessels (*arrowheads*).
F Superselective injection of the more posterior frontal polar branch reaches the
portion of the malformation with deep venous drainage (*arrowheads*). The *curved
arrow* points to the subtracted cast of the first embolized pedicle

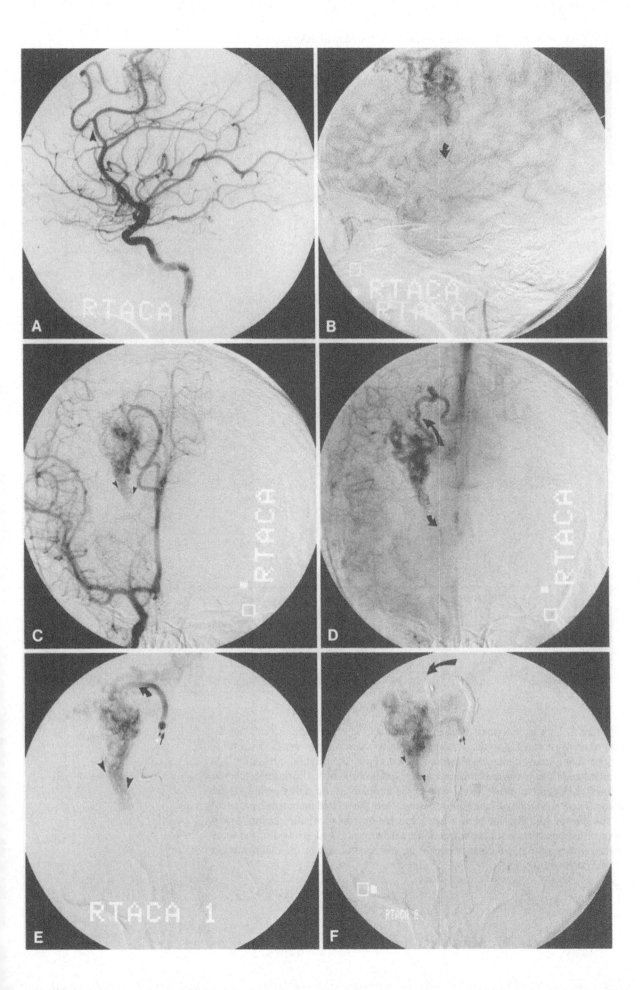

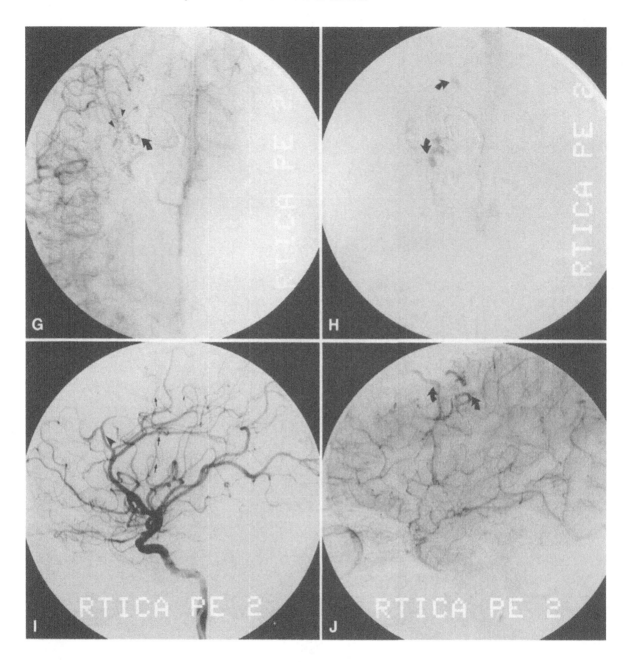

Fig. 3.20. G Late arterial phase of the postembolization study demonstrates stagnation of contrast material in the nidus of the malformation (*arrowheads*) with some venous filling (*curved arrow*). **H** More delayed phase; the cerebral circulation has emptied and there is stagnation in the venous outflow of the malformation (*curved arrows*). **I** Postembolization lateral view of the internal carotid artery in midarterial phase. There is no filling of the malformation. Note the dilated main trunk proximal to the sites of embolization (*arrowhead*) and the opercular middle cerebral artery branch just posterior to the malformation (*small arrows*). **J** Late phase of the same injection shows the stagnant, slow emptying, venous drainage of the malformation (*curved arrows*)

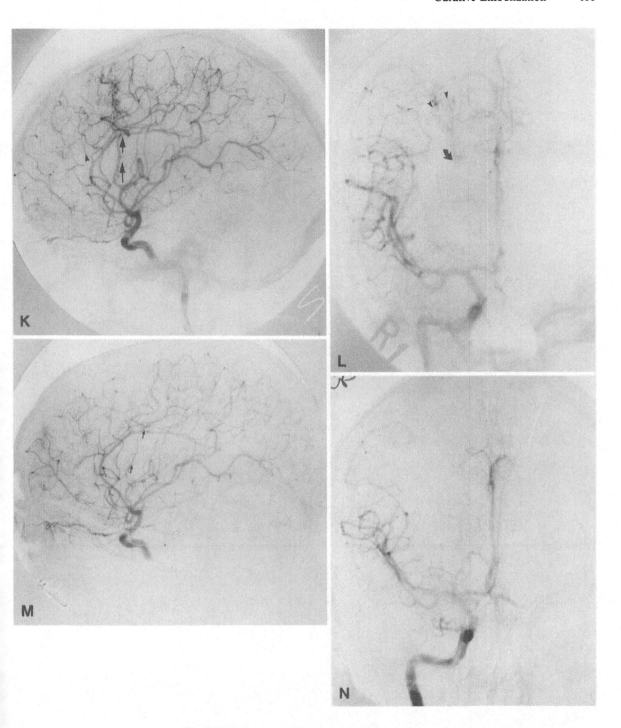

Fig. 3.20. K 3 A month follow-up angiogram demonstrates the diminution of caliber in the previously embolized main trunk (*arrowhead*) but compensatory hypertrophy of the opercular branch (*arrow*) demonstrated in **I** (*small arrows*). **L** Frontal view of the same injection demonstrates a patent nidus at the leptomeningeal border (*arrowhead*) and deep venous drainage (*curved arrow*). **M, N** Postoperative follow-up angiogram shows return to normal caliber of the opercular branch (*small arrows*). Removal of the malformation was possible in 3 h

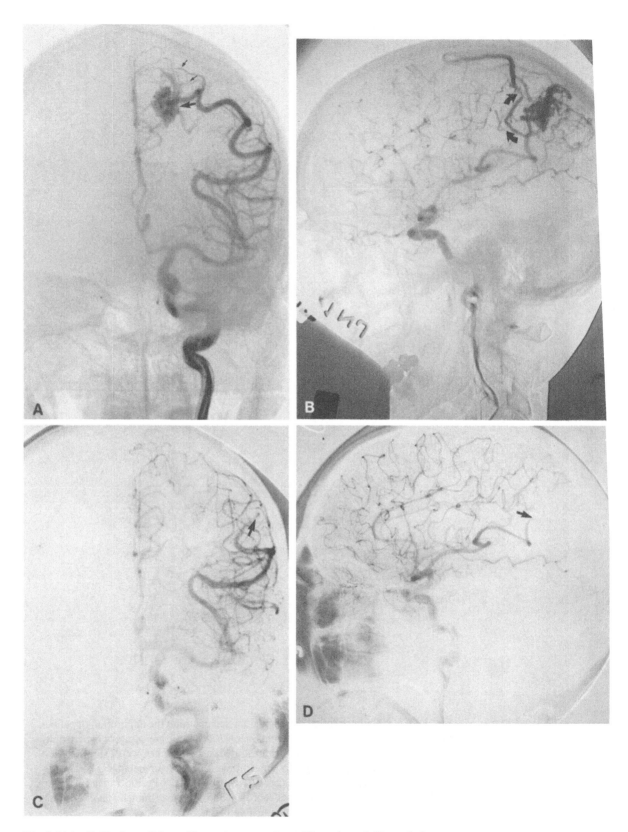

Fig. 3.21 A–F. Single pedicle malformation, complete obliteration. **A** Frontal view of the left internal carotid artery in arterial phase demonstrates a single dominant pedicle (*arrow*) with two long anastomotic arteries (*small arrows*) originating from the same trunk. **B** Late phase of the left internal carotid artery in lateral projection demonstrates outflow restrictions in the venous drainage of the malformation (*curv-*

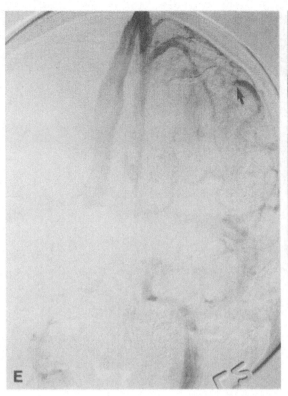

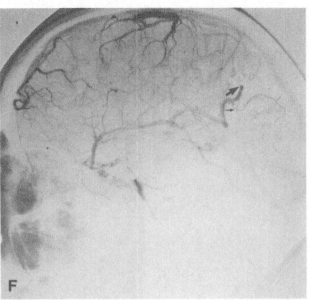

ed arrows). **C** Frontal and **D** lateral mid-arterial phase after embolization demonstrates no filling of the malformation and the stump of the trunk embolized (*arrow*). **E** Frontal and **F** lateral views of the postembolization angiogram in late phase. There is no filling of the malformation and stagnation in the stump of the embolized pedicle (*arrow*). Note preservation of the normal parietal branch (*small arrow* in **F**)

This statement fails to consider that most patients referred for embolization have very large lesions in difficult locations. If one considers large lesions with supply from multiple sources (anterior, posterior, and middle cerebral arteries and perforators), the incidence of complete obliteration is close to zero. However, in lesions supplied by one or two pedicles regardless of location, complete obliteration can be attained, over 95% of single pedicle lesions including those very distally located (Fig. 3.21) or in critical areas (Figs. 3.13, 3.19, 4.32). With advances in technique, overall complete occlusion in the last 3 years has exceeded 20% of all lesions.

When discussing complete obliteration by embolization, we must also consider that many patients with extensive malformations are still in the process of treatment and it may take several years to reach the limits of what can be accomplished by embolization. As our capabilities evolve, complete intravascular occlusions will become more frequent. The important question as to the long-term efficacy of complete embolization and its stability is as yet not known; our preliminary experience with follow-up angiograms at 2 years (Fig. 3.19) is no different than angiograms at 6 months. In other words, those patients in whom recanalization or repermeation had not occurred in a 6 month control study showed no interval change at a 1 or 2 year control angiogram. In addition, none of the patients in whom complete occlusion was accomplished with acrylic embolization have had a hemorrhage or delayed deterioration of their neurological condition.

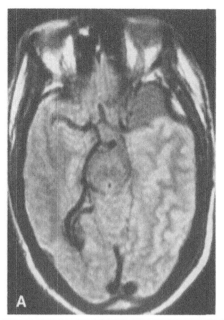

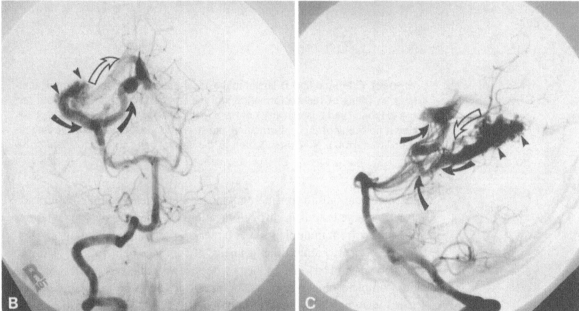

Fig. 3.22 A–F. Monopedicular malformation in the distribution of the optic radiations. **A** Axial MRI demonstrates the malformation and its venous drainage in the region of the optic radiations. **B** Frontal and **C** lateral subtraction angiograms of the right vertebral artery demonstrate the posterior temporal vascular malformation (*arrowhead*) with its venous drainage medially (*open curved arrow*) and deep towards the basal vein of Rosenthal and vein of Galen (*curved arrows*). **D** Lateral cast obtained under flow control. **E** Immediate postembolization left vertebral angiogram demonstrates complete obliteration of the malformation. Note the stump of the embolized pedicle (*arrow*). **F** A cut film angiogram 20 m later demonstrates retrograde thrombosis of the stump (*arrow*)

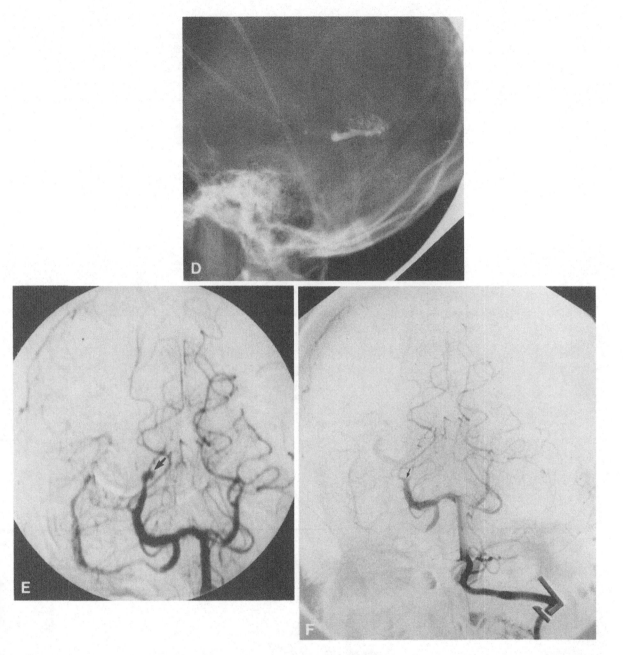

In malformations involving the optic radiations or when the surgical approach carries a high probability of optic radiation damage, embolization is the first line of treatment (Fig. 3.22). If incomplete, radiosurgery or surgery will then be considered.

In some patients with malformations located in (surgically) difficult or inaccessible areas, embolization is done to convert a large lesion into one that can then be treated by radiosurgery, further increasing the total occlusion rate (vide infra).

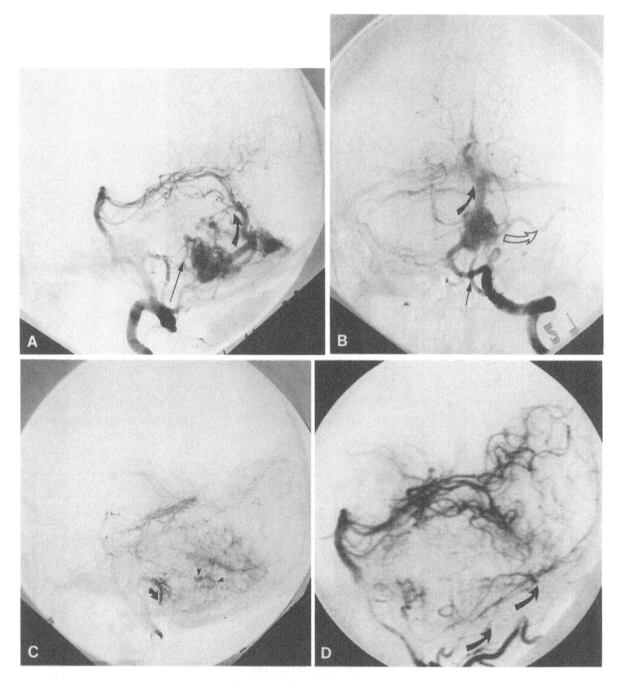

Fig. 3.23 A–E. Inferior vermian vascular malformation originally referred for pre-operative embolization. **A** Lateral and **B** frontal views of the left vertebral artery injection demonstrate an inferior vermian vascular malformation supplied by the left posterior inferior cerebellar artery (*arrow*), with venous drainage through the inferior vermian vein (*curved arrow*) and the great vein of the cerebellar fissure (*open curved arrow*). **C** Immediate postembolization control angiogram in late phase demonstrates the stump of the posterior inferior cerebellar artery (PICA) and some hypervascularity without filling of the draining vein(s) (*arrowheads*). **D** 6 A month follow-up angiogram; there is complete obliteration of the malformation with a collateral meningeal branch supplying a cerebellar artery (*curved arrows*). There has been regression of the proximal PICA. **E** Frontal view of the same injection, surgery was deferred in view of the long-lasting occlusion

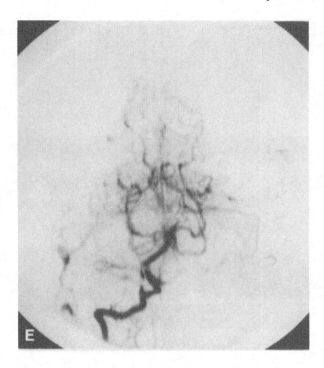

VII. Combination Treatments

Cure can be accomplished by a combination of two or more modalities, one of which usually being embolization.

1. Preoparative Embolization

Preoperative embolization has gained in popularity as an adjunct to surgical removal of BAVMs (Luessenhop and Rosa 1984; Wolpert and Stein 1975; Stein 1977, 1980; Hilal et al. 1975, 1978). In most centers, it is primarily used in large lesions or in those with high flow. In these cases the aim is to decrease bleeding, shorten operative time, and minimize the hemodynamic changes at the time of excision. The latter factor is felt by some to decrease the chances of NPPB.

Various materials have been proposed for preoperative embolization, including silicone spheres (Luessenhop and Spence 1960; Luessenhop et al. 1962, 1965, 1984; Kricheff et al. 1972; Wolpert and Stein 1975; Hilal 1975), polyvinyl alcohol particles injected transfemorally (Latchaw and Gold 1979), silk or polyethylene threads (Benati 1974, 1987), or a combination of agents such as collagen and alcohol mixtures (Dion et al. 1988; Metha 1984). In addition, following surgical exposure of feeding vessels at operation embolization with Gelfoam and iophendylate (Drake 1979), polyvinyl alcohol (Spetzler et al. 1987), or IBCA has been recommended (Cromwell and Kerber 1980). We feel that, with the availability of variable stiffness microcatheters and acrylics, at present there is no place for these modalities.

Both of us perform embolizations with acrylic material, with the aim of complete obliteration. In preoperative situations, if complete obliteration is accomplished the operation is postponed. If at 6 months follow-up the occlusion is confirmed at angiography, surgery is not performed (Fig. 3.23);

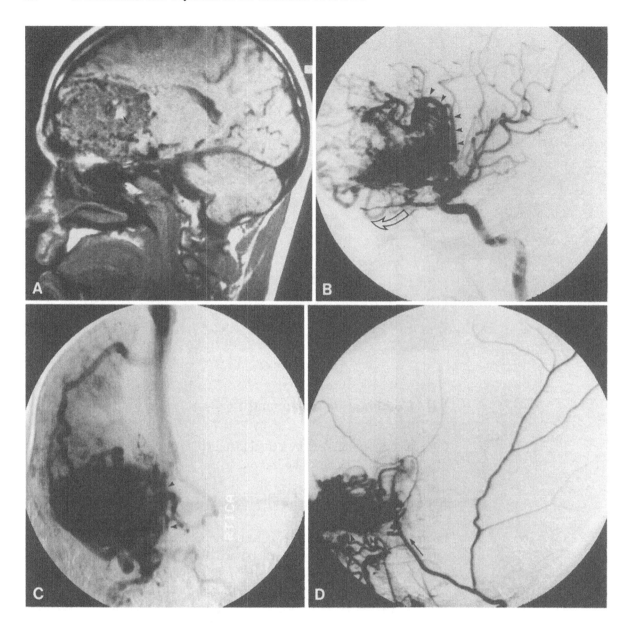

Fig. 3.24 A–H. Combined treatment, preoperative embolization. **A** Sagittal MRI demonstrates a large, right frontal, vascular malformation extending posteriorly and medially. Note the intralesional thrombosis (*small arrow*). **B** Lateral digital subtraction angiogram of the right internal carotid artery demonstrates the posterior margin of the malformation (*arrowheads*) and poor opacification of the inferior frontal arteries (*open curved arrows*). **C** Late phase of the right internal carotid artery in frontal view demonstrates the medial extension of the malformation (*arrowheads*). **D** Right external carotid artery supply via the middle meningeal artery (*arrow*) and ethmoidal arteries (*arrowheads*). The external carotid artery was embolized with acrylic material (*not shown*). **E** Right internal carotid artery injection after embolization of the most posterior medial aspect of the malformation (*arrowheads*). At the time of operation this represents a good landmark for the surgeon. Note better filling of the anterior inferior frontal arteries (*curved arrow*). This supply is easily reached surgically. **F** Frontal view after embolization showing a significant decrease in vascularity. **G** Lateral and **H** frontal subtraction angiograms 3 weeks after surgical excision. Note the persistent dysplastic anterior cerebral artery (*arrowheads, left*) and no filling of the malformation

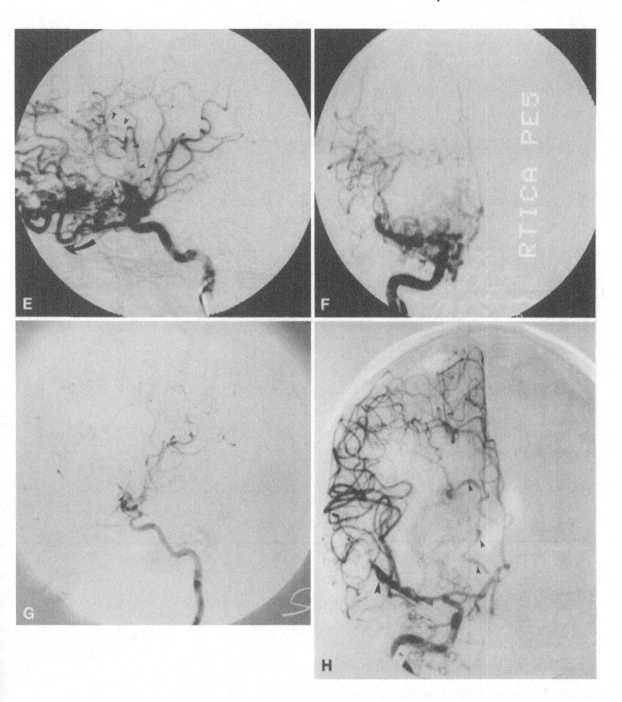

if embolization is incomplete surgery is done. No problems result from the presence of intravascular acrylic (mainly the newer *n*-butyl-cyanoacrylate, NBCA), the material being ideally suited for preoperative embolization (see Table 4.2). The low rate of complications in our experience justifies preoperative embolization of surgically accessible lesions.

The strategy of preoperaative embolization should consider the surgical operative approach. The deepest feeder(s) (posterior and anterior cerebral arteries or perforators) are embolized first; embolization of the vessels at the margins of the malformation, primarily if abutting a functionally important area, is also performed if possible (Fig. 3.24). Embolization can thereby assist in determining the plane of dissection, guided by the black

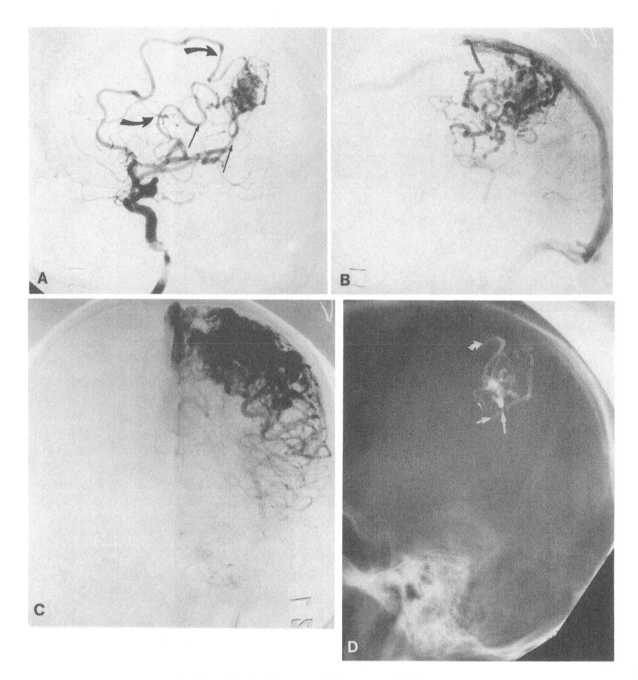

Fig. 3.25 A–I. Relatively small nidus with significant overlying venous drainage. **A** Lateral angiogram of the left internal carotid artery in mid-arterial phase demonstrates a vascular malformation supplied by the anterior cerebral artery (*curved arrow*) and middle cerebral artery (*arrows*) with a relatively small compact nidus. **B** Late phase of the same injection in lateral projection demonstrates prominent cortical venous drainage. **C** Frontal view in midarterial phase of the left internal carotid artery illustrating the cortical venous drainage in the surface of the brain, making dissection of the feeders and nidus more difficult. **D** Lateral and **E** frontal plain radiograms demonstrate the radiopaque cast of the malformation's anterior cerebral artery (*curved arrow*) and middle cerebral artery contributions (*arrows*). **F** Postembolization control angiogram in frontal projection demonstrates only a small amount of supply remaining from the anterior cerebral artery (*arrowhead*) with its persistent venous drainage (*curved arrow*). **G** Late arterial phase in lateral view demonstrates significant stagnation in the embolized middle and anterior cerebral arteries (*small arrows*). **H** Venous phase of the same injection. Note the stagnation of contrast material in the middle cerebral artery (*small arrows*), nidus (*arrowheads*), and draining veins (*curved arrow*)

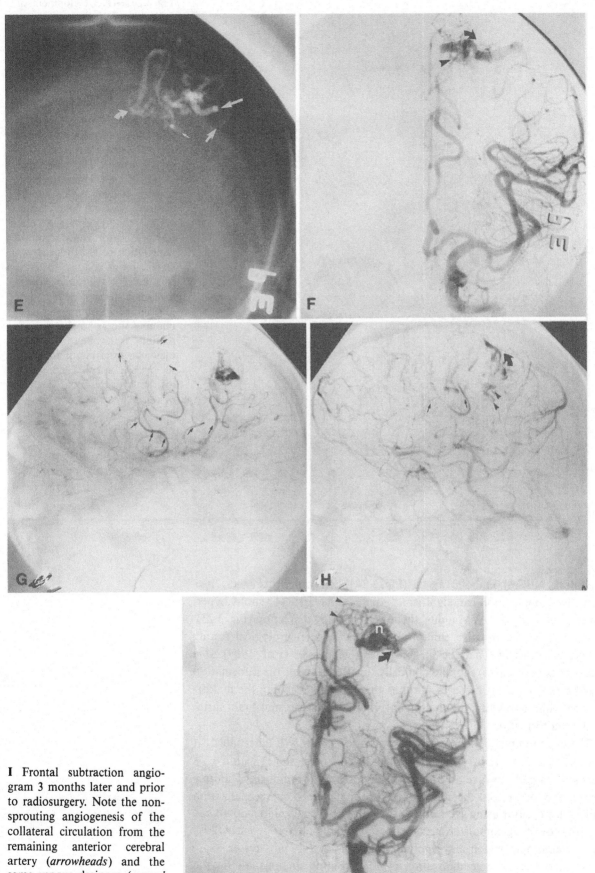

I Frontal subtraction angiogram 3 months later and prior to radiosurgery. Note the nonsprouting angiogenesis of the collateral circulation from the remaining anterior cerebral artery (*arrowheads*) and the same venous drainage (*curved arrow*). The nidus, however, remains the same (*n*)

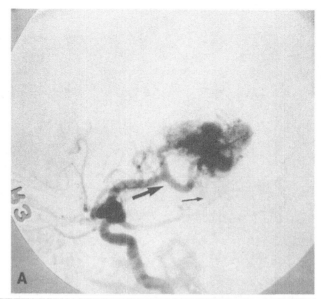

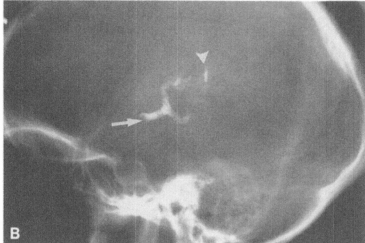

Fig. 3.26 A–F. Development of collateral circulation (nonsprouting angiogenesis). **A** Lateral view of the right internal carotid artery demonstrates a temporal vascular malformation supplied by a markedly hypertrophied middle cerebral artery branch (*arrow*) and an additional contribution from the posterior choroidal artery (*small arrow*). The malformation is of high flow with fistulization. **B** Lateral view of the postembolization plain film shows the radiopaque cast (*arrow*), with only limited penetration to the nidus. Note stagnation of contrast material in a draining vein (*arrowhead*). **C** Immediate postembolization angiogram demonstrates remaining supply to the malformation from more anterior opercular branches of the middle cerebral artery. There is significantly better opacification of normal cerebral arteries

(tantalum NBCA) embolic agent (Fig. 3.24 I). In other instances, preoperative embolization can significantly reduce the cortical venous hypertension overlying the AVM nidus, thereby facilitating dissection (Fig. 3.25).

As part of preoperative embolization, functional neurological testing during the procedure may be of assistance (Duckwiller et al. 1989). If a feeding vessel (indirect) supplies clinically functional tissue the information may be used by the surgeon to "prune" the branches reaching the malformation while preserving the main trunk that supplies normal brain distal to the malformation.

The ideal timing of preoperative embolization is not well determined. It appears best to embolize (in large malformations, last stage) within 1–3 weeks of surgery, to take advantage of any delayed thrombosis. The time frame also minimizes the development of collaterals or recanalization which may occur if using agents other than acrylic. The local hemodynamic benefits following embolization may be unfavorably altered by early (2–3 days) craniotomy, which may apply new local and regional stresses.

When the result of embolization is nonsprouting angiogenesis in the region of the AVM, a feature usually occurring secondary to proximal oc-

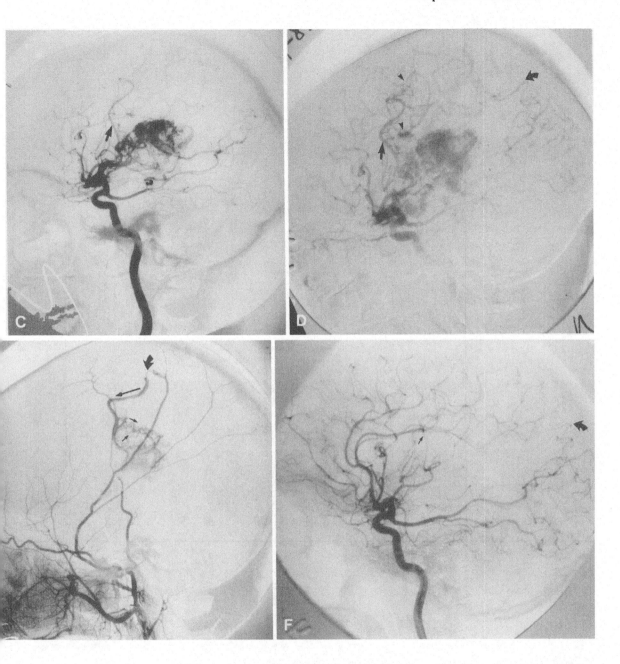

D 3 years later; note the hypertrophy of the more anterior opercular parietal branch of the middle cerebral artery (*arrow*, compare to **C**) and the development of nonsprouting angiogenesis from collateral circulation (*arrowhead*). This type of radiographic appearance is difficult to differentiate from nidus but was not present before (compare to **C**). Also note hypertrophy of leptomeningeal collaterals from the posterior and middle cerebral arteries (*curved arrow*). This type of neovascularization (*arrowhead*) may make surgical excision more difficult. **E** Lateral view of the external carotid artery at the same time as **D** demonstrates a meningeal to pial anastomosis (*curved arrow*) filling a middle cerebral artery (*long arrow*) which in turn supplies the malformation via long anastomotic arteries (*small arrows*). This supply was not present in the original angiogram (same time as **A**) suggesting nonsprouting angiogenesis in the collateral circulation secondary to remaining arteriovenous shunt. **F** Postoperative angiographic control approximately 6 months after surgery demonstrates regression in the caliber of the middle cerebral artery (*small arrow*) and leptomeningeal collaterals from the posterior to the middle cerebral artery (*curved arrow*) and regression of the nonsprouting angiogenesis and collateral circulation (*arrowheads* in **D**)

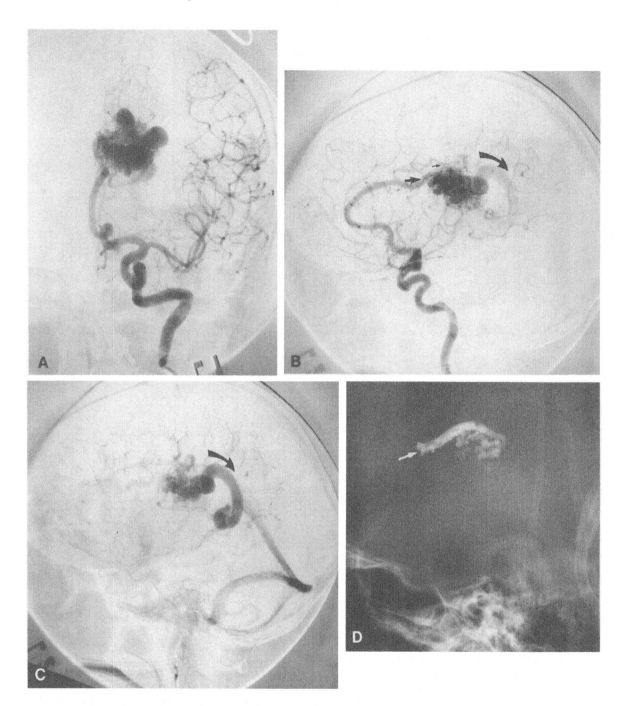

clusion, surgical resection becomes more difficult. Another surgical difficulty produced by embolization or larger caliber vessels is the development of adventitial angiogenesis (see Chap. 1). Both phenomena develop in a few weeks time and have occurred only when part of the shunt remained (Fig. 3.26).

Fig. 3.27 A–P. Preradiosurgery embolization in a patient with recent hemorrhage. **A** Frontal and **B** lateral subtraction angiogram of the left internal carotid artery demonstrating a midline corpus callosum vascular malformation supplied by the pericallosal artery (*arrows*). **C** Note the venous drainage towards the medial atrial vein (*curved arrow*). **D** Radiopaque cast of the main pericallosal artery embolized (*arrow*). **E** Frontal and **F** lateral postembolization control angiograms of the left internal carotid artery demonstrating supply to the malformation via the second pericallosal branch showing supply "en passage" (*arrow*). There has been significant reduction in the nidus. **G** Vertebral artery injection; there is some contribution from the posterior pericallosal artery (*small arrow*)

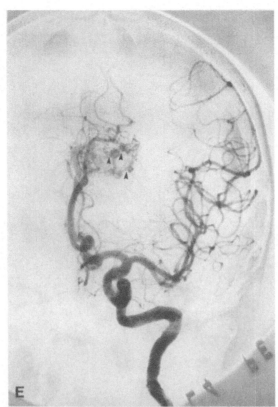

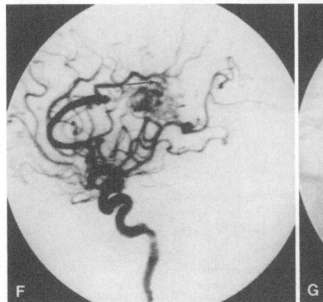

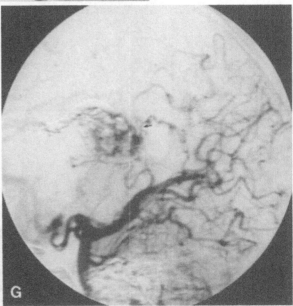

2. Radiosurgery and Embolization

When planning embolization prior to radiosurgery, the goal is to reduce the lesion to a size treatable by that modality, i.e., to leave an open malformation no larger than $20 \times 30 \times 40$ mm (Steiner 1985) (Fig. 3.27). The data reported by Steiner on the results of radiosurgery for small AVMs are impressive; however, there appears to be no protection against repeated hemorrhages in these patients until the lesion has completely thrombosed, a pro-

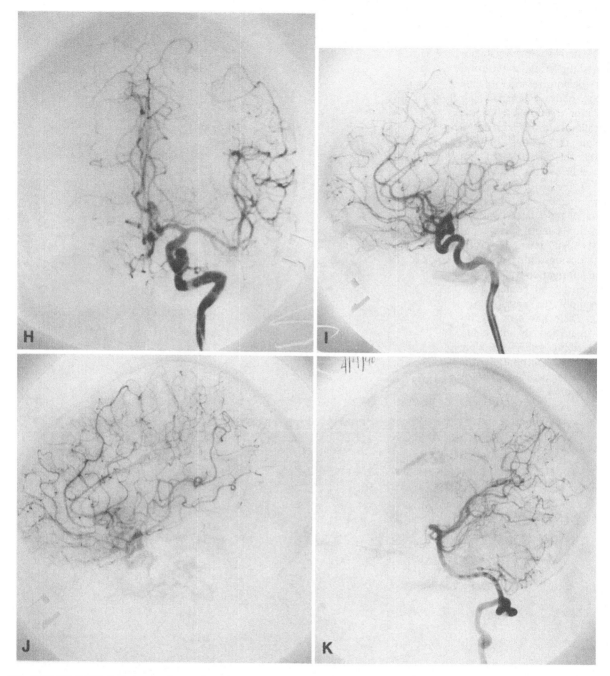

Fig. 3.27. H, I, J, K Left internal carotid and vertebral artery studies showing the thrombosis of the malformation 22 months after radiosurgery with the gamma knife. **L** Coronal and **M** sagittal MRI examinations prior to treatment demonstrating the nidus of the malformation (*arrowhead*) and its venous drainage (*curved arrow*). **N** Control MRI scan 6 months after the radiosurgery shows decrease in the size of the nidus (*arrowhead*) which correlates with the decrease in size of the draining vein (*small curved arrow*). **O** Axial MRI at the level of the centrum semiovale done at the same time as **N**, demonstrating some bright signal (*white arrows*) representing white matter edema secondary to the radiosurgery. This type of edema, if clinically manifested, responds readily to low dose corticosteroids. **P** Coronal scan at 22 months showing no gross evidence of flow by MRI. This correlated with the angiograms demonstrated in **H, I, J,** and **K**

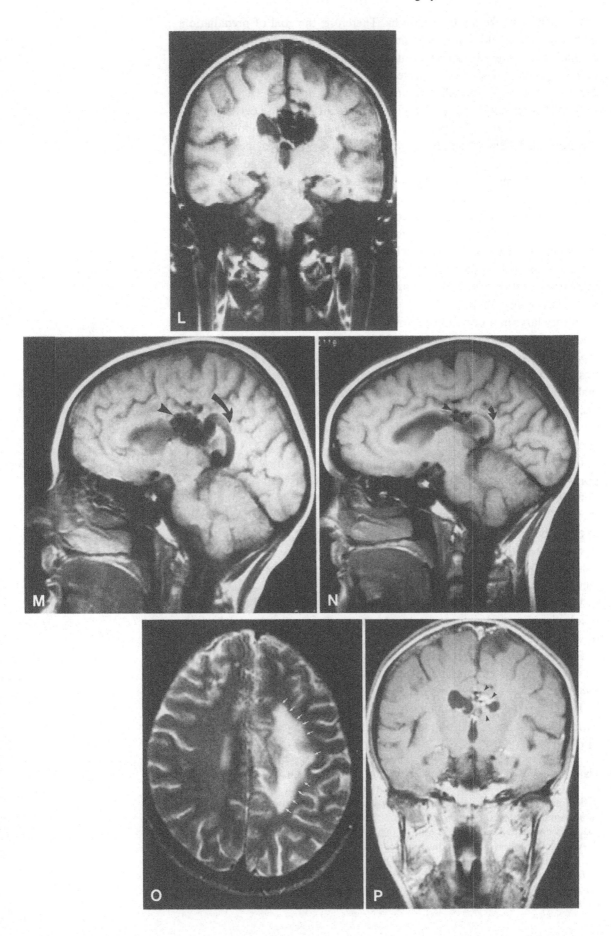

cess which may take up to 24 months. Therefore, the goal of preradiation embolization, in addition to reducing the size, is to stabilize the lesion by occluding the nidus, an arterial aneurysm, venous pouches, etc. This stabilization attempts to give some protection in the latency period, following radiation but before complete thrombosis has occurred.

In AVMs which have bled, those lesions in difficult surgical locations, and those which are of appropriate size for radiosurgery, embolization is recommended. Embolization in these instances will provide (at least theoretically) some protection. When radiation is performed after embolization of small malformations it appears prudent that the occluded portion be included in the radiation field (Fig. 3.28).

When planning embolization prior to radiosurgery, it is imperative that nonabsorbable or nonrecanalizing materials are used. Silicone spheres, polyvinyl alcohol particles, coils, "cocktails," or acrylics used in a "push" or other fragmented mode of injection should be avoided, as the likelihood that recanalization will occur is high (Vol. 2, Chap. 1, see Recanalization and this volume, Chap. 4).

In very large malformations, in which embolization is incomplete, every effort should be made not to leave the open portions of the lesion as separate patchy areas of incomplete occlusion. In such cases, it may be impossible to deliver sufficient radiation to produce thrombosis. In such large malformations, embolization is planned to leave one or more areas of compact arteriovenous shunting, each one less than $20 \times 30 \times 40$ mm. If more than one area is left, each focus is radiated as a single malformation (Fig. 3.29).

In patients in whom radiotherapy is planned but who have a dural component to the lesion, embolization of the meningeal (surface) supply is warranted, as this represents a source of difficulty for gamma radiation therapy. The difficulty arises from the proximity of the meningeal supply to the bone and scalp. We have seen cases in which the pial supply reduces in size (or even thromboses) after radiotherapy, while the dural contribution enlarges. Here, embolization can be done after radiotherapy to produce complete obliteration.

The combination of embolization, radiosurgery, and neurosurgery can obtain significant advantages that none of the techniques alone may be able to accomplish (Fig. 3.30).

Finally, radiotherapy can be used to thrombose a feeder that could not be reached by the endovascular route, thus completing treatment (Steiner 1987).

The long-term effect of radiated malformations, alone or in combination with embolization, is still unknown and caution is suggested, particularly in children.

Fig. 3.28 A–E. Combined treatment. **A** Lateral subtraction angiogram of the internal carotid artery on the left demonstrates a malformations in Broca's area (same patient as in Fig. 4.4). **B** Later phase angiogram after embolization demonstrates a small remaining nidus (*arrowhead*). **C** Later phase; there is some stagnation in the nidus (*arrowheads*) but there is still filling of the draining vein (*curved arrow*). **D** At 6 month follow-up the nidus remains patent (*arrowheads*). **E** Later phase of the same injection. The nidus is still visualized with increased filling (*arrowheads*) of the remaining deep venous drainage (*curved arrow*). In such cases embolization gives early protection. The radiosurgery in this size malformation should probably include the entire nidus with the embolized portion

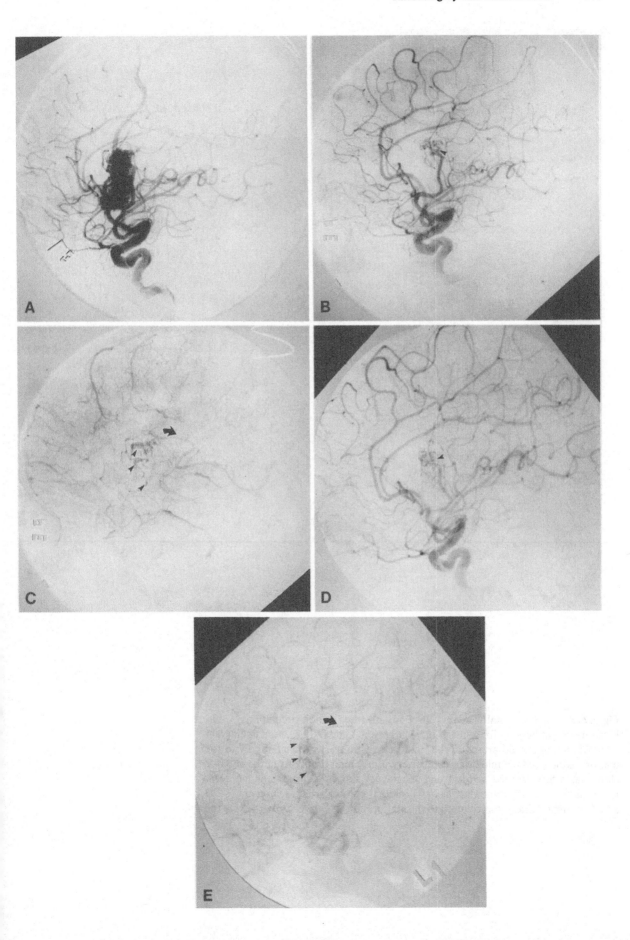

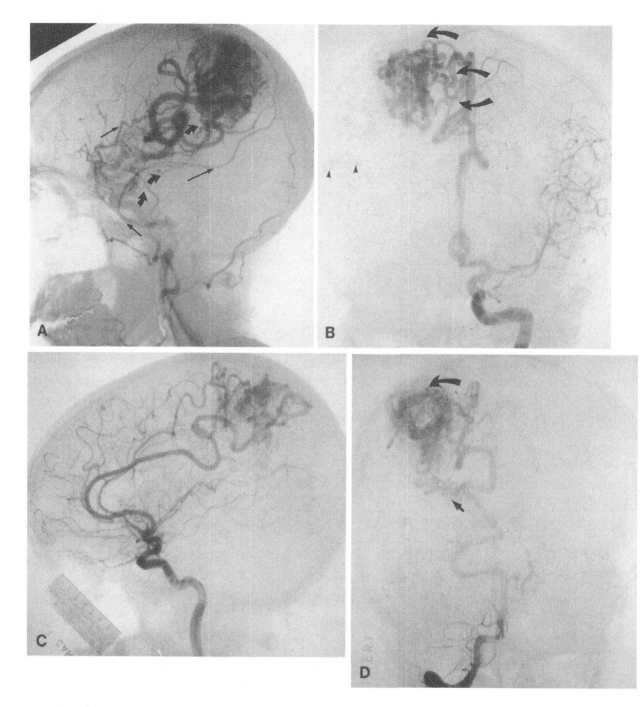

Fig. 3.29 A–M. Large malformation involving all three major circulations. Combined treatment by embolization and radiosurgery. **A** Lateral subtraction angiogram of the common carotid artery on the right demonstrates significant supply to the malformation from the middle cerebral artery. Additional supply from the anterior choroidal artery (*curved arrows*) and meningeal supply (*arrows*) can be seen. **B** Frontal view of the contralateral (*left*) internal carotid artery demonstrates the anterior cerebral artery contribution to the malformation (*curved arrows*). Note the

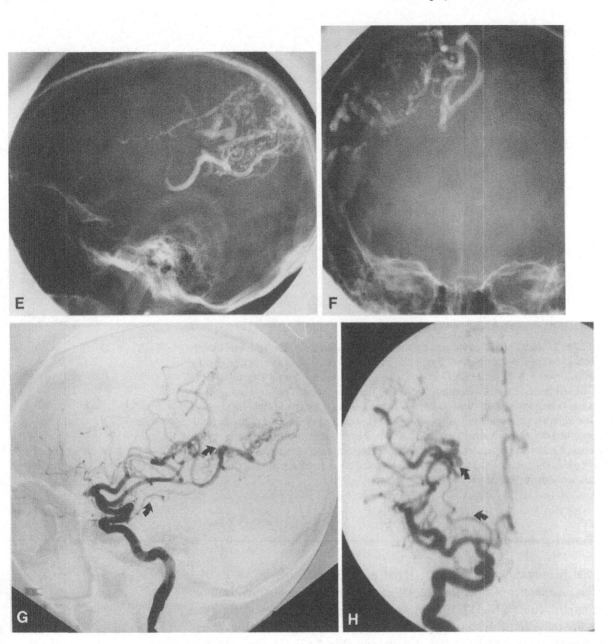

extent of the malformation from the middle cerebral artery (*arrowheads*). **C** Lateral
view of the left internal carotid artery demonstrates the medial and anterior portion
of the malformation (compare to **A**). **D** Frontal view of the right vertebral artery
injection demonstrates supply to the malformation at the choroidal level (*arrow*)
and distal posterior cerebral artery (*curved arrow*). This represents the medial
posterior extension of the malformation. **E** Lateral and **F** frontal plain radiograms
demonstrate the radiopaque cast of the malformation using high volume acrylic embolization. **G** Lateral and **H** frontal subtraction angiograms after embolization demonstrate the significant reduction in the supply to the malformation. Note the persistence of the anterior choroidal artery supply to a small nidus (*curved arrows*)

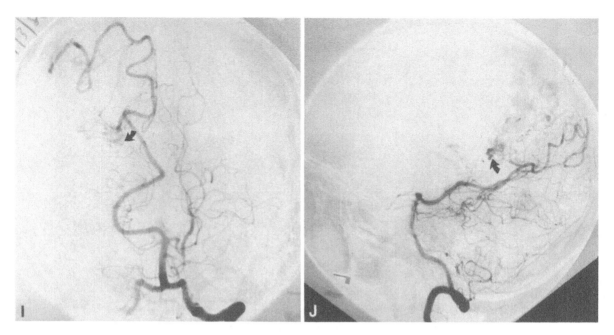

Fig. 3.29. I Frontal and **J** lateral postembolization angiograms of the vertebral artery injection on the left demonstrate the remaining medial portion of the malformation (*curved arrow*). **K** Lateral and **L** frontal views of the right internal carotid artery, and **M** left internal carotid injection with a stereotactic frame. The large malformation has been converted to two small fields of radiation (*I, II*). The *I* field is supplied by the anterior choroidal and a branch of the posterior cerebral artery; the *II* field is supplied by the remaining contribution of the middle and anterior cerebral arteries. Each nidus is treated as a separate malformation (radiosurgery performed by Prof. L. Steiner). The radiosurgery is targeted to the remaining arteriovenous shunt without including the collateral circulation (*II*)

3. Partial Treatment

Partial permanent treatment is reserved for those patients in whom the various modalities of management, either alone or in combination, cannot accomplish cure. A backup strategy is therefore proposed in an attempt to stabilize the lesion. Such a strategy is geared towards a morphological target or clinical objective such as relief of symptoms (Fig. 3.12), closure of an anatomical weakness (Figs. 3.5–3.7), or relief of venous hypertension (Figs. 3.1, 3.10). It is important that, when partial treatment is proposed, no compromise to potential future treatment results.

As previously stated there is no place for partial surgical intervention, partial radiosurgery, or partial embolization with nonpermanent agents; therefore, partial targeted treatment by embolization is reserved for the use of permanent agents such as liquid acrylics (IBCA and NBCA).

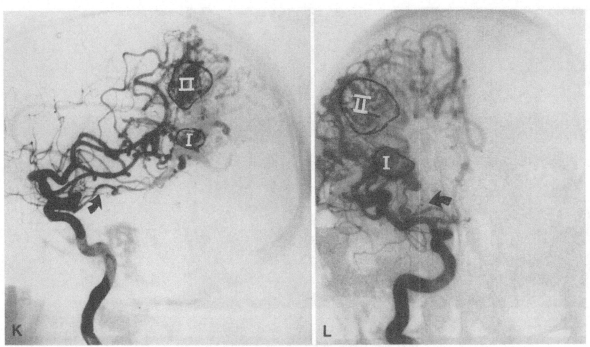

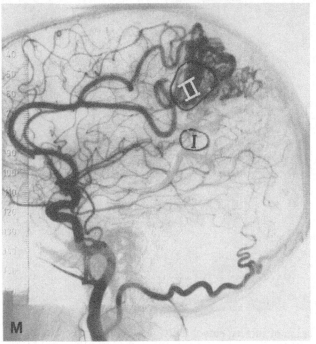

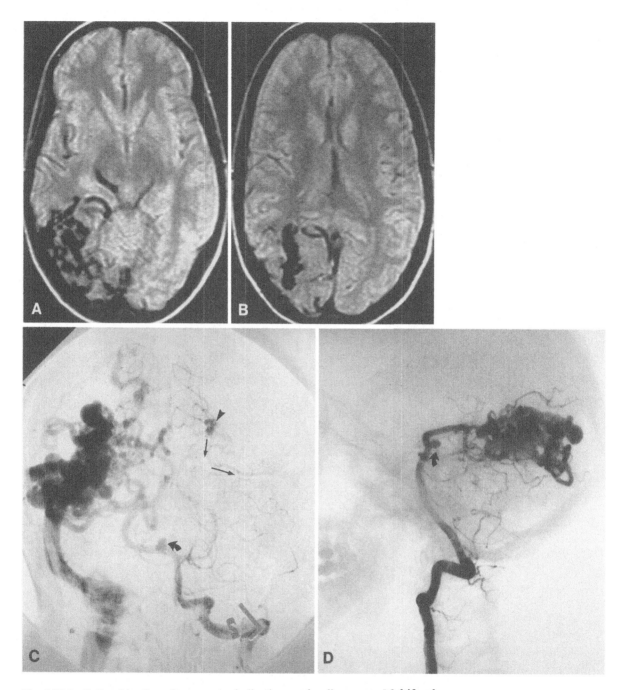

Fig. 3.30 A–J. Combination of surgery, embolization, and radiosurgery. Multifocal vascular malformation with a larger occipital malformation on the right side, a smaller lesion on the left, and an enlarging P1 aneurysm. **A** and **B** Axial MRIs demonstrate the malformation on the right occipital region. No vascular lesion is discernible on the left. **C** Frontal and **D** lateral subtraction angiograms of the left vertebral artery injection demonstrate an enlarging aneurysm on the P1 segment (*curved arrow*). There are two malformations; the larger one is on the right occipital region supplied by the posterior cerebral artery and the smaller malformation is on the contralateral (left) side. The left malformation (*arrowhead*) has independent venous drainage (*arrows*). **E** Lateral and **F** frontal plain radiograms of the skull demonstrate the large volume NBCA cast obtained (the aneurysm was clipped prior to embolization because of its relatively rapid enlargement). **G** Frontal and **H** lateral subtraction angiograms of the left vertebral artery demonstrate marked reduction in the malformation from the right side

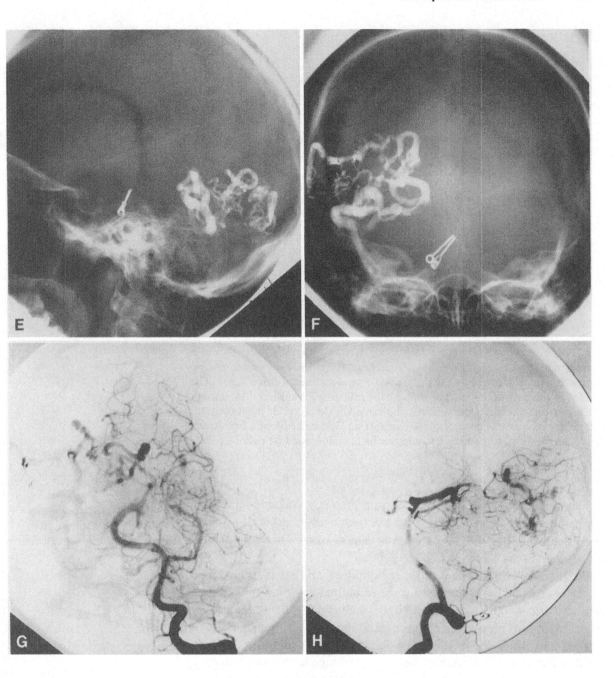

4. Intraoperative Embolization

Intraoperative embolization developed from the frustration of early experiences with superselective embolizations in the early 1970s. Drake (1979) described the embolization of a posterior cerebral artery which was exposed surgically; an arteriotomy was performed and a small catheter was advanced. Drake used Gelfoam particles soaked in iophendylate, either palliatively or preoperatively. Cromwell and Harris (1980) modified the technique and used softer Kerber tubing and IBCA, and Spetzler et al. (1987) reported on the use of polyvinyl alcohol as part of surgical excision of large AVMs.

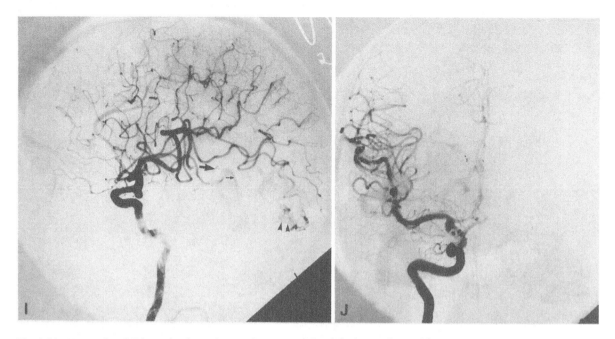

Fig. 3.30. I Lateral and **J** frontal subtraction angiograms of the right internal carotid artery demonstrate the stumps of the embolized vessels (*arrows*) with some remaining malformation supplied by the distal middle cerebral artery (*arrowheads*). The strategy in this patient consisted of clipping the enlarging P1 aneurysm by conventional surgical techniques, followed by embolization of the right side malformation, and radiosurgery of the remaining right side. If no field defect occurs from treatment, the malformation on the left side can be then addressed by radiosurgery

The technique is only rarely needed with presently available superselective catheterization capabilities. It has not been used by either of us in the last 7 years but may still have a place in centers where transfemoral techniques are not available.

Pitfalls exist during intraoperative embolization, and one must be certain of the course of flow in the vessel to be embolized so as not to confuse a feeding artery with an arterialized draining vein. Intraoperative angiography is of great value. Doppler ultrasonography, although useful, is less accurate. In AVMs in which the dominant venous drainage is superficial, the draining veins usually overlie the feeding arteries and dissection prior to arteriotomy may be difficult. In selected patients, however, this technique can be curative.

Intraoperative embolization may be used after the limits of transcutaneous techniques have been reached, or it may precede transfemoral embolization. In the latter case, it is done in an attempt to convert a lesion supplied by more than one circulation into a malformation supplied by only one.

5. Timing of Embolization

Concerning the timing of embolization following hemorrhage from the AVM, there is no general consensus or specific guidelines that must be followed, as the rebleed rate in the immediate posthemorrhagic period is relatively low (probably in the 6% range in the first 6 months) (Perret and

Fig. 3.31. Vasospasm following arteriovenous malformation hemorrhage. Vasospasm is infrequent and only has been encountered in 2 out of more than 500 patients. Left internal carotid artery angiogram demonstrates spasm in the supraclinoid carotid (*long arrow*) and in the calllosal marginal arteries (*small arrows*)

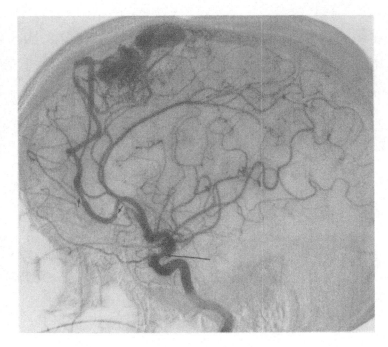

Nishioka 1966; Crawford et al. 1986). In contrast to bleeding from an aneurysm, vasospasm is a rare occurrence in BAVMs that have bled (2 in over 500 treated by both authors) (Fig. 3.31). If rapid deterioration occurs in the immediate postictal period, it is most likely related to mass effect from a hematoma, a situation requiring surgical removal usually without manipulation of the AVM. Embolization after a hemorrhagic event is usually postponed until the patient is in optimal condition. In small lesions readily accessible to endovascular embolization, endovascular obliteration may be performed in the acute period following the angiographic study (Fig. 3.19).

The development of vasospasm during cerebral navigation in the management of BAVMs is infrequent in our experience and has occurred only when endovascular manipulation were done close to the time of the original bleed.

6. Staging Embolization

Staging embolization is usually done in large malformations or when the delay is expected to let a small feeder enlarge in order to facilitate future catheterization. There is no apparent increased risk in leaving a part of a malformation patent, even if a large or high-flow portion is occluded. Therefore staging in large malformations may be advantageous from a technical and hemodynamic viewpoint.

Staging is advisable in patients in whom a deficit or other complications occur. The embolization is then resumed when the deficit has cleared. If no complication occurs, a second or additional procedure can be repeated within a day or two. Staging is also recommended when a large amount of contrast material has been used. If none of the above circumstances exist and if the lesion can be completely obliterated in one session, there is no

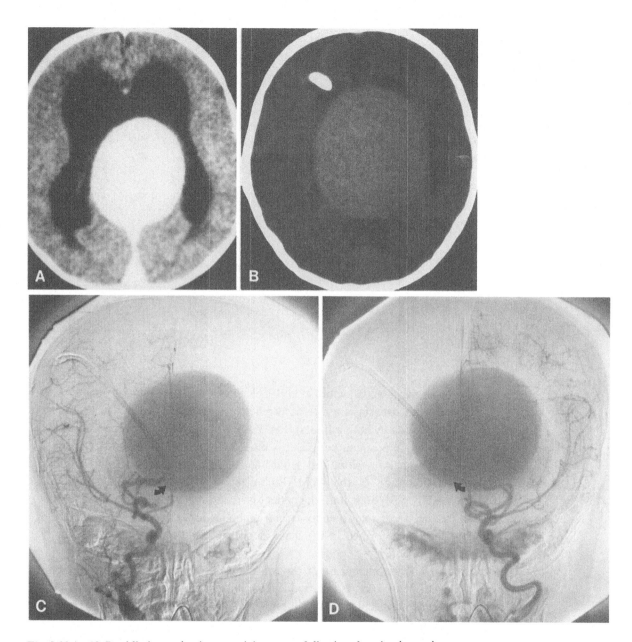

Fig. 3.32 A–N. Rapidly increasing intracranial pressure following shunting in a vein of Galen aneurysmal malformation (VGAM). **A** Axial CT scan after intravenous administration of contrast material demonstrates the aneurysmally dilated medial vein of the prosencephalon producing ventricular enlargement. **B** After shunting the fontanels bulge and the intracranial pressure is raised secondary to "ex vacuum" enlargement of the midline aneurysmal vein. **C** Frontal subtraction angiogram of the right common carotid artery injection and **D** left internal carotid artery injection demonstrate mural fistulas in the wall of the aneurysmal vein (*curved arrows*). **E** Digital subtraction angiogram injection of the right posterior, medial choroidal artery demonstrates the mural fistula (*arrowhead*). **F** Superselective catheterization of the left posterior medial choroidal artery after the right side has been embolized.

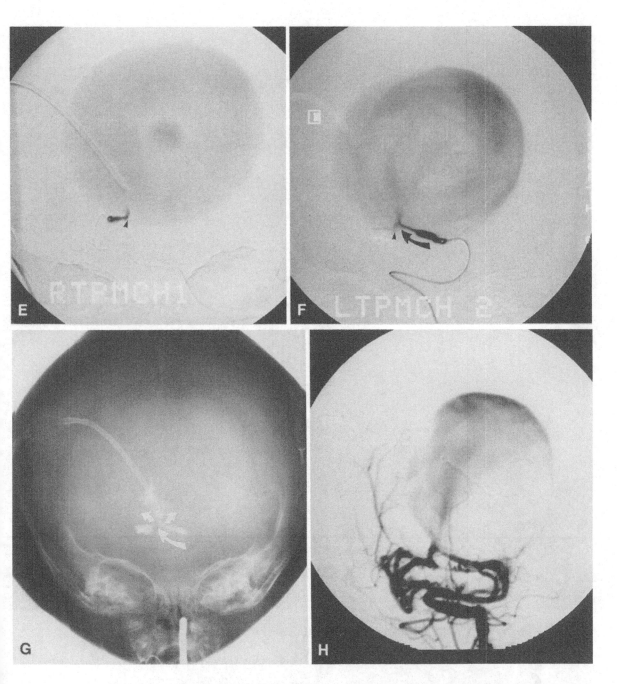

Note the area of fistulization to be partially diluted (*arrowhead*) with the dominant flow coming from the left posterior medial choroidal artery (*curved arrow*). **G** Post-embolization plain radiogram shows the cast of the left posterior medial choroidal artery (*long curved arrow*) with filling of the right side, which was producing the dilution (compare to **F**) and the "mushrooming" of the acrylic column as it enters fistula (*small curved arrows*). **H** Immediate postembolization frontal view of the left vertebral artery injection demonstrates still some shunting and marked stagnation of nonopacified blood in the large vein

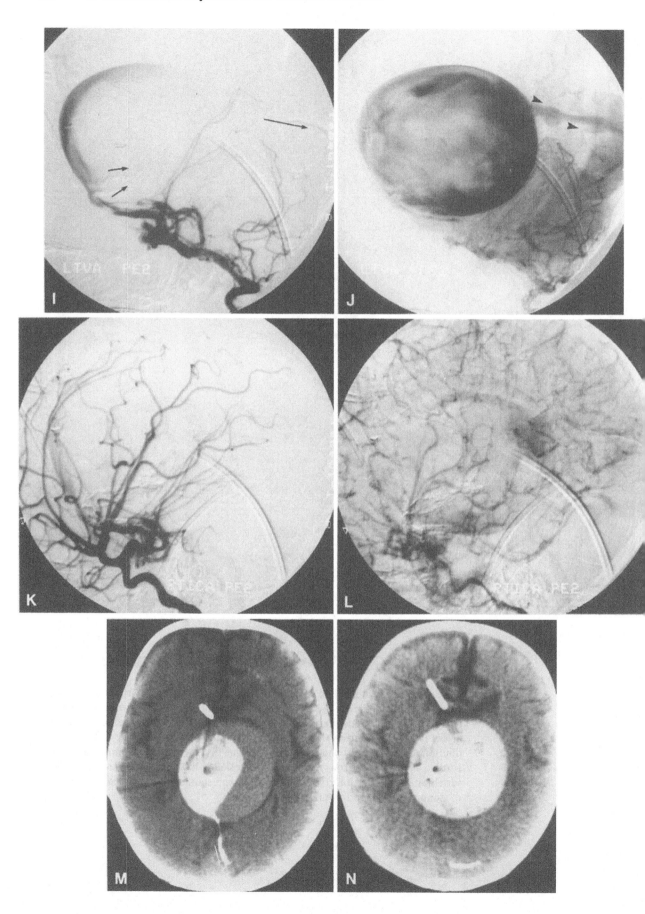

need for staging. No NPPB has been observed by either author despite occlusion of large high-flow AVMs or AVFs.

Staging is of utmost importance and value in the very young patient with a delicate cardiovascular state, in which careful monitoring of fluids and contrast material is imperative (see Chap. 5).

7. Emergency Embolization

There are few indications for emergency embolization. A significant exception includes the newborn or very young patient in high output congestive heart failure (see Chap. 5), rapidly progressive CSF disorders, or a rapidly enlarging head circumference secondary to enlargement of a vein of Galen after ventricular shunting is performed and which results in acute increased intracranial pressure (Fig. 3.32).

Emergency embolization may be needed at the time of the actual procedure if a vessel ruptures and is discussed in the following chapter in the management of complications of CNS embolization.

Urgent need for embolization may arise when the preliminary study demonstrates a pseudoaneurysm or enlarging aneurysm in a feeding artery (Fig. 3.18). Embolization should probably not be delayed in the presence of a venous aneurysm not present in a prior examination (Fig. 3.8), i.e., a venous pseudo aneurysm (Fig. 3.7).

Other instances requiring emergency intervention may relate to preoperative embolization in the presence of an acute hematoma in a sick patient in whom embolization may permit evacuation of the clot without risk of rebleed from the AVM; however, surgical evacuation of the clot is the priority. Only if expeditious embolization can be done at the same time is embolization warranted. In general, early rebleeding is an exceptional situation which does not force early endovascular intervention. Recovery from hemorrhagic insult may, in fact, be compromised by aggressive, early, endovascular intervention.

◄ **Fig. 3.32. I** Postembolization of the left vertebral artery in lateral projection showing the radiopaque glue at the site of the fistula (*arrows*) and extension into the narrow falcine sinus (*straight arrow*). **J** Late phase of the same injection. Note the diluted contrast material due to the large amount of stagnant blood in the aneurysmal vein and poor filling of the falcine sinus (*arrowheads*). **K** Midarterial and **L** late phases of the right internal carotid artery in lateral projection after embolization show further thrombosis of the fistulization. **M** CT scan within the first 24 h after embolization shows partial thrombosis of the aneurysmal vein with some acrylic material seen in the falcine sinus (*white arrow*). Note the significant decrease in the size of the aneurysmal vein. **N** Axial CT scan 1 week after **M**. Note complete thrombosis of the aneurysmal vein

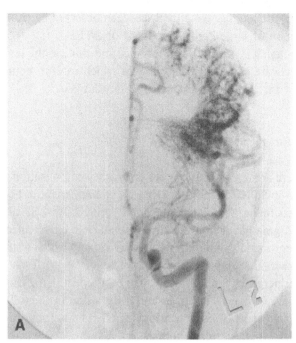

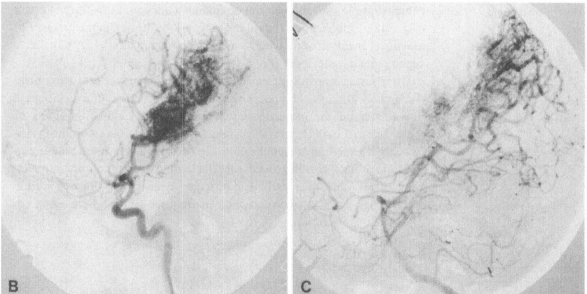

Fig. 3.33 A–C. Ill-defined vascular malformation without distinctive weakness in the angioarchitecture. There are no good predicles for embolization, and the amount of collateral circulation vs nidus is difficult to distinguish. **A** Frontal and **B** lateral subtraction angiograms of the left internal carotid artery and **C** lateral view of the left vertebral artery. Note the amount of vascularization which is difficult to distinguish from true malformation. There is relatively slow filling of the venous part of the malformation. This represents a technical limitation of embolization

VIII. Contraindications for Treatment

In general the major contraindication for treatment of a BAVM is the absence of an indication for treatment. More specific contraindications exist in patients in whom the goal of treatment cannot be achieved, e.g., no cure in an asymptomatic patient or the inability to catheterize the pedicle harboring an arterial aneurysm.

When there is a technical failure either to reach the desired pedicle or to achieve distal catheterization, it may be prudent to desist and try in another session when the goal can usually be achieved.

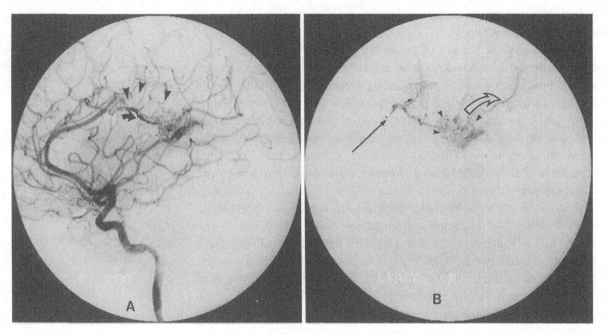

Fig. 3.34 A, B. Anatomical limitation. **A** Lateral digital subtraction angiogram of the right internal carotid artery after embolization of a midline malformation. The pericallosal supply has been embolized and is subtracted (*arrowheads*). Note remaining malformation supplied by a small pericallosal branch (*curved arrow*). **B** Superselective injection of the anterior cerebral artery. Note the anatomical limitation for embolization. There is a normal branch to the singular gyra (*small arrow*). There is supply to the malformation in vessels "en passage" (*arrowheads*) and supply to normal brain distally (*open curved arrow*). Embolization of this pedicle would result in occlusion of normal cerebral arteries

In patients in whom obvious brain damage has occurred or in whom congestive heart failure with severe liver dysfunction and prerenal azotemia is present (see Chap. 5), treatment options must be carefully evaluated before proceeding.

With the present technology some treatment is possible in the great majority of patients; an additional limitation still includes ill-defined vasculature where it may be impossible to distinguish between malformation and nonsprouting angiogenesis or collateral formation (Fig. 3.33). Anatomical limits may be imposed on portions of a malformation thereby preventing complete treatment (Fig. 3.34).

IX. Embolization

In this section we will analyze our results of embolization from data gathered since 1979 and their relation to the evolution in technical advances that has occurred in the intervening period.

Prior to 1982, the available techniques consisted of free, flow direct particulate agents, primarily silicone spheres, which, although relatively safe and easy to use (Luessenhop and Rosa 1984; Kricheff et al. 1972; Hilal 1975; Wolpert et al. 1975, 1981), are very ineffective in reaching the nidus of the malformation. Such agents result in proximal vessel occlusion without protection against future hemorrhage, a situation analogous to vessel ligation (see Vol. 2, Chap. 1).

The beginning of acrylic embolization was limited by the difficulty in using the Kerber calibrated leak silicone balloon (Kerber 1976). Balloon unreliability produced various complications, particularly overinflation resulting in vessel rupture (Berenstein and Kerber 1980). The fast polymerization time of IBCA carries the high likelihood of gluing the catheter into the vessel wall or may result in proximal vessel occlusion without proper penetration into the AVM nidus. The effect in the latter situation is analogous to "ligating" the feeder proximally, not much different than with silicone spheres.

The introduction of iophendylate by Cromwell (1980) as a retardant in IBCA polymerization time improved our technical ability to penetrate into the AVM nidus. Nonetheless, it was not until the use of latex calibrated leak balloons (Berenstein and Kricheff 1979; Debrun et al. 1982) that a more reliable and reproducible embolization technique became available. Cerebral navigation, however, was still dependent on very soft flow-directed microcatheters that required pressure chambers to introduce them into the circulation (Vol. 2, Chap. 1).

The more recent availability of variable stiffness microcatheters and steerable microguide wires (Jungreis et al. 1987; Kikuchi et al. 1987) represents a major breakthrough in technical advancement. In 1989, a new generation of acrylics, including the homologue N-butyl-cyanoacrylate (NBCA) (Berenstein 1989; Brothers 1989), was introduced. With its lower bonding strength and lesser fragmentation at time of injection, NBCA permits better penetration with less risk of catheter gluing and better control at the time of injection (see Chap. 4). The ability to reach the cerebral circulation without balloon propulsion adds safety, since there is no risk of balloon overinflation and rupture of a vessel. The ability to inject acrylic material without the need for balloons to close high-flow fistulas (VGAMs) (see Chaps. 4 and 5) without pulmonary embolization also decreases overall risk. Good permeation of the AVM nidus without a balloon is possible.

If calibrated leak balloons are used with NBCA, the risk of catheter gluing is minimal, larger volumes of NBCA can be injected, and therefore better results can be obtained with a continuous column (with less autologous blood clot mixture) (see Vol. 2, Chap. 1, Recanalization) (Fig. 3.30).

X. Complications of Embolization

When analyzing our complication rates, it becomes apparent that they relate to both increased experience and the added safety of more recent techniques (Table 3.6).

In our experience prior to 1982 (AB, 1977–1982), 44 adult patients were treated: there were six deaths (13.6%), five of which were related to vessel rupture with the Kerber silicone balloon and one immediately after use of polyvinyl alcohol. Two (4.5%) severe complications occurred in this group, one from vessel rupture, the second from iatrogenic embolization.

Between 1983 and 1985, of 47 adult patients that were embolized, there was one death (2.1%) and two severe deficits (4.2%). In addition, in 22 neonates or infants with high-flow AVFs, two lethal pulmonary embolizations

Table 3.6. Complications of embolization in 482 patients (New York University and University of Paris, 1983–1990)

Patients	n	(%)
Deaths	8	(1.6)
Severe deficits	7	(1.4)
Mild deficits	27	(5.6)
Transient deficits	53	(10.9)
Technical	7	(1.4)

Table 3.7. Complications from embolization (New York University)

	1977–1982 n (%)	1983–1985 n (%)	1985–1990 n (%)	Total n (%)
Patients	44	47	188	279 (100)
Deaths	6[a] (13.6)	1 (2.1)	1 (0.5)	8 (2.8)
Severe deficits	2 (4.5)	2 (4.2)	3 (1.5)	7 (2.5)
Mild deficit[b]	6 (13.6)	6 (12.7)	17 (9.0)	29 (10.3)
Transient deficits	11 (25)	7 (14.8)	20 (10.6)	38 (13.6)

[a] One intraoperative embolization.
[b] Mild deficit represents a mild aggravation of a previous deficit, which does not change the patient's lifestyle, or an expected deficit in visual field.

Table 3.8. Mild deficits from embolization (New York University and University of Paris, 1983–1990)

Patients	482
Quadrantanopsia	8 (30%)[a]
Hemianopsia	10 (37%)[a]
Sensory deficit	3 (11%)[a]
Motor deficit	6 (22%)[a]
Total	27 (5.6%)[b]

[a] Percentage of mild deficits.
[b] Percentage of all patients.

occurred, one in a neonate with a VGAM and one in an infant with multiple fistulas of the middle cerebral artery (see Chap. 5).

Between 1985 and 1990, 188 adult patients were treated with the newer techniques. The complications in this population included one death (0.5%) and three severe deficits (1.5%). No pulmonary complications occurred in an additional 25 pediatric patients with high-flow fistulas. A significant improvement in safety over earlier techniques is therefore apparent (Berenstein et al. 1989) (Table 3.7).

In the combined series of both authors, 482 adult patients treated from 1983 to 1990 (Table 3.8), death related to the procedure (within 1 week) occurred in eight patients, for a mortality rate from embolization of 1.6%. Of these, four occurred within the first 24 h (0.8%). Permanent deficits occurred in 34 patients (7%), of whom 7 (1.4%) had severe deficits and 27 (5.6%) had mild (defined as expected deficits, such as field cuts, or aggravation of a preexisting one, none of which prevent the patient from returning to their previous lifestyle) (Table 3.8).

Technical complications since 1977 (in over 1000 procedures) occurred in seven patients and included five catheters that became glued, all with IB-CA, and two vessel dissections, one in the internal carotid artery and one that was intracerebral guidewire-related and without permanent sequelae.

XI. Conclusions

To properly assess embolization as a therapeutic modality at this stage is difficult, as not sufficient time has elapsed for long-term follow-up.

The usefulness of embolization prior to surgical excision is clear (Stein et al. 1975; Wolpert and Stein 1975; Wolpert et al. 1981; Luessenhop and Rosa 1984; Spetzler et al. 1987 and others). Although various techniques and embolic agents are reported as useful, we believe that the low risk of NBCA embolization justifies its use exclusively (Vol. 2, Chap. 1; this volume, Chap. 4 and this chapter).

Prior to radiosurgery, embolization is able to reduce the volume of most large malformations, making them suitable for treatment by this modality. The long-term evaluation of the effects of these two modalities is still in the evolving stages. In malformations small enough for radiosurgery that have bled and are not surgically accessible, embolization with permanent liquid can occlude the weakness in the angioarchitecture (arterial aneurysm in the nidus, pseudoarterial or venous aneurysms, etc.). Such occlusion may last throughout the latency period of radiation. The use of particulate agents in these situations, in our opinion, has no place in the management of such patients (see Combination Treatment).

Embolization as the sole form of treatment is usually done in a selected group of patients, usually those with large malformations, malformations in inaccessible areas, or in nonsurgical candidates. This group is therefore left with the choice of either medical management or palliative embolization.

Complete obliteration at present is usually not possible in large BAVMs with multiple pedicles and circulations involved. In contrast, AVMs with a single pedicle have a 95% chance or better of anatomical cure regardless of location. Malformations with several feeders can also be obliterated in an ever increasing number of patients. The percent occlusion has no meaning, as many patients are in the process of being treated and treatment may take years to reach completion.

As stated above, if complete obliteration can be accomplished by embolization alone, it will be the only form of treatment. In the over 100 patients in whom complete anatomical obliteration of the AVM has been accomplished by both authors, as judged in a follow-up angiogram of at least 6 months, none have rebled or deteriorated neurologically.

In patients that have bled and in whom complete anatomical cure is not possible, the long-term incidence of rebleeding is still difficult to assess the decreased rate of rebleeding in partially embolized malformations, improvement in seizure control, and stabilization of neurological deteriroation appears favorable (see above, this chapter, Sect. III.4). The evolution in our understanding of the angioarchitecture, as it relates to the natural history of an individual patient (Lasjaunias et al. 1986), permits a better approach to lesions that cannot be completely eradicated by embolization or combination treatments (Chaps. 1 and 2). The present risks of liquid acrylic embolization in BAVMs are a 1.6% mortality and a 1.4% severe morbidity. We believe these risks to be significantly less than the risk of no intervention in symptomatic untreated lesions that carry a cumulative 1% mortality per year and 1.7% significant morbidity per year. These risks pertain regardless of the mode of presentation (Ondra 1990).

CHAPTER 4

Technical Aspects of Surgical Neuroangiography

I. Introduction

The general principles of therapeutic endovascular embolization described in Vol. 2, Chap. 1 apply for the brain, the spine, and the spinal cord and its dural covers. Patient preparation, preoperative medications, anesthesia, puncture site, and the use of introducer sheaths are similar. Specific aspects of angiography and embolization in the brain, spine, and spinal cord, as they apply to the various pathologies or to particular situations, will be discussed.

The techniques for catheterization and embolization of the CNS, as performed by the authors, will be discussed in detail. However, it is imperative that extensive training and experience is gained prior to attempting these procedures in the clinical setting. The risks in properly trained hands are minimal, but in the untrained individual tragic consequences can occur. For proper training a laboratory setting is best, with the use of animal experimentation (TerBrugge et al. 1989; Lee et al. 1989) or in vitro training models (Kerber and Flaherty 1980; Bartynski et al. 1987).

Based on our experience with over 500 patients treated for brain arteriovenous malformations (BAVMs) with over 2500 vessel occlusions, we believe that safety is related to proper preparation, planning, and experience.

II. Patient Preparation

In general, no specific preoperative medications or measures are required prior to endovascular embolization of cerebral or spinal lesions, with the exception of those related to anesthesia, such as 6 h fasting, mild sedation, and atropine in case emergency endotracheal intubation is required.

Of importance is the discussion as to the details of the procedure, including its risks, goals, and alternative modes of treatment, with the patient and his or her family. The objective of the procedure and the possibility of additional treatment (multiple stages, shunting, postembolization surgical resection, or radiation) must be planned and discussed in advance (Chap. 3).

Preoperative clinical assessment includes a detailed neurological examination and neuropsychological testing for fine cortical functions (which not infrequently are impaired in patients otherwise thought of as "neurologically intact"). Preliminary EEG testing is not needed for the procedure but may be important as part of a complete neurological evaluation.

The prophylactic use of Ca^{2+} channel blockers to prevent cerebral vasospasm has been advocated by some investigators (Merland and Reizine 1987; Picard 1988, unpublished data); however, vasospasm during cerebral

Table 4.1. Perioperative measure differences

	Berenstein	Lasjaunias
Corticosteroids	−	+
Foley	+	−
Arterial line	+	−
Systemic hypotension	+	−
Lower blood pressure	±	±
Heparinization	+	+
Electrophysiologic monitoring	+ (spinal)	−
Amobarbital	+ (spinal)	−
	± (brain)	−

navigation has not been a problem in our experience, and Ca^{2+} channel blockers are not used by us for that purpose. Prophylactic steroids prior to the procedure are not routinely used (see Corticosteroids).

III. Perioperative Care

Perioperative care relates to the general measures during the actual procedure and will vary depending on the team (Table 4.1), the technique to be used, and the lesion to be treated. These measures will be discussed with the description of the techniques and lesions.

1. Corticosteroids

In general, corticosteroids are not used as a prophylactic measure but may be used acutely after a complication. Steroids may be of more value in posterior fossa and spinal cord lesions than in supratentorial malformations. The use of corticosteroids as part of the management of acute stroke is very controversial. It may, however, be of assistance in the edema that follows a hemorrhagic complication (mass effect).

One of us (PL) routinely uses postoperative corticosteroids as an antiedema agent. Dexamethasone (Decadron, 8 mg IV is given) during the procedure as soon as the embolization is started and is repeated every 8 h for 3 days (it is given p.o. as soon as tolerated), followed by tapering off over 3 days. Appropriate prophylactic antacids are used to prevent GI complications.

2. Anticonvulsants

Endovascular embolization neither produces seizures nor increases their frequency (Table 3.3). Therefore, anticonvulsant medications are used only in patients who have had previous seizures, an intracerebral hematoma, or subarachnoid hemorrhage or in those patients already on anticonvulsants or with EEG evidence of possible epileptogenic activity. In such patients, we maintain the anticonvulsant doses but no additional doses are given for the procedure. If complete obliteration of the malformation is obtained and confirmed, the patient is followed for 1 year clinically. If no seizure activity occurs in the intervening year, a repeat EEG is performed. If potential epileptogenic activity is not present, the anticonvulsant medication is tapered off and eventually discontinued.

3. Puncture Site

The femoral approach is routinely used; direct carotid or vertebral puncture is not needed. In high-flow lesions, e.g., BAVMs, brain arteriovenous fistulas (BAVFs), vein of Galen aneurysmal malformations (VGAMs), if the venous approach is to be used, direct jugular puncture is contraindicated. Direct puncture of the jugular vein presents a higher risk and may compromise the venous drainage. The femoral venous approach is safe and easy.

4. Anesthesia

The role of anesthesia includes the overall monitoring of the patients physiologic and metabolic status. This includes not only the level of consciousness but all other physiologic functions, including input and output, blood pressure control, degree of anticoagulation, and, when needed, reversal of anticoagulation. A close cooperation and familiarity with the procedure by anesthesia personnel is required for optimal results.

In general, neuroleptic analgesia is preferred, as described in Vol. 2, Chap. 1. It permits easy intraoperative neurological monitoring. In very young patients or those that are uncooperative, general anesthesia is preferred. If electrophysiologic monitoring is planned, neuroleptic anesthesia is used, avoiding inhalation agents. Nitrous oxide (NO_2) is never used during intravascular procedures in view of the risk of air bubble expansion and embolization (see Vol. 2, Chap. 1).

5. Input and Output Monitoring

One of us (AB) routinely used a Foley catheter to monitor urinary output and to prevent bladder distention and retention. In case of emergency treatment or if surgery will follow, an indwelling catheter is already in place. If no Foley catheter is used, bladder evacuation is accomplished at the end of the procedure, prior to compression of the groin and after reversal of heparinization.

6. Blood Pressure Monitoring

If pharmacological manipulation of the systemic blood pressure is planned, an arterial line or use of the newer, noninvasive, blood pressure monitoring cuffs is advisable. One of us (AB) almost routinely uses blood pressure control during and immediately after occlusion, especially in high-flow lesions and in very young children.

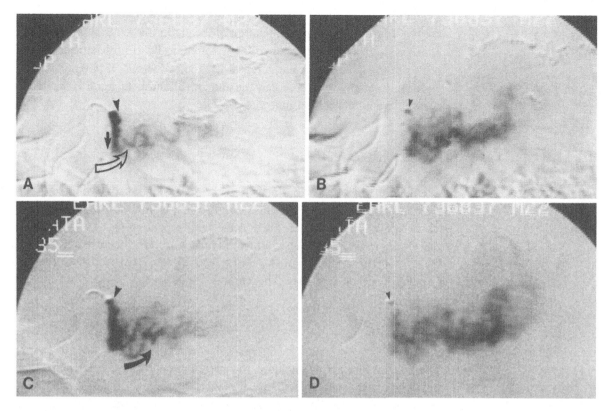

Fig. 4.1 A–D. Use of hypotension in brain arteriovenous malformations. **A** and **B** Under normotensive conditions (135/95 mmHg), injection of a middle cerebral artery demonstrates poor flow control. **A** Lateral digital subtraction angiogram with the balloon (*arrowhead*) inflated produces only limited flow arrest (*arrow*), with dilution (*open curved arrow*) from another pedicle. The balloon has been deflated (*arrowhead*) with rapid washout of the contrast material best appreciated fluoroscopically. **C** and **D** Under hypotensive conditions (BP 70/35 mmHg). **C** With balloon inflation (*arrowhead*), note the significantly better opacification of the malformation without dilution (*curved arrow*). **D** Following balloon deflation there is slow emptying of the malformation with significantly better opacification of the malformation. An appreciable difference in circulation time is noted under fluoroscopy

Controlled hypotension is usually done with a nitroprusside drip. In very young children, lowering of the blood pressure can be easily and expeditiously done with high dose inhalation agents. Blood pressure control may be of value in the immediate postocclusion period (especially if an aneurysm is proximal to the embolized territory or if a very high flow pedicle has been occluded). The systolic blood pressure is not permitted to rise above the baseline and preferably is kept 10–20 mm Hg less. As an alternative blood pressure may be lowered with Ca^{2+} channel blockers such as nicardipine. This is given as a loading dose of 1 mg IV bolus and repeated up to 2–4 mg/h, aiming for a 20%–30% reduction of the baseline blood pressure.

Lowering the systemic blood pressure may permit better penetration into the nidus of the AVM, as flow through the AVM is dependent on the systemic blood pressure (Fig. 4.1) (see Chap. 3, Hemodynamic Basis of BAVMs).

An arterial line may also be advantageous in young children or infants to permit easy accessibility in repeated measuring of blood gases. In addition, a central venous line may be necessary if hypotensive medication will be given for a long period of time or if significant amounts of fluid will be used. Central venous pressure monitoring is especially useful in the infant with cardiac problems or in the older patient (AB).

One of us (PL) seldom uses blood pressure control, either during the actual occlusion or in the immediate postocclusion period. We both agree that the most important aspect of blood pressure monitoring is to prevent abrupt systolic blood pressure elevations at the time of embolization or immediately after occlusion when the mean pressure in the occluded feeder increases (Duckwiller 1989; Jungreis and Horton 1989).

Elevation of the baseline blood pressure may be of assistance in children when the femoral pulse is not optimally palpated. Any decrease in blood pressure in this situation is usually secondary to the anesthesia itself. Permitting the patient to become lighter will usually be sufficient to raise the blood pressure and increase perception of the pulse. Rarely, a small dose of ephedrine may be needed to improve the pulse perception. In theory at least, short increases in blood pressure may assist in flow guided distal catheterization and may be attempted in rare occasions (less important with the newer variable stiffness microcatheters). The use of Doppler guidance may also facilitate puncture in small children.

7. Heparinization

Systemic heparinization is recommended when using coaxial catheter assembly systems or when using balloons, either of the calibrated leak, detachable, or nondetachable variety. Heparinization in these circumstances is to prevent fibrin clot aggregation between catheters and/or balloons. Preliminary PT, PTT, and, if available, activation coagulation time (ACT) (Scott et al. 1986) are obtained and are used as guidelines for protamine dosage when heparinization is to be reversed.

Two techniques of heparinization can be used:

1. A bolus loading dose of 50 U/kg, with a continuous maintenance IV infusion of up to 500 U/kg over 24 h. When using this technique, there is no need for additional heparin in the liquids used for continuous perfusion between coaxial catheters or in the sheath at the arteriotomy site.
2. If heparin is used in the flushing solution, in the various perfusion lines between coaxial catheters, and at the sheath site (2000 USP/1000 ml of 2.5% D/W in children, and 4000 USP/1000 ml of 5% D/W in adults), a loading dose is usually not necessary unless cerebral navigation is immediately started, in which case a loading dose of 1000–1500 USP is given as a bolus. No heparin is used in children or neonates, if noncoaxial system are employed, or if treating a postoperative or postictal emergency.

At the end of the procedure protamine sulfate is used routinely to reverse heparinization. If hemorrhage occurs during the procedure, immediate reversal is performed. In such patients the dose is determined by calculating the amount of heparin given per unit time, per coagulation time, or simply by the activated coagulation time (ACT) value (see Vol. 2, Chap. 1).

8. Angiographic Investigation

a) Radiographic Filming

The technical aspects of radiographic filming in the CNS circulation vary depending on available angiographic equipment, the use of a conventional film-screen combinations (FSC), digital subtraction angiography (DSA), or a combination of both. The rapid improvements in digital technology should eventually surpass FSC in the near future. At present FSC has better lines/mm resolution and DSA has better contrast resolution.

The filming sequence for a specific territory (brain, spine, spinal cord) will be addressed as it applies in the various chapters. Individual variations as to films per second, volume of contrast material for injection, etc., are less important than consistency in the technique used, which will permit the detection of physiologic abnormalities in static images.

b) Contrast Material

The newer generation of nonionic agents are well suited for selective and superselective angiography as they are less neurotoxic than ionic agents; they should probably be used routinely. As to the best agent, there appears to be no major differences in commercially available contrast materials. Hopefully in the future a less expensive nonionic agent will be introduced.

For FSC a 60% iodine concentration is used; for DSA a 30% iodine concentration is employed. It is important that the volume and time of injection for both FSC and DSA are the same to obtain comparable results.

Specific volumes to be injected will be addressed as they apply to a specific investigation (internal carotid artery, common carotid artery, vertebral artery, etc.). Injection volumes are standardized at the beginning of the diagnostic exploration, with adjustments made as to size of vessel injected, patient size, fluoroscopic assessment of flow, etc.

IV. Functional Evaluation

A variety of tools are presently available for functional evaluation prior, during, and after endovascular procedures (Berenstein et al. 1984b; Hacke 1983), including continuous monitoring using EEG to assess tolerance to occlusion of major vessels such as the internal carotid artery. This method primarily relates to changes in delta wave activity. The use of EEG monitoring during internal carotid artery occlusion was first suggested by Sundt 1979, 1981) and although useful, it is not absolute and is only another approach to measuring tolerance to sacrifice of a major vessel (Vol. 2, Chap. 1). Monitoring may be done under both normotensive conditions and under relative hypotension (Pile-Spellman unpublished). This is done in an attempt to compensate for changes that occur in a control situation under sedation in the resting position, as compared to possible orthostatic changes. Cerebral blood flow studies using xenon-133 or PET scanning, if available, may be more accurate (see Vol. 2, Chap. 1).

1. Somatosensory Evoked Potentials

SEP monitoring in cerebral embolization has significant limitations and may even be confusing. It may have limited applications in patients in whom the procedure is done under general anesthesia. SEP is of potential assistance in patients who have a lesion in the thalamus, perirolandic area, or brainstem. The role of SEP or brainstem-evoked potentials may expand in intracranial procedures as more experience accumulates (Berenstein et al. 1984b; Hacke et al. 1983; John et al. 1989).

In spine and spinal cord lesions SEPs are routinely used by one of us (AB) and are felt to be very sensitive in detecting potential dangers. The addition of pharmacological testing, with the intra-arterial injection of amobarbital, adds further reliability and safety (see Vol. 5, Chap. 1, Spinal Cord Arteriovenous Malformations, Figs. 1.58 – 1.60) (Berenstein et al. 1989).

2. Pharmacological Testing

a) Amobarbital

During cerebral and spinal cord embolization, a major risk is the occlusion of functionally important tissue. This complication is best avoided by a solid knowledge of functional anatomy, the careful analysis of the preliminary selective and superselective angiograms, very distal catheterization (as close as possible to the nidus), and meticulous technique to avoid reflux. In some cases, the ideal point of catheterization may not be achievable, and one must identify the more proximal point of catheterization where safe occlusion can be performed. This must be done with the knowledge that the ideal morphological result may be more difficult to obtain from the more proximal position. Between these two locations is the "security" area of embolization (Fig. 4.2).

In instances when a normal branch is visualized or when in doubt as to the functional significance of a pedicle, a provocative functional test using 50 – 75 mg of amobarbital (Amytal) (Wada and Rasmussen 1960; Berenstein et al. 1984b; Horton and Dawson 1988) may clarify the importance of the tissue irrigated by that specific artery. Development of neurological deficit represents a contraindication for embolization at that position. In that case, either more distal catheterization, preferably beyond normal branches, is achieved or an alternative route is chosen. If no normal vessels are visualized, provocative testing may give a false sense of security. Hemodynamics in high-flow lesions may give an inaccurate picture. As the contrast materials or amobarbital is injected, it may travel only to the high-flow channels of the AVM, bypassing adjacent normal tissue. The dynamics that occur during the injection of the embolic liquid agent are different; the first portion of the column of acrylic will polymerize, rerouting the additional, still liquid, embolic agent to other areas not opacified by the contrast material or infused by the amobarbital. Thus, the injection of amobarbital in this circumstance is potentially misleading. In addition, multiple injections of amobarbital can result in a sleepy noncooperative patient, in whom monitoring is more difficult.

Despite these constraints, in spine and spinal cord embolization, in which perforating vessels may be smaller than the ability of the X-ray equipment

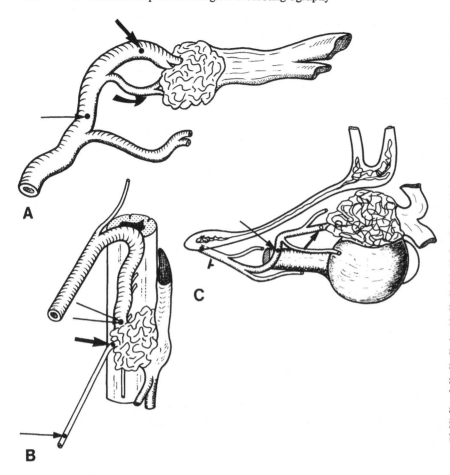

Fig. 4.2 A–C. Security point in brain, spinal, or ophthalmic embolization. **A** Pedicle feeding an arteriovenous malformation (AVM) demonstrates a dominant pedicle to the malformation (*broad arrow*) and a secondary feeder (*curved arrow*). The ideal point of embolization (*broad arrow*) would be in the major feeder and a similar point in the secondary feeder. However, the security point is at the origin of the common trunk (*long arrow*). **B** A spinal cord AVM supplied by a radiculomedullary artery. The ideal point of embolization is represented by the *broad arrow*, the security point is at a more proximal position (*long arrow*). Also note that the ideal and security points in the venous system in the spinal cord are the same (*double long arrows*). **C** The ideal point (*broad arrow*) and security point (*long arrow*) in an ophthalmic artery embolization

to resolve them, intra-arterial amobarbital (Amytal) combined with SEP monitoring often adds further reliability and safety (Berenstein 1984).

As part of the preoperative (embolization, surgery) investigation, the need may arise to determine hemispheric dominance for speech (left handed individual, speech difficulties in a right sided AVM, etc.). In these patients a Wada test may be an important part of assessing the risks of treatment of the AVM. When an (intracarotid) amobarbital test is done in a patient harboring an AVM, the amobarbital should be first injected into the hemisphere not harboring the high-flow lesion. This is designed to prevent a falsely negative test as the amobarbital (175–400 mg) may be "sumped" selectively through the malformation, thereby bypassing normal ipsilateral speech areas.

Electrophysiologic and pharmacological testing do not guarantee safety or better results and are not a replacement for anatomical knowledge and recognition of normal territories. One of us (PL) has not used neither since 1986 without added morbidity or mortality (Chap. 3, Tables 3.6, 3.7).

b) Xylocaine

Xylocaine has been used for functional testing of peripheral nervous tissue supplied by the external carotid artery (Vol. 2, Chap. 1). In CNS patients, Takahashi (presented at Val D'Isere 1990) has used it to test axonal function. Only cardiac xylocaine can be used in the CNS, but we have not used it.

V. Catheters and Delivery Systems

A brief review of the various devices that have permitted superselective cerebral catheterization is in order.

1. Flow Guided Microcatheters

The first devices available included flow guided microcatheters, originally described by Dotter et al. (1972). However, for cerebral navigation, it was not until Kerber's development of the calibrated leak microballoon catheter that reliable and reproducible, superselective, flow controlled catheterization of cerebral arteries was feasible (Kerber 1976). This microcatheter is shown in Chap. 1, Fig. 1.7A of Vol. 2. The introduction of this very soft microcatheter into the circulation required a propelling chamber (Pevsner 1977; Pevsner and Doppman 1980) or similar device in view of its very supple shaft (Vol. 2, Chap. 1, Fig. 1.8A, B). Although these catheters entered the cerebral circulation, inflation of the distal balloon was frequently needed. The silicone balloons were unreliable, with only approximately 20% – 25% of balloons usable. Another drawback of this system was the lack of hysteresis or memory of silicone, resulting in a defective balloon carrying the risk of overinflation and vessel rupture.

Advancements in the technique occurred in the late 1970s and early 1980s with the introduction of a Debrun latex calibrated leak balloon. In this system, a hole was made at the distal tip of the balloon (Vol. 2, Chap. 1, Fig. 1.7B) (Berenstein 1978; Debrun et al. 1982b), which was then attached to Kerber tubing or similar soft tubing such as Siltane (Ingenor Medical Systems, Paris, France) or Pursil (Balt Medical Systems, Paris, France). The use of these soft tubes, which in conjunction with the propelling chamber permitted a more reliable microballoon, aided cerebral catheterization (see Vol. 2, Chap. 1). This system at present is not employed by either author. It has been replaced by the new generation of variable stiffness microcatheters which have revolutionized the ability for distal cerebral navigation.

2. Variable Stiffness Microcatheters

A major revolution in superselective catheterization occurred with the development of variable stiffness microcatheters. The concept of variable stiffness and variable size selective and superselective catheters has been introduced earlier (Berenstein et al. 1983). These early model catheters could reach only distal branches of the external carotid artery but could not be introduced into the brain (see Vol. 2, Chap. 1, Fig. 1.3B). The development of 1–3 French variable stiffness microcatheters (Kikuchi et al. 1987) opened a new horizon in selective catheterization of the brain and spinal cord. These catheters permit cerebral navigation without the use of cumbersome systems. They can be used with steerable microwires or with calibrated leak balloons at their tip for more distal catheterization to obtain flow control, flow reversal, or flow arrest. The variable stiffness principle combines torque control with flow guided navigation.

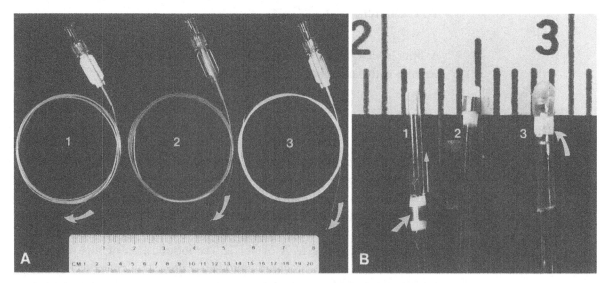

Fig. 4.3 A, B. Variable stiffness microcatheters. Various sized Tracker microcatheters are available. **A** (*1*) Tracker 10 with an internal diameter (ID) at the tip of 0.014 inches (0.35 mm) and outer diameter (OD) at the tip of 0.027 inches (0.69 mm). (*2*) Tracker 18 with an ID at the tip of 0.020 inches (0.51 mm) and OD at the tip of 0.036 inches (0.92 mm). (*3*) Tracker 25 with ID at the tip of 0.027 inches (0.69 mm) and OD at the tip of 0.049 inches (1.25 mm). Curved arrow points to the radiopaque tip. **B** Close-up view of various distal ends. (*1*) "extended" tip. (*2*) Conventional Tracker 18. (*3*) Tracker with a calibrated leak detachable microballoon (*curved arrow*). The arrow in *1* points to the radiopaque marker

The microcatheters manufactured by Target Therapeutics (San Jose, CA) are called Tracker catheters (Fig. 4.3) and can be obtained in a variety of lengths and sizes. For cerebral navigation in adults, the 150 cm catheter with a 25–30 cm distal soft end seems best to us; a radiopaque tip marker permits easy fluoroscopic monitoring of its position and progression (Fig. 4.4). One of the main advantages of these variable stiffness catheters, the ability to use guide wires intracranially (Fig. 4.5), gives the possibility of torque control and steerability (see Microguide Wires). If a calibrated leak balloon is deemed necessary, the balloon is hand mounted (see Calibrated Leak Balloons) (Fig. 4.3 B, 4.17).

Another model of variable stiffness microcatheter is the Mini-Torquer microcatheter manufactured by Ingenor (Fig. 4.6) (Garcia-Monaco et al. 1990 b). This catheter has the advantage of being softer in the distal end, thus permitting navigation through more tortuous vessels. It is radiopaque throughout and the more proximal shaft is stiffer than the Tracker catheter. The proximal stiffness carries several advantages. The catheter can be used alone without a guiding catheter, a feature of importance in newborns or young children (Fig. 4.7). When tortuousness and loops are encountered, such as in the cervical or cavernous carotid arteries, the vessel loop can be straightened by pulling back on the catheter (Fig. 4.8). In adults, loops can be corrected with the combination of the Mini-Torquer and the guiding catheter (Fig. 4.9) (Garcia-Monaco et al. 1990 b). The Mini-Torquer is primarily used without a balloon, although one can easily be placed. The catheter has a slightly dilated radiopaque tip which permits fluoroscopic monitoring and gives the Mini-Torquer some degree of flow guidance.

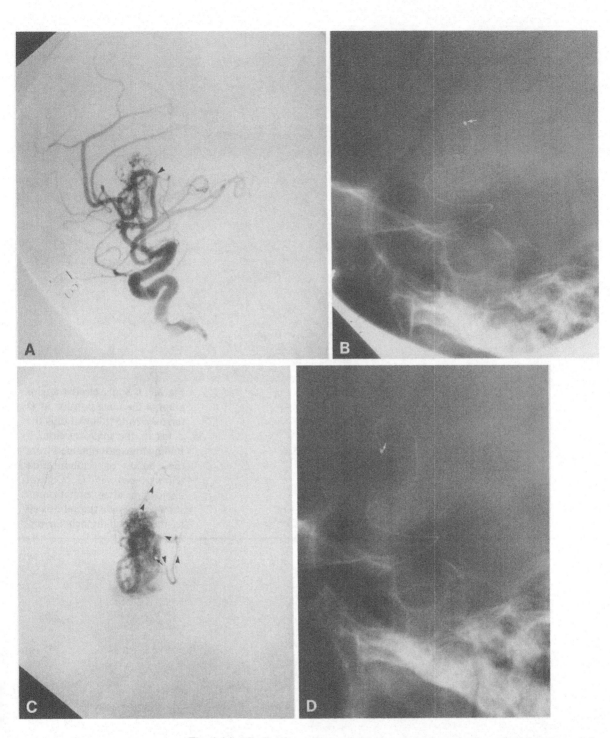

Fig. 4.4A–G. Tracker microcatheter in cerebral navigation. Same patient as in Fig. 3.28. **A** Lateral view of the left internal carotid artery in early phase shows a small malformation in Broca's area. The safety point was felt to be beyond the normal branch to the midtemporal gyrus (*arrowhead*). **B** Tracker 18 advanced to the level of the normal branch (*arrow*). **C** Superselective angiogram at this level demonstrates filling of the normal branch (*arrowheads*). **D** Plain lateral view of the distal advancement of the microcatheter to a safer position (*arrow*). Variable stiffness microcatheter assembly systems permit accurate and easy minor advancements or withdrawal of the catheter tip

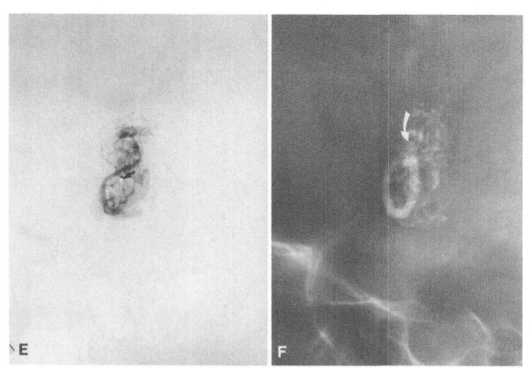

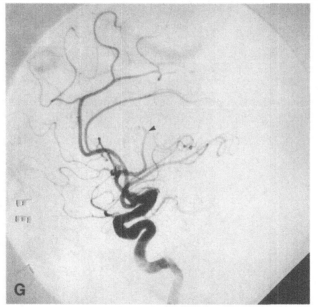

Fig. 4.4. E Superselective angiogram at the same position as **D** (*arrow*). Note filling of only the nidus of the malformation. **F** Radiopaque cast obtained from the point of embolization (*curved arrow*). **G** Control angiogram after embolization shows retrograde thrombosis up to the normal branch (*arrowhead*)

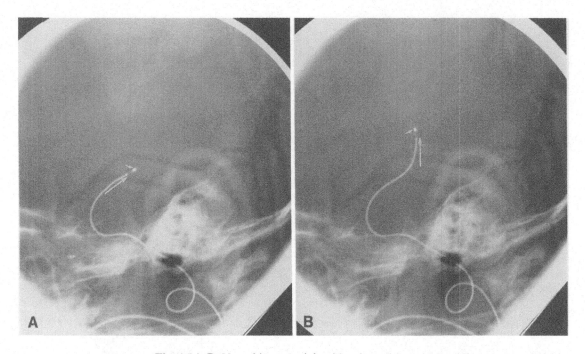

Fig. 4.5 A, B. Use of intracranial guide wires with variable stiffness microcatheters. **A** Lateral 100 mm spot plain film shows the variable stiffness microcatheter entering the posterior communicating artery from the ipsilateral carotid approach. Note the radiopaque tip marker (*arrow*) and the position of the microguide wire (*long arrow*). **B** Further advancement of the catheter wire assembly into the posterior medial choroidal artery

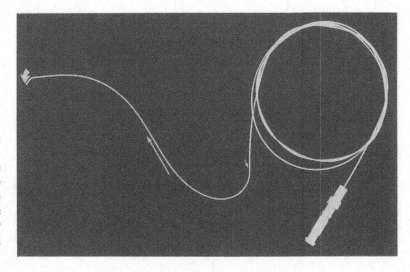

Fig. 4.6. Variable stiffness Mini-Torquer. This microcatheter is used with a stylet for introduction. The transition from the rigid catheter (*arrow*) to the very soft portion (*long arrow*) is usually 20 cm long. A gentle curve (*curved arrow*) is usually best for cerebral navigation and is formed under steam

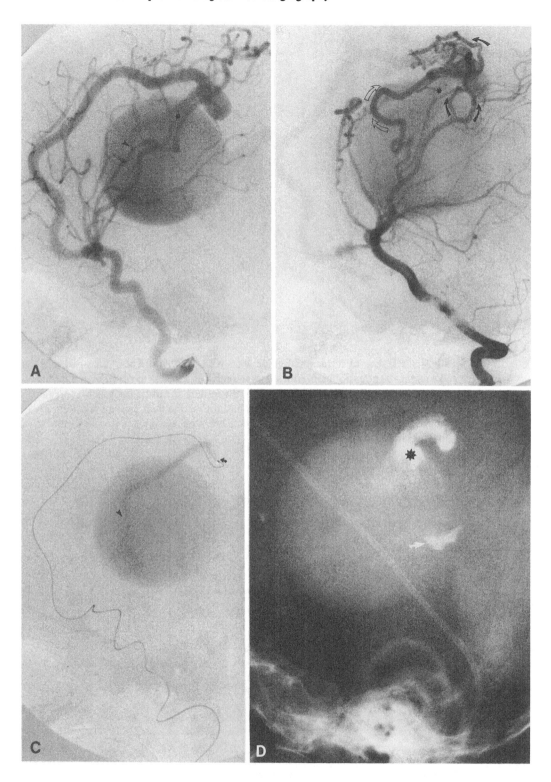

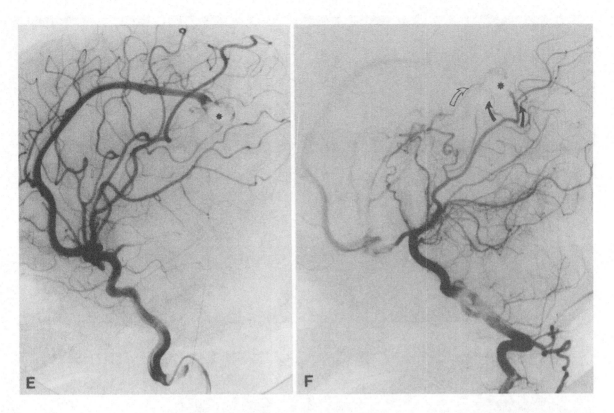

Fig. 4.7 A–F. Mini-Torquer used without guiding catheter. This is best in newborns or young infants. **A** Lateral view of the right internal carotid artery demonstrates hypertrophy of the anterior cerebral artery supplying two mural fistulas (* and *arrowhead*). **B** Lateral view of the left vertebral artery demonstrates hypertrophy of choroidal arteries (*curved arrows*) with indirect filling of the malformation. **C** Lateral view of superselective catheterization, using the Mini-Torquer, of the choroidal branch of the anterior cerebral artery (*curved arrow*). Note the "sump" effect with opacification of only one fistula (*arrowhead*). **D** Plain film of the radiopaque cast primarily in the more proximal fistula (*) and in the narrow outflow of the venous obstacle (*arrow*). **E** Postembolization control angiogram of the right internal carotid artery shows occlusion of the fistula (*). **F** Control vertebral artery injection confirms the obliteration of the fistula and regression of the collateral circulation without the need of treating these vessels. The same arrows correspond to the same branches as seen in **B**. Note that even the subependymal supply has regressed. (Also see Fig. 5.34)

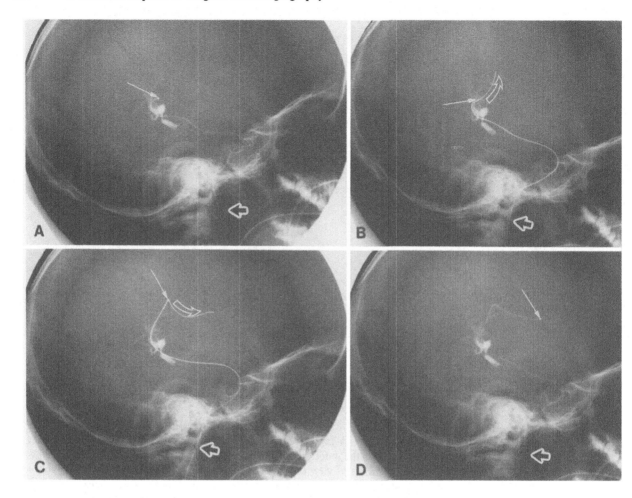

Fig. 4.8 A – D. Progressive catheterization with a Mini-Torquer system and guide wire in a patient with a choroidal type vein of Galen aneurysmal malformation. Note the disappearance of the carotid kinking (*arrow*) during manipulation of the devices. By gently pulling back on the catheter, the carotid curves can be straightened (*broad arrow*) subsequently permitting more distal advancement of the guide wire (*curved open arrow*); the microcatheter tip (*small arrow*) is then advanced. Prior to acrylic deposition, excess catheter should be avoided

Catheterization with the Mini-Torquer can be facilitated by preshaping the catheter with a right J-curve as it is advanced into the circulation (Fig. 4.10). The J-curve prevents the catheter from entering small or proximal vessels (basilar tip, ophthalmic, C1, posterior inferior cerebellar artery, etc.). Once the desired vessel is entered, flush injection through the catheter straightens the tip and more distal catheterization can be done (Fig. 4.10F). When using microguide wires, coating the wire with silicone spray is recommended to reduce friction between the wire and the inner lumen of the catheter. As the intracranial circulation is reached, the wire is progressively withdrawn to prevent kinking the soft distal end. Mini-Torquer catheters come with 20, 25, or 30 cm distal soft ends for more distal catheterizations.

A third type of microcatheter is the Magic microcatheter manufactured by Balt (Rufenacht and Merland 1986c, d). It performs similar to the Mini-Torquer but with limited guide wire compatibility (Fig. 4.11).

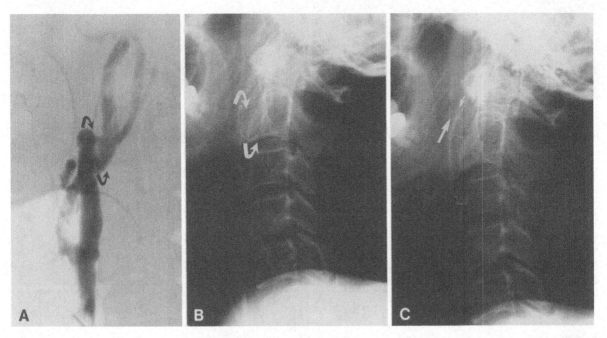

Fig. 4.9 A–C. Adult patient with an AVM and marked tortuosity. The ability to straighten out the curve with a coaxial assembly maneuver is shown. **A** Lateral view of the common carotid artery demonstrates the marked tortuosity of the internal carotid artery (*bent arrows*). **B** Mini-Torquer passing through the tortuous carotid (*bent arrows*). **C** By retracting the Mini-Torquer (*small arrow*) and advancing the 5 French introducer (*large arrow*) the tortuous loop is straightened

For cerebral catheterization the Mini-Torquer and Magic Variable stiffness microcatheters are provided with a stylet or rigid wire to facilitate introduction into the vascular system. In most instances, they are used with an outer catheter that has a lumen of sufficient diameter to permit the coaxial introduction of the microcatheter with or without a balloon. In newborns or very young children, however, they maybe used alone or with a 4F outer catheter. In such instances the microcatheter is loaded backwards, prior to introduction into the circulation. As the tip of the catheter exits the introducer sheath, the stylet must be withdrawn to prevent damage to the vessel or the catheter. Withdrawal of the stylet is done under a closed water system to prevent the accidental introduction of air. Air entry is prevented by submerging the microcatheter in a saline-filled container, by continuous drip irrigation at the hub as the stylet or microguide wire is being withdrawn (Fig. 4.12) (Choi 1990), or by using a Y-adaptor (see Vol. 2, Chap. 1). If backflow exists, it will assist in backbleeding the air.

Other versions of variable stiffness catheters can be assembled including the one manufactured by Pacific Medical Co., San Diego, CA, utilizing a proximal stiff polyethylene 2F shaft and a distal Kerber silicone tubing to which a Kerber latex calibrated leak balloon is attached (Fig. 4.13).

The softer the distal segment the further and more complex the vascular structures that can be negotiated. Laminar flow in vessels has a parabolic profile of velocity (see Chap. 3), with its maximum in the center and decreasing peripherally. The flow propelled microcatheters therefore tend to

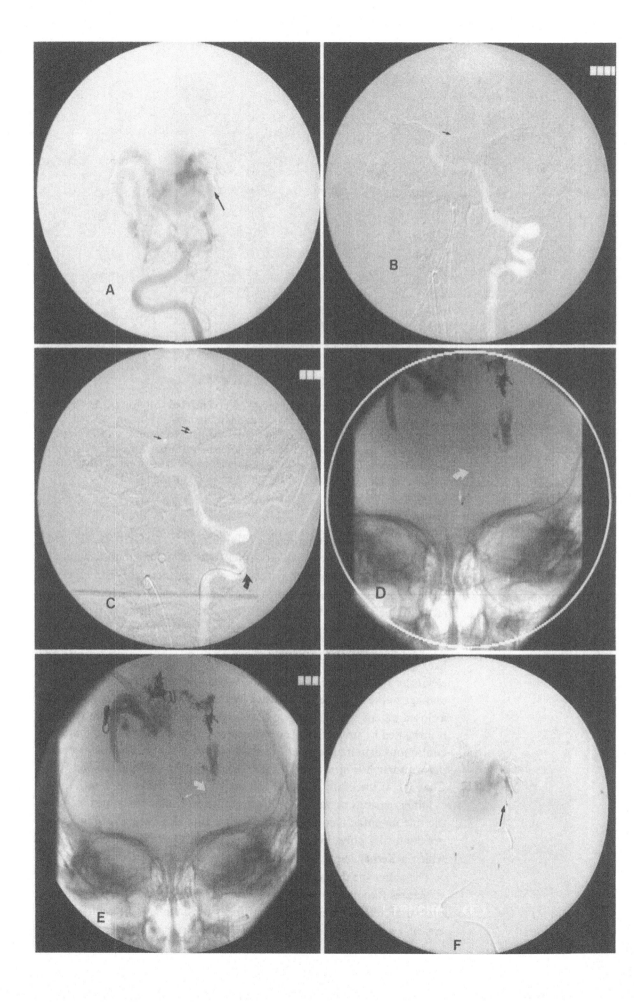

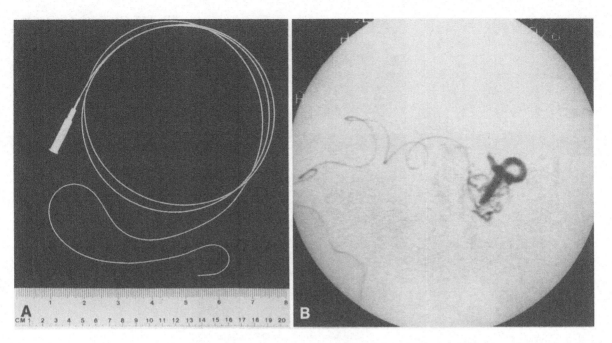

Fig. 4.11 A, B. Magic variable stiffness microcatheter. **A** Very supple distal end of this microcatheter makes its performance similar to that of the Mini-Torquer. **B** The catheter is useful for very tortuous and distal catheterizations, such as this distal middle cerebral artery branch

◀ **Fig. 4.10 A–F.** Magic navigation with guide wire support and with a tight J-curve in the distal catheter tip. **A** Frontal view of the left vertebral artery, intermediate phase after embolization, demonstrates remaining supply to a choroidal vein of Galen aneurysmal malformation from bilateral choroidal arteries. The goal of catheterization is the left medial choroidal feeder (*arrow*). **B** Frontal digital subtraction angiography road mapping technique demonstrates the tip of the microcatheter (*arrow*) and the marked tortuosity of the left vertebral artery at C2. **C** Guide wire assistance towards the vertebral loop (*curved arrow*) permits further advancement of the microcatheter tip with the original position (*arrow*) and the further advancement (*double arrow*) shown. **D** In view of the tortuosities in the vertebral artery, the catheter cannot be advanced further shaping a tight J-curve to the distal portion of the microcatheter (*curved arrow*) is used for advancement. The J is at the level of the basilar bifurcation preventing the catheter tip (*arrow*) from entering the small perforators (see **A**). **E** Frontal view after further advancement entering the proximal P2 segment (*curved arrow*). Note the catheter tip (*arrow*) as the J (*curved arrow*) is still formed. **F** After forceful injection of contrast material the J-curve is straightened and the tip of the microcatheter has entered the desired choroidal vessel (*arrow*)

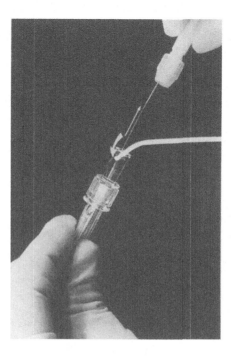

Fig. 4.12. Continuous irrigation of saline is done with a vessel dilator (*curved arrow*), while the microguide wire is being withdrawn (*arrow*) to prevent air bubbles. (Courtesy of Dr. Choi)

advance in the center of the cerebral arteries. As the nidus of the malformation or fistula is being reached and the flow becomes turbulent, spontaneous advancement is less likely. On occasion, one may fluoroscopically see the transmitted turbulence at the tip of the catheter, as the nidus or venous outflow is reached.

Variable stiffness microcatheters can be shaped with steam, which further facilitates navigation especially when the anterior cerebral artery or the posterior communicating artery is being negotiated. There are several maneuvers that can assist in directing a variable stiffness microcatheter. Manual compression of the opposite carotid artery while attempting to enter the anterior cerebral artery is sometimes helpful. The approach from the contralateral internal carotid artery to reach the anterior cerebral artery, curving the catheter, flush injection, or a combination of maneuvers may also be necessary. When using these catheters, contrast material injection may displace the very flexible tip causing it to accidentally enter another vessel; therefore careful and initially very gentle injections are made.

The great flexibility of the variable stiffness microcatheter can permit the use of more than one system to change flow hemodynamics (Fig. 4.14) or to catheterize difficult curves. Systems can be also combined to reverse flow or permit better penetration.

A modification of these catheters is the addition of a short distal segment (2 mm) of a more rigid Teflon tubing, which is used to mount of detachable balloon. The mounting system is similar to the Serbinenko-Debrun type, using a latex thread (see Vol. 2, Chap. 1), or a latex valve (Fig. 4.15) (Bressel 1981, unpublished data; Rufenacht 1986b). These modified catheters are very effective for high-flow fistulas such as CCFs or intracranial vessel occlusion.

A double-lumen version with an exchange inner chamber, the Moret catheter, is available and is used in the treatment of aneurysms in which a

Fig. 4.13 A–C. Kerber variable stiffness microcatheter (VSMC). **A** The microcatheter is assembled with a 2F polyethylene tubing and a tantalum impregnated 1 F silicone Kerber microcatheter (*curved arrows*). A Kerber calibrated latex balloon is placed in the tip (*arrow*). **B** Frontal and **C** lateral plain films of a very distal posterior cerebral artery catheterization with a Kerber VSMC (*arrow*)

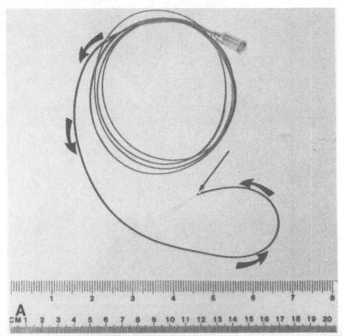

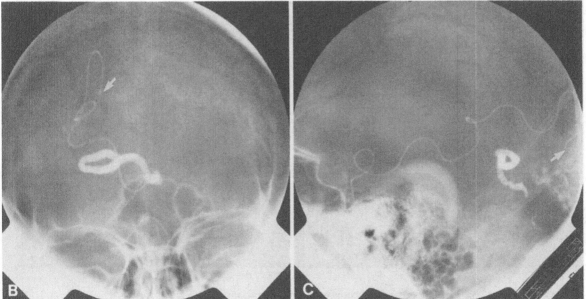

polymerizing substance in the balloon is desired (see Vol. 2, Chap. 1 and Vol. 4, Chap. 3). Variable stiffness technology can be incorporated for the construction of angioplasty catheters (Berenstein and Engel, unpublished data) (see Angioplasty of Cerebral Arteries, Vol. 5, Chap. 3).

Variable stiffness microcatheters can be used in catheterization of normal or non-high-flow arteries (Fig. 4.16) or retrograde venous catheterizations (Fig. 4.30) with a great degree of accuracy and will probably be of major importance in future endovascular procedures such as evaluation and treatment of epilepsy, investigation of cerebral function, treatment of cerebral ischemia and even tissue transplants.

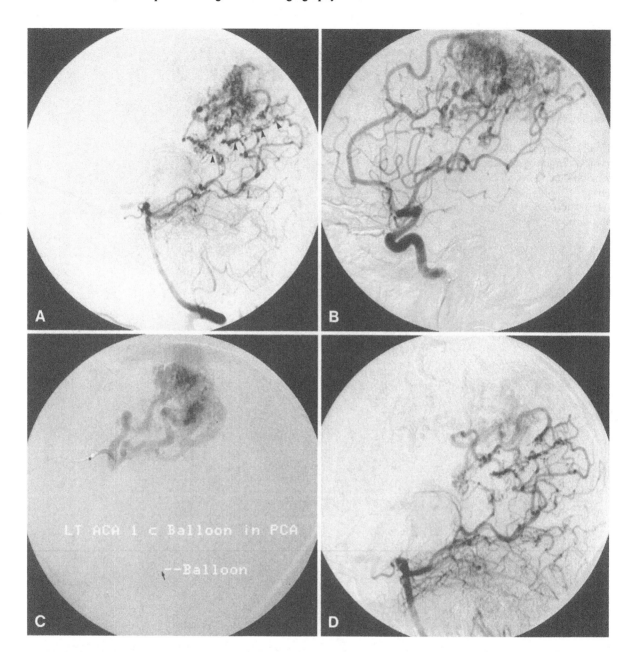

Fig. 4.14 A – D. Two variable stiffness systems to produce flow modifications. **A** Lateral subtraction angiogram (DSA) of the left vertebral artery. There is indirect filling of the AVM from the posterior cerebral artery (PCA) via leptomeningeal collaterals (*arrowheads*). **B** DSA of the left internal carotid artery. **C** Lateral DSA of the left anterior cerebral artery (ACA) injection with temporary balloon occlusion of the posterior cerebral artery (*arrow*). **D** Left vertebral artery injection after embolization via the ACA. The posterior cerebral artery was temporarily occluded while the acrylic was injected into the AVM via the ACA. Note the significant decrease in nidus field by the PCA (compare to **A**)

Fig. 4.15 A–F. Variable stiffness microcatheter (Mini-Torquer or Magic) with an extended tip for detachable balloons. The 2 mm Teflon extended tip (*black arrow*), where the latex valve is introduced (*white arrow*), may be of variable sizes (*white arrows* in **B**). Additional valves can be mounted on a larger Teflon cylinder (*open white arrow* in **B**) for placement of the valve in the extended tip of the microcatheter (**C**). **C** Mounting of an additional valve. The extended tip (*arrow*) is introduced into a hollow Teflon tubing, where the valve is mounted. The valve is then transferred to the extended tip (*white arrow*). **D** The balloon is then mounted over the valve (*arrow*). **E** The excess latex is cut with microscissors (*curved arrow*). **F** The latex piece acts as a sealing valve in the balloon after detachment (*arrow*)

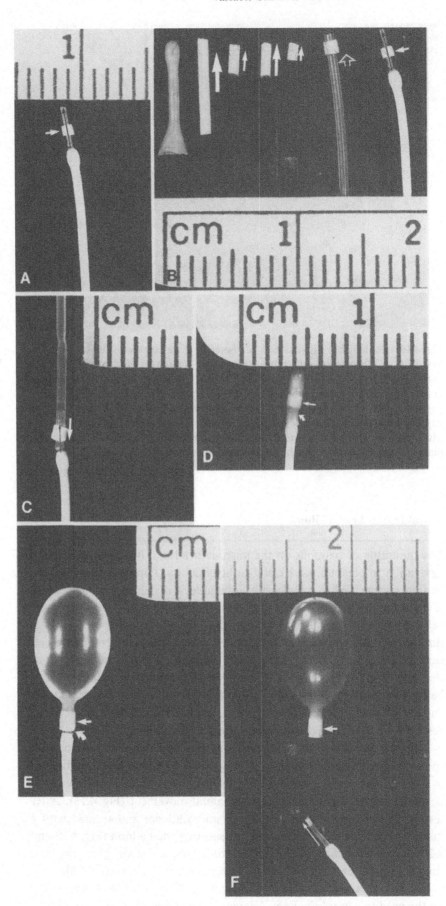

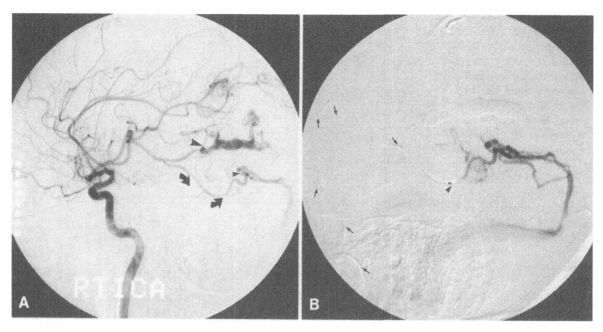

Fig. 4.16 A, B. Variable stiffness microcatheter in distal superselective catheterization of a middle cerebral artery in a patient with malignant glioblastoma without high flow. Same patient as in Vol. 5, Fig. 3.26. **A** Lateral digital subtraction angiogram of the right internal carotid artery shows the tumor with arteriovenous shouting (*arrowheads*) and small caliber, non-high-flow middle cerebral artery (MCA) supply (*curved arrows*). **B** Superselective catheterization of the posterior temporal MCA branch (*curved arrows* in **A**). The microcatheter (*arrows*) is of similar diameter as the MCA. Note the tip of the microcatheter (*arrowhead*)

3. Calibrated Leak Balloons

The mounting of balloons on the microcatheter can be useful in cerebral navigation to obtain a more distal catheterization, improved flow control, or flow reversal. When a balloon is to be used, a distal injection capability is created with a calibrated leak. The term "calibrated leak" refers to a small valve or hole in the tip of a balloon that permits inflation and leakage through the balloon (see Vol. 2, Chap. 1) (Kerber 1976). For cerebral navigation we prefer a small, soft, thin, oval latex balloon configuration such as the Balt 1 or Colibri (Fig. 4.17). This results in a reliable calibrated leak balloon that will grow less than 1 – 3 mm in diameter, thus minimizing the chance of vessel rupture. The oval, thin, latex balloon will best adapt to the vessel size, shape, and configuration, even at a sharp vessel loops.

The leak can be created in various manners. We prefer to make it prior to mounting the balloon using a sewing needle. Various sized needles are available to accomplish the desired hole size (Fig. 4.17). The balloon must be punctured in the center to prevent lateral movement (Fig. 4.18). After testing, the balloon is mounted on the microcatheter and secured with a hand tied latex thread. This method of securing the balloon (Fig. 4.19 and 4.20) permits its detachment from the catheter if accidentally glued in place, thus permitting catheter withdrawal (Berenstein and Kricheff 1978).

The hole creating the calibrated leak can be of different sizes, depending on the need to control the flow. A larger leak will permit more distal injec-

Fig. 4.17. Microballoons of different sizes and shapes made out of thin latex. The numbers refer to increased sizes: *0,1,3,* and *5* are oval balloons. Two different sizes of balloons that are longitudinal when inflated (Colibri, *c,C*) (Balt, Paris, France) are shown. Different sized needles are used to make the leak (*white arrows*)

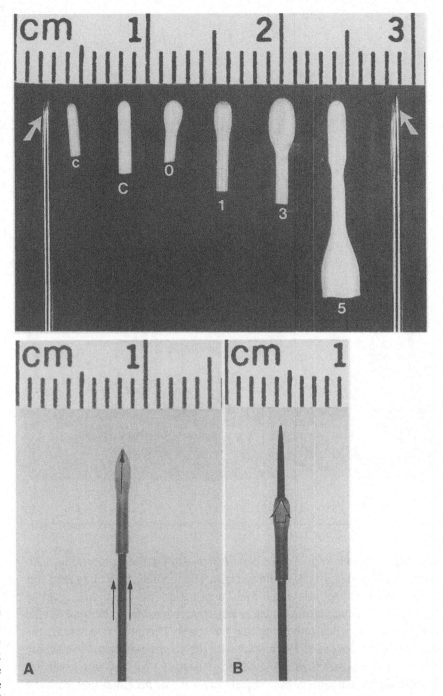

Fig. 4.18 A, B. Making the calibrated leak on the balloon. **A** A sewing needle (*double arrows*) is used to purse the apex of the balloon (*arrow*). **B** The hole is made at the center of the balloon to create the calibrated leak (*arrow*)

tion prior to balloon inflation (Fig. 4.21). In very high flow fistulas, a small leak that inflates the balloon prior to allowing distal flow of embolic material may provide better flow control (Fig. 4.22).

If, for example, the goal of embolization is the maximum permeation of a larger territory, use of a balloon with a relatively large distal opening permits distal penetration of acrylic in the beginning of the deposition with the balloon deflated. This is followed by balloon inflation and complete flow arrest later in the injection. The lack of flow creates a final continuous col-

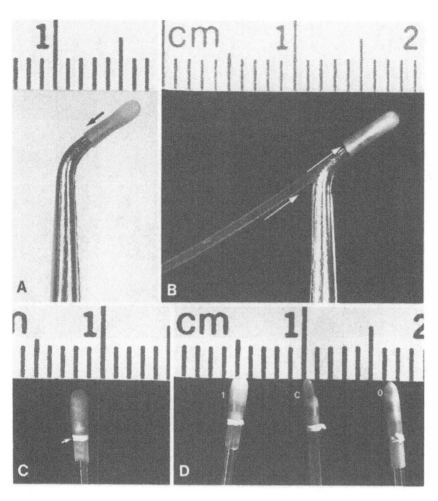

Fig. 4.19 A – D. Balloon mounting. A The balloon (*arrow*) is mounted on an angle forceps. B The forceps is opened to permit introduction of the microcatheter (*arrows*). C The balloon is then secured with a latex thread (*arrow*) proximal to the radiopaque marker of the Tracker catheter. D Various models and sized balloons are utilized (see Fig. 4.17). The latex thread will permit detachment of the balloon if it becomes adherent to the vessel wall

umn injection which fills the feeding pedicle distal to the balloon (Fig. 4.23) (see Vol. 2, Chap. 1, IBCA Embolization). The theoretical advantage of this type of injection includes initial distal penetration into the nidus, aided by flow in the feeding pedicle. There is less fragmentation of the final acrylic column, thus more effectively sealing the vessel. This process decreases the amount of autologous blood mixture with the acrylic cast, thereby lessening the theoretical possibility of delayed recanalization (Vol. 2, Chap. 1, see Recanalization). In addition, by complete blockage of proximal flow with the balloon, flow reversal can be accomplished and any distal normal branches can be preserved (see Flow Controlled Cerebral Embolization, this chapter).

The major disadvantage of using a balloon is the risk of rupturing a small perforator branch vessel. To avoid inadvertent rupture of a small ves-

Fig. 4.21 A – E. Calibrated leak microballoon. A At the beginning of injection the ▶ leak should be large enough to permit infusion (*arrow*) without balloon inflation. B Increased pressure increases the flow rate of injection and starts the balloon inflation (*arrow*). C Further pressure of injection permits infusion with balloon inflation (*arrow*). D Larger oval balloon are in a Tracker microcatheter. Arrow shows the calibrated leak. E Colibri longitudinal balloon. The balloons shown in D and E also used for angioplasty (see Vol. 5, Chap. 3)

Fig. 4.20 A–D. Mounting of a calibrated leak balloon in a very soft (Mini-Torquer, Magic, Kerber) tubing. **A** The balloon is mounted as illustrated in Fig. 4.19A. **B** Ligatures are placed in an 18 gauge Teflon sheath (*arrows*). **C** The balloon (*broad arrow*) and microcatheter (*long arrow*) are advanced into the Teflon sheath. The ligature (*arrow*) is then threaded towards the balloon collar. **D** The ligated balloon is now secured in the microcatheter and can be detached if needed

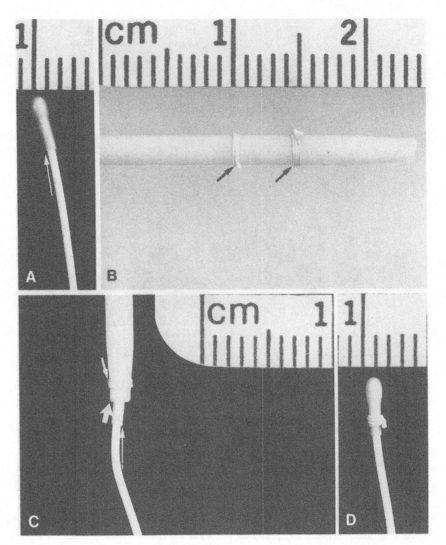

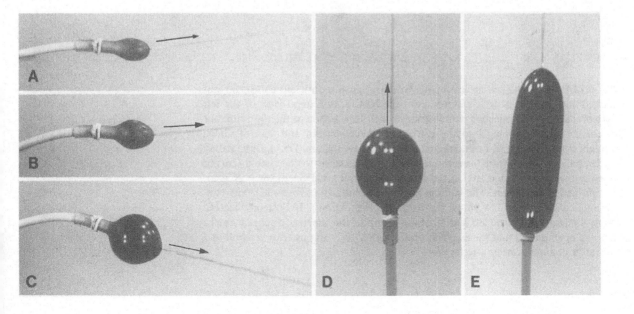

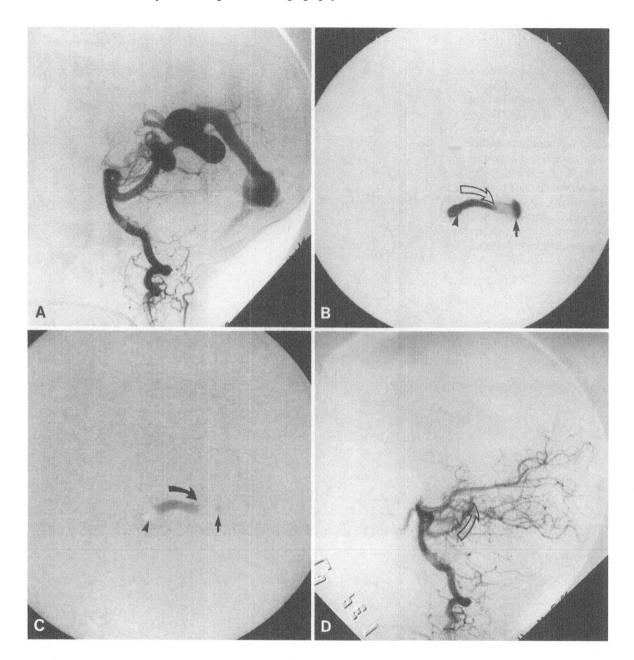

Fig. 4.22 A–D. High-flow arteriovenous fistula in an 8 month old child who was treated with calibrated leak balloon and pure NBCA. **A** Lateral view of the left vertebral artery (VA) injection demonstrates a high-flow fistula of the right superior cerebellar artery draining into the precentral cerebellar vein and vein of Galen straight sinus complex. **B** Lateral digital subtraction angiogram (DSA) of the fistula under balloon flow arrest (*arrowhead*). Note the entrance to the fistula (*curved open arrow*) and the fluid level at the venous sac (*arrow*). **C** DSA of the NBCA injection under flow arrest. The balloon has been withdrawn (*arrowhead*). The continuous column of NBCA enters the fistula (*curved arrow*). **D** Postembolization control angiogram of the left VA. Note the stump of the superior cerebellar artery (*curved open arrow*) and the excellent opacification of both posterior cerebral and posterior communicating arteries

Fig. 4.23 A–G. Calibrated leak embolization in a continuous column with flow control. **A** Lateral view of the right internal carotid artery in early arterial phase demonstrates two opercular branches of the middle cerebral artery (*arrows*) supplying a vascular malformation. **B–E** Progressive injection of contrast material in a continuous column manner under flow arrest. **B** Injection prior to balloon (*arrow*) inflation; **C** with balloon inflation (*arrow*). **D, E** Note filling of the malformation with flow control and without dilution in a continuous column manner

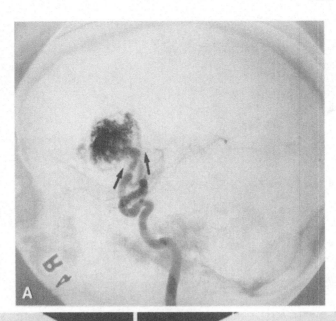

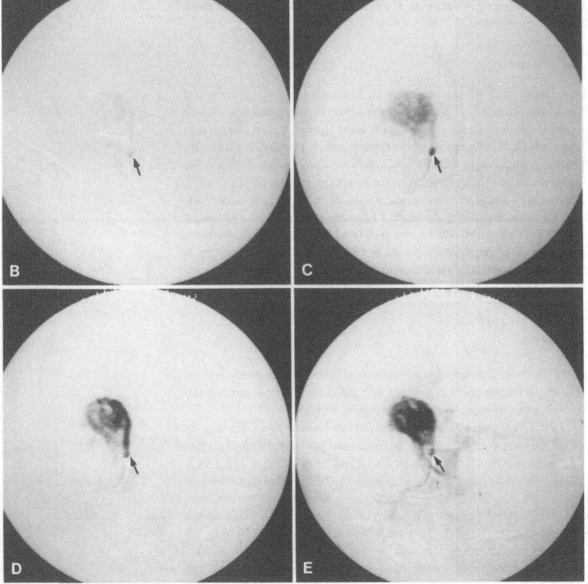

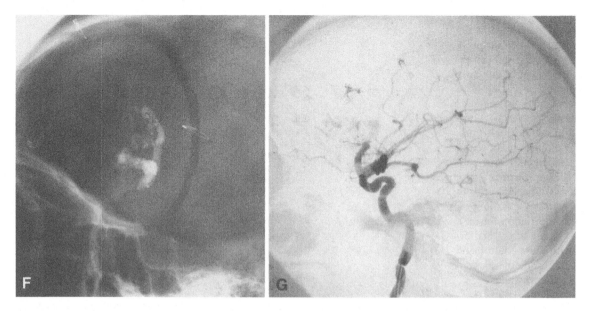

Fig. 4.23. F Radiopaque cast obtained. **G** Immediate postembolization study shows significant obliteration of the malformation

sel, initial injection of contrast material is always done very gently and without balloon inflation. If the tip of the balloon is in a small branch, one will clearly see the contrast material as it exists the catheter. If the tip is in a larger branch, rapid washout of the contrast material is noted, often with no visible contrast material, as the fast flow washes it away. At this point it is safe to inflate the balloon by more forceful injection.

Moret uses a small leak and complete flow control to permit the slow progressive injection of larger volumes of acrylic into the nidus, a technique that we have used with good results. The need for a balloon that inflates early during injection, however, results in a higher risk of vessel rupture. A trend towards nonballoon navigation and embolization is however more accepted as a safer technique.

4. Microwires

One of the greatest advantages of variable stiffness microcatheters is the ability to use microguide wire assistance, in addition to torque control and flow assisted navigation, in distal intracranial locations.

If the microcatheter cannot be advanced, variable stiffness microguide wires (Jungreis et al. 1987), similar to those used in coronary angiography, can be employed (Figs. 4.5, 4.14, 4.24, 4.10 C and Vol. 2, Chap. 1, Fig. 1.4 C).

Microwires from 0.010 inches (0.25 mm) to 0.018 inches (0.46 mm) in diameter with distally increasing flexibility are available. The proximal portion is made of stiff stainless steel which then tapers distally. The stainless steel is welded to a distal (3–9 mm), very soft, tapered platinum tip (0.024–0.23 mm diameter) obtaining further distal flexibility (Fig. 4.24).

This very soft microwire can be used with a straight or a simple curve in its distal end (Vol. 2, Chap. 1, Fig. 1.4 C). The wire can be easily steered with

Fig. 4.24 A, B. Microguide wires of different softness and flexibility. **A** *a, b*, and *c* represent 0.016 variable stiffness wires; *ft*, flexed tip with increased flexibility; *S*, seeker guidewire is the softest. Torque is best with the stiffer wires. **B** Curved microguide wire through the Tracker microcatheter allows steering

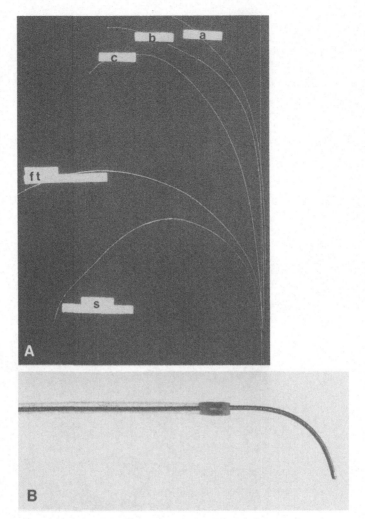

1:1 torque control. The guide wire curve will permit engagement of difficult curves such as the anterior cerebral artery (Fig. 4.25) and, once engaged, the proximal stiffness assists in advancing while the soft distal tip prevents vessel damage. If one observes buckling of the tip, the guide wire is slightly withdrawn and rotated to prevent reentering the undesired branch (Fig. 4.26). Variable stiffness microcatheters (Tracker type) are not dependent on high-flow conditions to reach their desired locations. Their ability to be steered also permits catheterization of smaller feeders at will. The use of these catheters, in conjunction with digital fluoroscopy and road mapping, have significantly improved our ability for superselective navigation in the cerebral circulation (Fig. 4.27).

As mentioned above, when using microguide wires, advancement is best with a J-curve to prevent entering more proximal small vessels (ophthalmic, C1, posterior inferior cerebellar artery, basilar tip, etc.) (Fig. 4.28). In addition a J-curve can be used in a "sidewinder" fashion. In this technique the curved wire is initially passed beyond the vessel to be catheterized and then, by withdrawing the system, the desired artery is engaged.

The ability to superselectively catheterize cerebral arteries with a high degree of accuracy permits a more functional approach to studying patients

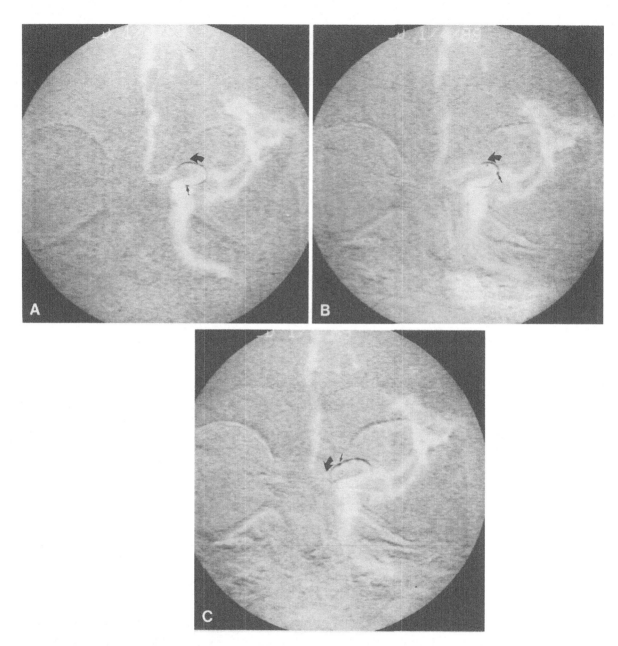

Fig. 4.25 A–C. Guide wire through balloon catheterization of the anterior cerebral artery. **A** Frontal projection of a digital subtraction angiogram road mapping image demonstrating the tip of the microcatheter (*small arrow*) at the supraclinoid internal carotid artery. The curved microguide wire as it enters the A1 segment (*curved arrow*) is shown. **B** The microguide wire is held at that position by gently withdrawing it as the microcatheter (*arrow*) is advanced, engaging the origin of the anterior cerebral artery. **C** Once the catheter has entered the A1 segment, both catheter and wire are advanced jointly, with the guide wire as a lead. Note position of the catheter tip in the distal A1 segment (*arrow*)

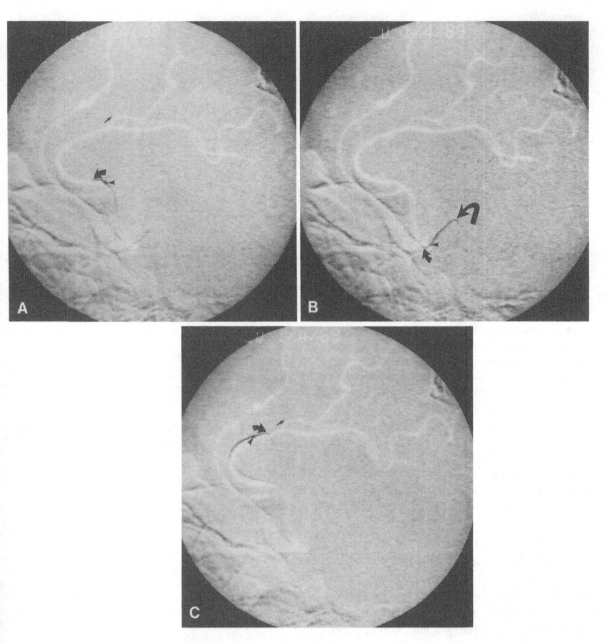

Fig. 4.26 A–C. Same patient as in Fig. 4.25. Lateral digital subtraction angiogram road mapping demonstrating the progressive advancement of the catheter wire assembly in the pericallosal artery. **A** The microcatheter has entered the A2 segment (*arrowhead*). The tip of the guidewire has a small curve and is leading the microcatheter (*curved arrow*). As the catheter is advanced, the buildup of tension against the wall of the more proximal vascular segments (*bent arrow*) assists in determining the degree of pressure that can be safely applied in progressive forwards advancement. Afterwards relaxation of the system may further forward advance of the microcatheter. **B** Further advancement of the catheter guidewire assembly. Note the microwire (*curved arrow*) which has been torqued to obtain further access into the artery, and is pointed downwards to avoid entering a more proximal bifurcation (*arrow*). **C** Advancement of the catheter guide wire assembly system beyond the genu of the corpus callosum. Note the guide wire pointing downwards (*curved arrow*) to enter the desired vessel avoiding the normal artery (*arrow*). The arrowhead in **B** and **C** is the tip of the microcatheter

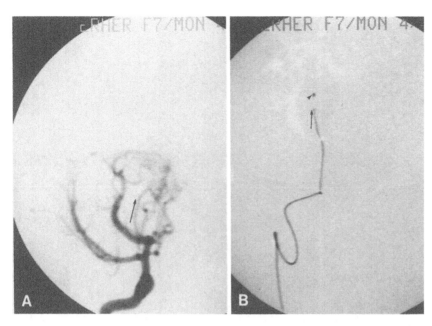

Fig. 4.27 A, B. Catheterization of small non-high-flow vessels with the use of road mapping and steerable guide wires. **A** Frontal view of the right internal carotid artery demonstrates supply to a vein of Galen aneurysmal malformation. The goal is to enter an anterior thalamo-performating artery (*arrow*). **B** Road mapping with the microcatheter and guide wire in the desired position. Tip of catheter is marked by the *arrowhead*. The guide wire (*arrow*) is withdrawn as the catheter is advanced

with vascular disease. It also permits a more superselective angiographic study and allows pressure monitoring prior to and after the occlusion of vessels (Lasjaunias et al. 1986; Duckwiller et al. 1989; Jungreis and Horton 1989).

When superselective angiography is the main goal, a high-flow Tracker catheter with slightly thicker walls and diameters is available that permits rates of injection of up to 3 ml/s (Tracker 25, Fig. 4.3).

The wire is soft enough to pass through a calibrated leak balloon without damaging it. The guide wire through balloon technique is very useful in cerebral angioplasty (see Vol. 5, Chap. 3) (Fig. 4.29).

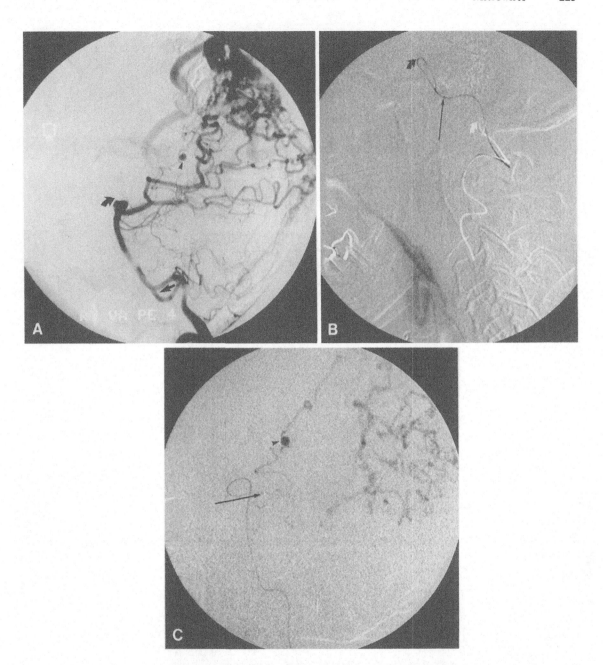

Fig. 4.28 A – C. Technique for J guide wire advancement. **A** Lateral digital subtraction angiogram of the right vertebral artery demonstrates a tortuous vertebral artery (*arrow*) and basilar tip (*curved arrow*). Note the small arterial aneurysm (*arrowhead*). **B** The catheter guide wire assembly system is advanced through the basilar tip with the J in the guide wire formed (*curved arrow*). Note the original position (*white curved arrow*) as both the catheter (*long arrow*) and J-shaped guide wire (*curved arrow*) advance through the basilar tip. **C** After the basilar curve has been passed, the J-curve is straightened. The tip of the microcatheter (*long arrow*) is pointing towards the small choroidal artery feeding an arterial aneurysm (*arrowhead*)

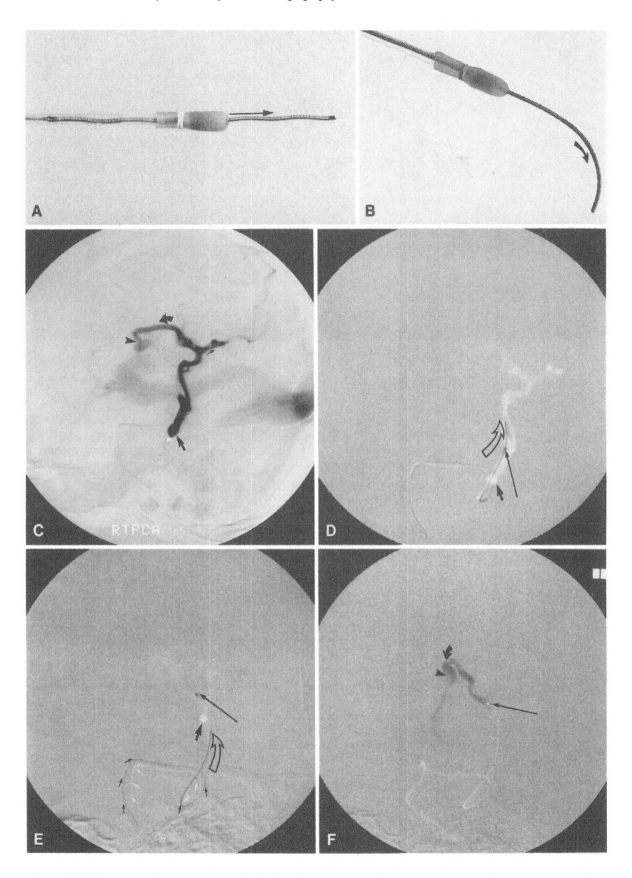

VI. Embolic Agents in Cerebral and Spinal Embolization

1. Particulate Agents

Particulate agents were used prior to the availability of liquid agents (Luessenhop et al. 1965, 1977; Kricheff et al. 1972; Hilal et al. 1978; Woppert et al. 1981). One of us (AB) used silicone spheres and polyvinyl alcohol (see Vol. 2, Chap. 1) at the beginning of his experience. Both agents are still used by many investigators. At present neither of us use either agent, except for rare instances if no other possibility exists. The disadvantage of particulate agents includes the inability to distally penetrate the nidus of the malformation, resulting in proximal vessel occlusion. In our experience, the long-term results of such proximal occlusions show no improvement over the natural course of BAVMs as it relates to rebleeding rate. In some centers particulate agents are used as the main embolic agent in preoperative devascularization (Hilal 1975; Wolpert 1975; Hieshima 1987) or during intraoperative embolization (Drake 1979; Spetzler et al. 1987).

In the spine and spinal cord, particulate agents, including reabsorbable particles or coils, may be used to protect normal territories or to redirect flow when superselectivity cannot be accomplished (see Vol. 2, Chap. 1 and Embolization of Spine and Spinal Cord, Vol. 5, Chaps. 1, 2).

1) Polyvinyl Alcohol Foam (PVA): (See Vol. 2, Chap. 1).
2) Silicone Spheres (SS): (See Vol. 2, Chap. 1)

The long term result with SS have been disappointing, and at present we do not use this embolic agent (see Chap. 5).

Fig. 4.29 A–F. Microguide wire through balloon technique. Same patient as in Fig. 3.9. **A** Guide wire through calibrated leak balloon technique (*arrow*); also used for cerebral angioplasty. **B** Curved guide wire through balloon for steering. The curved guide wire (*curved arrow*) must be passed through the balloon prior to curving. **C** Posterior cerebral artery contribution to a temporal vascular malformation (fistula). Lateral digital subtraction angiogram (DSA) of the posterior cerebral artery on the right. Note the inflated balloon (*arrow*) at a distance from the temporal branch supplying the fistula (*curved arrow*). Note the fistula site (*arrowhead*). Also note a normal parietal branch (*small arrow*). **D** A road map mask with the inflated balloon (*arrow*) at the starting position as shown in C. The guide wire with a gentle curve has been passed beyond the balloon (*open curved arrow*) and is pointing towards the desired feeder. Note the tip of the microcatheter (*long arrow*) that has been advanced. **E** As the catheter has entered the desired pedicle a road map is obtained at that position with the balloon inflated (*arrow*). The guide wire is then withdrawn proximal to the balloon (*open curved arrow*) for support and the microcatheter is advanced entering the desired pedicle (*long arrow*). Note the difference between the catheter position in the original mask at the basilar and posterior cerebral arteries (*small white arrows*) and the position where the microcatheter abuts against the vessel wall and can be advanced by torque (*black small arrows*). **F** NBCA cast obtained. DSA image after the microcatheter has been removed (*long arrow*). Last image hold of the acrylic cast of the desired pedicle (*curved arrow*). The fistula site (*arrowhead*) and a small amount of acrylic in the draining vein, without fragmentation of the NBCA column, are shown. (Compare to preembolization angiogram, Fig. 3.9B and postembolization, Fig. 3.9I)

a) Silk

Surgical silk as an embolic agent was introduced by Benati et al. (1987) and has been used by others, alone or in combination with other embolic agents, for preoperative embolization or to close single-hole fistulas (Eskridge and Hartling 1989; Halbach et al. 1989a, b). It is both biocompatible and easy to inject through small catheters. Its main value appears to be in obtaining thrombosis when other particulate agents (coils, Avatine, etc.) fail and distal catheterization for liquid deposition cannot be achieved. We have had limited experience with silk in cerebral embolization but have found it useful when using the venous approach to dural AVMs (Halbach et al. 1989a, b).

b) Coils

The general principles and indications for coils have been discussed in Vol. 2, Chap. 1. However, newer versions of microcoils that can be introduced through variable stiffness catheters have widened their application. Coils come in multiple sizes and configurations. For embolization with microcatheters they are made of soft platinum, often with added fibers of Dacron or silk to enhance their thrombogenicity (Fig. 4.30) (Target Therapeutics, San Jose, CA; Cook Inc., Bloomington, IN) (Graves et al. 1989; Hilal et al. 1988). The primary indications for coil embolization involve the transvenous approach, such as in dural AVMs (Halbach et al. 1989) or vein of Galen fistulas (Dowd et al. 1990) (Fig. 4.31), or some aneurysms (Hilal unpublished) (Vol. 5, Figs. 3.11 and 3.15). Coils may be useful as a mechanical buffer to retain more thrombogenic agents such as silk (Young 1988) or acrylic and reduce the chances of distal migration (Berenstein et al. 1990). To better seal the fistula, a coil is placed first; the catheter is then advanced distal to the coil. The coil will then slow the flow (Fig. 4.32).

A major disadvantage of coil embolization is the risk of changes in the catheter tip position as the coil exits the catheter. Coil extrusion can be accomplished with a coil "pusher" (Target Therapeutics, San Jose, CA), with saline liquid injections, or a combination of both. The important aspect of coil extrusion is stability, i.e., to not change the catheter position. At present, once a coil is placed it cannot be retrieved. As newer designs of detachable coils using electrolytic or mechanical detachment promises to avoid this problem (Guglielmi, Marks, unpublished) (Fig. 4.30C) (see Vol. 5, Chap. 3). Coils used for the packing of aneurysms are discussed in Vol. 5, Chap. 3.

Fig. 4.30 A – C. Microcoils for cerebral embolization, at present are made of a very soft platinum wire and come in 0.015 inch (0.36 mm) and 0.010 inch (0.25 mm) gauges and in a multitude of lengths. **A** Various coils: *F*, flower; *T*, Target coil; *5*, Hilal 5 mm fiber coil; *3*, Hilal 3 mm fiber coil. **B** Target Therapeutics platinum fiber coils of various configurations, elliptical to straight. **C** Guglielmi detachable coils. Three different sizes GDC microcoils are available for electrothrombosis and can be detached by electrolysis

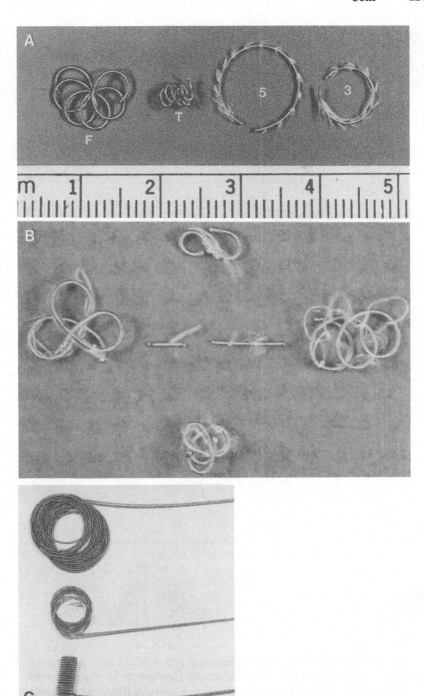

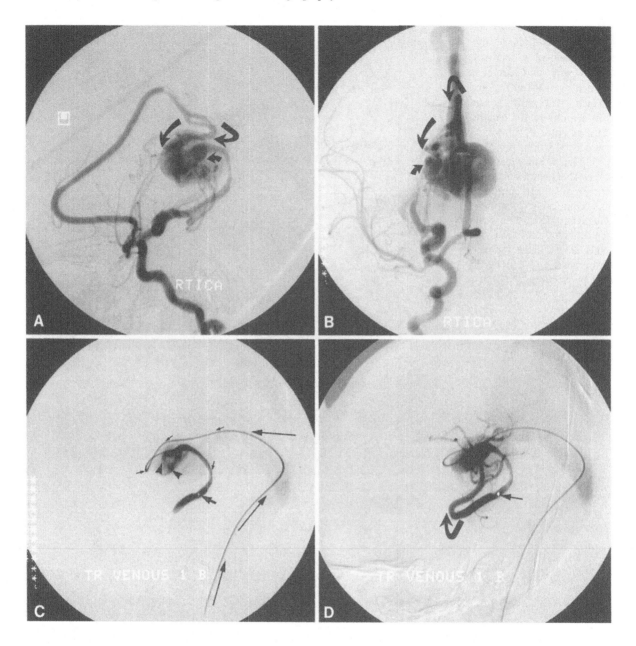

Fig. 4.31 A–R. Microcoils used in the management of a vein of Galen aneurysmal malformation by the transvenous and transarterial approach in combination with NBCA. **A** Lateral and **B** frontal digital subtraction angiogram (DSA) examinations of the right internal carotid artery demonstrate the choroidal branch of the anterior cerebral artery (*bent arrows*) entering a choroidal fissure vein (*curved large arrows*). Additional supply is seen from a posterior medial choroidal artery entering another fistulization (*small curved arrow*). **C** Lasjaunias 4F catheter (nontapered tip) introduced through the femoral vein up to the falcine sinus (*large arrows*) and coaxial introduction of a Tracker 18 (*small arrows*) obtaining superselective catheterization of the posterior medial choroidal artery on the right (*arrow*). Contrast material injection demonstrates in a retrograde manner two sites of fistulization (*arrowheads*).

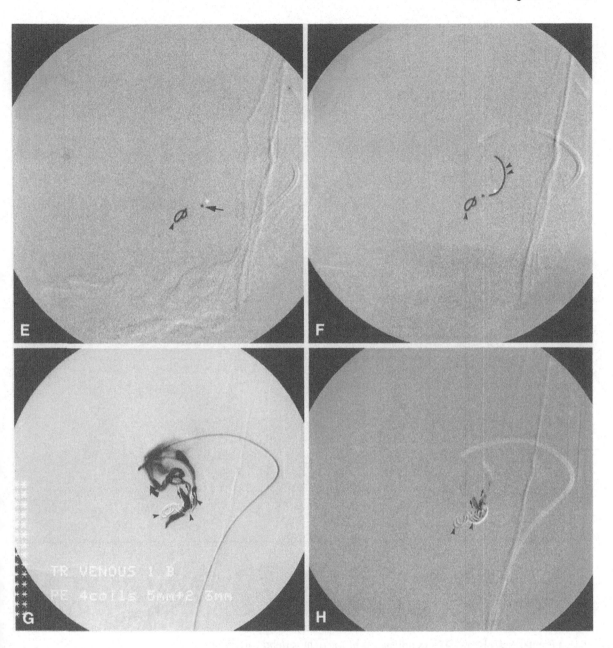

Compare with **A. D** Later phase of the same injection. The tip of the microcatheter (*arrow*) shows retrograde flow to a second choroidal artery (*bent arrow*) filling multiple normal branches. **E** DSA image of the progressive deposition of a 3 mm Hilal coil (*arrowhead*) which exits the tip of the microcatheter (*arrow*). **F** A second coil (*double arrowheads*) is still within the catheter shaft. The coils can be advanced with a "coil pusher" (Target Therapeutics) or more progressive injections of saline, which ever is more stable. **G** Four 5 mm and two 3 mm coils have been extruded (*arrowheads*). Contrast material injection demonstrates considerable slowing of flow and two additional fistulizations (*arrows*) entering a fissure vein (*curved arrow*). **H** Retrograde injection of NBCA to seal off this fistulizations (*small arrows*) around the microcoils (*arrowheads*)

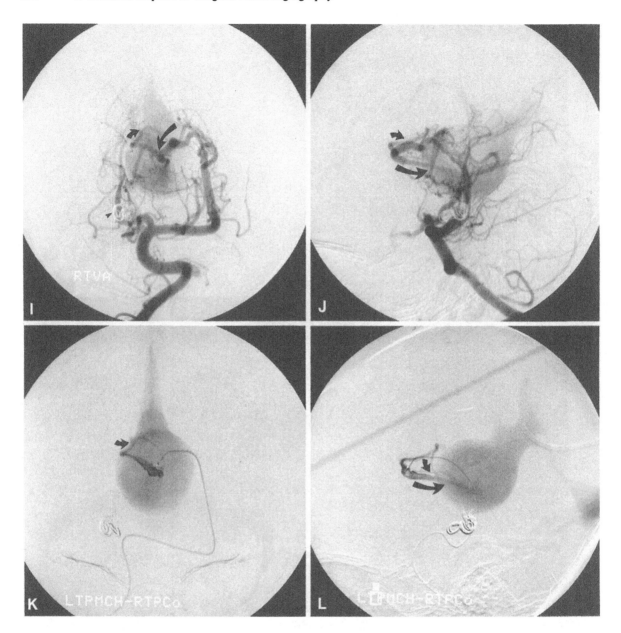

Fig. 4.31. I Frontal and **J** lateral DSA examinations of the right vertebral artery after embolization by the venous approach demonstrating a right side medial choroidal artery supply with two pedicles (*large curved* and *small curved arrow*). Note the previous coils on the right side (*arrowhead*). **K** Frontal and **L** lateral DSA examinations of the superselective injection of the left posterior medial choroidal artery (compare with **I** and **J**). Note the larger (*large curved arrow*) and smaller (*small curved arrow*) fistulizations with significant flow. **M** DSA image of the NBCA cast obtained after a transarterial coil (*arrowhead*) was extruded to slow down the flow prior to the NBCA injection. Note the NBCA deposition into the two fistulizations and entering the aneurysmal vein (*). **N** Lateral DSA of the superselective injection of the anterior cerebral artery in the same patient demonstrates the choroidal branch of the anterior cerebral artery reaching the fistula (*curved arrow*) and a normal branch to the singular gyrus (*small arrows*). The microcatheter tip (*long arrow*) could not

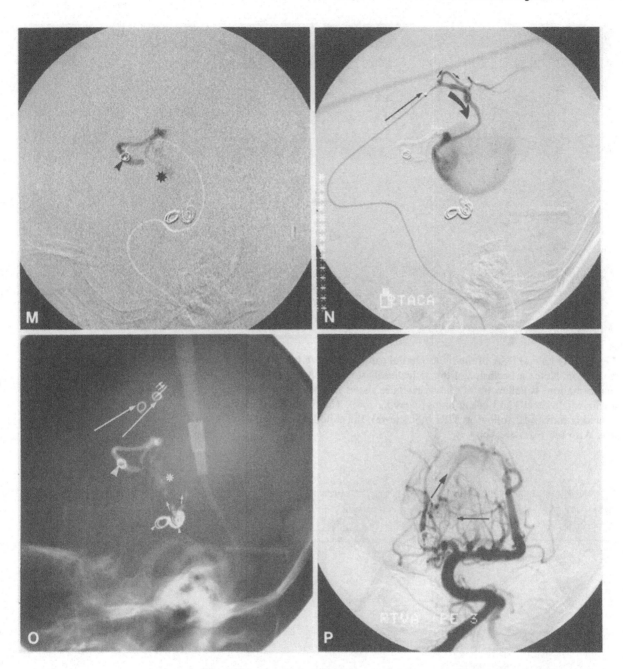

negotiate the curve towards the choroidal branch. **O** Plain film of the skull which demonstrates a straight Hilal microcoil in the proximal aspect of the normal anterior cerebral artery branch for protection (*double small arrows*). Two 3 mm curved coils are sealing the pericallosal supply (no acrylic was used because the coils produced proximal occlusion). Note the coils on the right choroidal side (*small arrowheads*) with the acrylic (*small arrows* and compare to **H**) and the embolization of the medial choroidal artery on the left (compare to Fig. **L** and **M**). There is acrylic on the venous side (*). **P** Frontal DSA of the right vertebral artery after embolization demonstrates almost complete obliteration of the malformation. There is minimal supply from a medial choroidal artery on the left (*long small arrow*) as it enters the fistulization (*long arrow*)

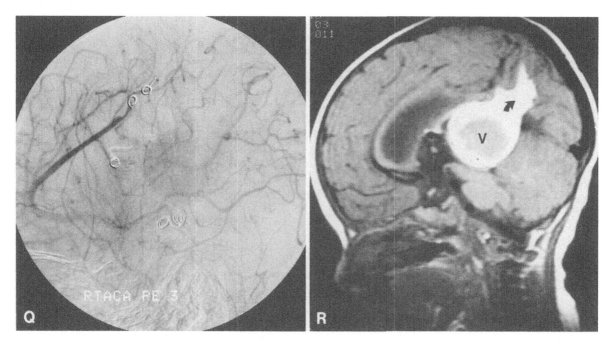

Fig. 4.31. Q Lateral DSA of the right internal carotid artery in late phase after embolization. Note the occlusion of the pericallosal artery supply and no filling of the malformation. **R** Follow-up MRI 3 weeks later shows complete thrombosis of the aneurysmal vein (*V*) and falcine sinus (*curved arrow*). The thrombosed vein disappeared in a one year follow up MRI (not shown), the child is normal at 3 years of age. Also see Fig. 5.36, Vol. 4

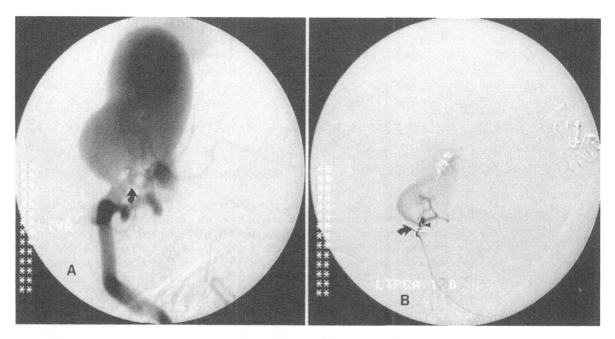

Fig. 4.32A,B. Coils and NBCA in the management of multiple high-flow fistulas. **A** Lateral digital subtraction angiogram of the left vertebral artery demonstrates multiple high-flow fistulas of the posterior cerebral artery. *Curved arrow* demonstrates one fistula. **B** A coil has been placed circumferential in the arterial side of the fistula (*curved arrow*). The tip of the microcatheter is distal (*arrowhead*). The flow is reduced to permit safer acrylic injection without proximal occlusion (see Fig. 4.31 O and Q)

2. Liquid Agents

a) Acrylates

Of the liquid embolic agents, the cyanoacrylates have been the agents of choice in the management of AVMs in both our experience and that of most investigators with extensive experience in the management of BAVMs. The isobutyl homologue isobutyl-2-cyanoacrylate (IBCA) (see Vol. 2, Chap. 1) was the first available to us (Zanetti and Sherman 1972; Kerber 1976; Berenstein and Kricheff 1979a, c) and is the one with which we have the longest experience and follow-up. More recently the *n*-butyl homologue *n*-butyl-2-cyanoacrylate (NBCA) has become available. The principles reviewed in Vol. 2, Chap. 1 with regard to techniques, mode of action, histotoxicity, etc., are the same for both agents. Specific characteristics of the *n*-butyl homologue will be discussed below.

N-Butyl-2-Cyanoacrylate

This newer homologue of the cyanoacrylates has been recently introduced for endovascular CNS embolization as a replacement for IBCA. Two commercial versions exist: *Histoacryl* was introduced in Germany for neural anastomosis and skin closure. It is the NBCA preparation presently used in Europe for endovascular embolizations. Two versions of Histoacryl are available: the "blue" version, intended for better visualization during nerve microanastomosis, and the "clear" version for skin application. One of us (PL) has used the "blue" version and finds it very similar to IBCA; in addition, at time of injection (even if without a balloon), there is less fragmentation and a more continuous column is obtained, resulting in a more complete cast of the embolized angioarchitecture.

Avacryl is the NBCA type being investigated in the USA (Berenstein et al. 1989; Brothers et al. 1989). In our experimentation in vitro, in dogs, and in humans we have found that shelf stability, reproducibility, ability to be sterilized, and setting time in vivo (with a 50% iophendylate mixture) are

Table 4.2. In vitro comparison between NBCA[+] and IBCA[++]

	NBCA[+]	IBCA[++]
Shelf stability	=	=
Sterilization	=	=
Spreadability	=	=
Wetability	=	=
Surface tension	20 dynes/cm^2	18 dynes/cm^2
Viscosity	2.66 CPS	2.40 CPS
Setting time	=	=
Integrity of the column	↑	→
Bond strength	7×10^3 g/cm^3	9.5×10^3 g/cm^2
Bond flexibility	↓	↑
Elasticity	↑	↓
Rigidity	↓	↑
Brittleness	↓	↑

+ These in vitro results apply to avacryl ® NBCA
+ + Ethicon ® IBCA

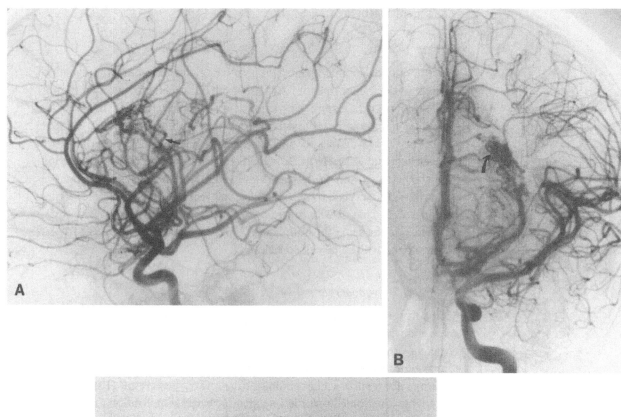

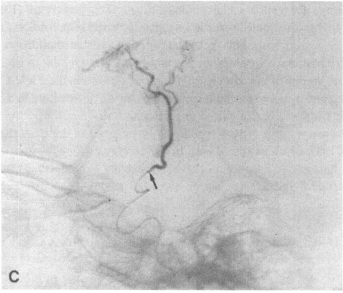

Fig. 4.33 A–E. NBCA and iophendylate combination (without tantalum powder) for low viscosity. **A** Lateral and **B** frontal preembolization angiograms of the left internal carotid artery demonstrate a small caudate lesion supplied by a lateral lenticulostriate artery (*arrow*). Note the small nidus in **B** (*curved arrow*). **C** Lateral subtraction angiogram of the superselective catheterization of the lenticulostriate artery (*arrow*) supplying the malformation. **D** Lateral and **E** frontal postembolization angiograms show complete obliteration of the malformation. Note the subtracted radiopaque cast (*arrowheads*)

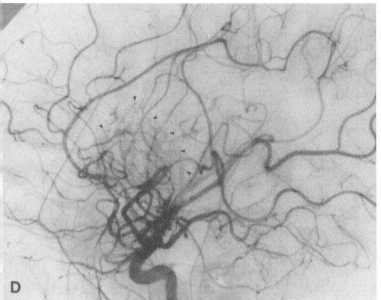

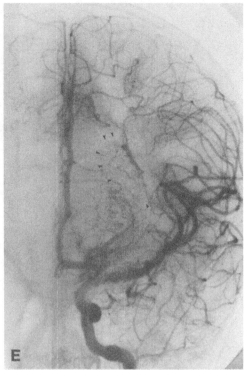

almost equal to IBCA (Table 4.2). Setting time in plasma was slightly longer for Avacryl. In addition, surface tension and viscosity are greater for Avacryl, resulting in better integrity and more uniformity of the acrylic column with less fragmentation. A significant lower bond strength was noted with this homologue. This feature offers a major advantage over IBCA, as gluing the catheter in situ is almost impossible. More time is available for deposition to obtain a better, more complete cast of the abnormality and seal of the embolized pedicle to prevent vessel rupture and to not glue the catheter. Bond flexibility, elasticity, rigidity, and brittleness were also less. Avacryl is more plastic, softer, and has a smaller shrinking factor than IBCA, all significant advantages in preoperative embolization. A single disadvantage of Avacryl arises from its slight increase in surface tension and viscosity, resulting in decreased penetration in small caliber vessels. This can be overcome, however, by reducing the amount of tantalum powder by replacing it with 0.5 g/ml of NBCA, decreasing the proportion of iophendylate, or using Lipiodol as a replacement for iophendylate. Alternatively tantalum may be omitted and 70% – 80% iophendylate mixed with 20% – 30% NBCA (Fig. 4.33). The overall performance of Avacryl is therefore superior to IBCA, and at present it is the cyanoacrylate homologue of choice for CNS and spinal cord embolization.

In general, a complete acrylic cast of the desired vascular tree is needed, as recanalization will occur if blood clot is left within or around the acrylic cast (Vol. 2, Chap. 1) (Fig. 4.34). Therefore, if contrast material is seen to surround the acrylic on postembolization injection, an additional acrylic deposition into the same pedicle is performed (Fig. 4.35).

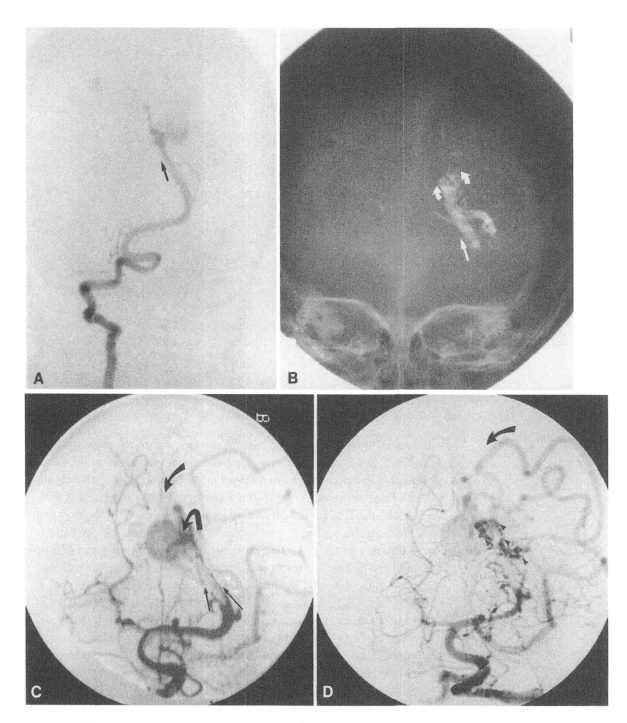

Fig. 4.34 A–D. Recanalization of cyanoacrylate. **A** Frontal view of the left vertebral artery early phase shows a prominent posterior artery (*arrow*) supplying two separate fistulas. **B** Frontal plain radiogram showing the cast of the posterior cerebral artery filling the beginning of both pedicles going towards the fistulas (*curved arrows*). **C** Immediate postembolization control left vertebral angiogram demonstrates contrast material still passing around the cyanoacrylate cast (*long arrows*). The fistula still fills (*bent arrow*). Note the additional middle cerebral artery contribution (*curved arrow*). **D** 3 year follow-up angiogram demonstrates irregular recanalization around the cyanoacrylate cast (*arrowheads*). Note increased diameter of the middle cerebral artery (*curved arrow*) and decrease in diameter of the posterior cerebral artery (compare to **C**)

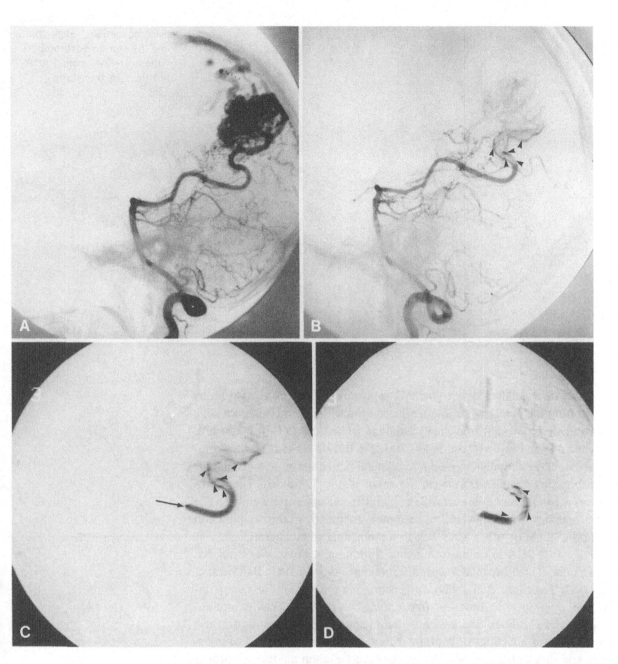

Fig. 4.35 A – E. Additional acrylic injection to prevent recanalization. **A** Lateral view of the left vertebral artery demonstrates the parietal branch of the posterior cerebral artery supplying the most posterior medial aspect of a left side malformation. **B** Immediate postembolization control angiogram of the left vertebral artery demonstrates contrast material passing around the acrylic cast (*arrowheads*). **C** Recatheterization of the posterior cerebral artery (*arrow*). Note the injection of contrast material around the acrylic cast (*arrowheads*). Although delayed thrombosis of this vessel with autologous clot is likely, there is also the possibility of recanalization as seen in Fig. 4.34. **D** Digital subtraction angiogram of the NBCA deposition using a low viscosity mixture. Note the penetration of the acrylic material (*arrowheads*)

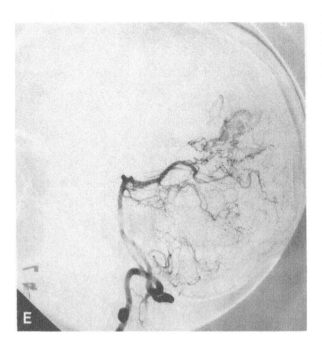

Fig. 4.35. E Final control postembolization angiogram. Note the retrograde thrombosis of the posterior cerebral artery until the first branching

Cases of recanalization of glue "disappearance" (Rao et al. 1989) may result from fragmentation of the acrylic column with intermixture of a large portion of blood clot and small amounts of acrylic (0.1–0.3 "push"). Recanalization has been seen in less than 2% of our patients and most incidents may actually represent collateral circulation (sprouting or nonsprouting angiogenesis) when the shunt is not eliminated. These processes are most prone to occur if the shunt is not completely closed. The later opening of feeding vessels is seen more frequently in the occipital and temporal lobes or other areas rich in leptomeningeal collaterals.

Prior to NBCA injection in humans, training and experience is needed in an animal or other model setup (Kerber and Flaherty 1980; Bartynski et al. 1987; TerBrugge et al. 1989). In general, due to the multiple factors involved in a specific situation (morphological goals, selectivity accomplished, vessel caliber, arteriovenous shunt hemodynamics, venous outflow, etc.), repeated injections of contrast material will guide the speed of injection and suggest the best NBCA-iophendylate-tantalum mixture for proper polymerization time and viscosity. All these factors are critical to achieve the best results and can only be developed from proper in vitro and in vivo training. The human factor and perceptions will permit the best choices.

When injecting without a balloon, it is recommended that the tip of the catheter be against the wall of the vessel and not in the center of the feeder. This will minimize distal migration of embolic agent through high-flow fistulas, taking advantage of the slower flow in the periphery of vessels (Fig. 4.36). Proper fluoroscopic equipment is a prerequisite to good results.

b) Iophendylate

Iophendylate (Pantopaque) acts primarily to retard polymerization of the IBCA or NBCA but also adds radiopacity. If decreased viscosity is required (small vessels, distal territory, tumor embolization), a 75% iophendylate

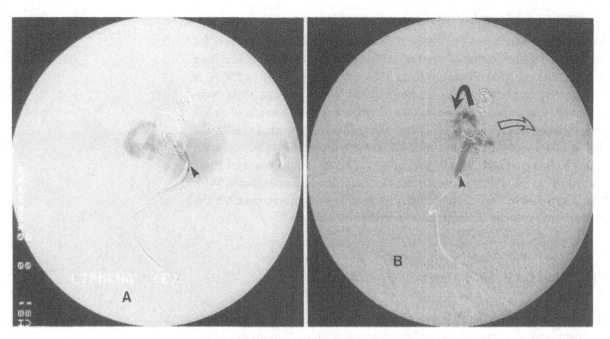

Fig. 4.36 A, B. High-flow fistula treated with NBCA injected without balloon. When injecting without a balloon, primarily in high-flow fistulas, the acrylic is mixed with tantalum powder alone or with no more than 0.2 ml of iophendylate per 1 ml of NBCA to permit rapid polymerization. In addition, the catheter tip should be against the vessel wall where the flow is slower. **A** Digital subtraction angiogram (DSA) in lateral projection of the superselective lateral view of the left posterior medial choroidal artery. Note the position of the microcatheter against the vessel wall. The injected contrast material layers against the blood vessel wall (*arrowhead*) with dilution of the parabolic central flow. **B** DSA cast obtained of NBCA with 0.2 ml of iophendylate per 1 ml of NBCA. Note the position of the original microcatheter which has been removed (*arrowhead*) and the distal portion of the injected pedicle and the site of fistulization (*bent arrow*) with a very small column of NBCA in the falcine sinus (*open curved arrow*). Note that the material has not fragmented. Previous pedicles had been embolized with coils and acrylic

25% NBCA mixture gives sufficient radiopacity such that tantalum may be omitted (Fig. 4.33).

c) Iodized Oil

Iodized oil (Lipiodol) chemically acts like iophendylate but has a lower viscosity, which can permit a better distal penetration of small vessels.

d) Ethanol

Ethanol, a cytotoxic agent, may be used alone, primarily in malignant tumors, or in combination with polyvinyl alcohol in a 20% – 30% concentration (see Vol. 2, Chap. 1, p. 40 and Vol. 5, Chap. 2, see Spinal Tumor Embolization). In BAVMs and SCAVMs we have not used it.

e) Avatine – Polyvinyl Alcohol-Ethanol Combinations

Various combinations of this "cocktail" have been introduced recently for preoperative embolization of cerebral AVMs (Fox et al. 1988). A variation is the addition of silk threads (Mehta 1989) as an alternative to IBCA in preoperative or preradiosurgical embolization. We do not use these combinations, as significant inflammation often occurs and recanalization has been reported. If this or any other embolic agent enters normal vessels, the risk of neurological consequences is the same but the long-term occlusion and therefore potential benefit appear less. The main advantage of these "cocktails" is the ability to use the same catheter in multiple pedicles. With todays variable stiffness microcatheters, the ability to catheterize CNS circulation and catheter reposition are not problematic.

VII. Flow Controlled Cerebral Embolization

Flow control refers to the ability to alter the flow characteristics in vascular territories and may represent a deliberate augmentation, diminution, or arrest of flow. It may be accomplished via a variety of techniques, including changes in systemic blood pressure, the use of calibrated leak balloons, occlusive, double lumen, balloon catheters, manual compression, rate of injection, etc. All share the aim of reaching a target and sparing normal tissue.

We originally introduced this concept in the embolization of the lenticulostriate arteries (Berenstein 1981) and the maxillofacial region (Berenstein et al. 1983) and then to the embolization of the rest of the craniofacial area using the collateral circulation (Lasjaunias et al. 1986; Vols. 1 and 2).

In the cerebral and spinal cord circulations, the complexity and small size of the vasculature, vitality of the tissue being supplied, and distal location within the vascular system require modification of some of the techniques described in the craniofacial area. Permanent mechanical rerouting of flow, for example (even temporary reabsorbable agents such as Gelfoam), is unacceptable in the CNS due to the sensitivity of CNS tissue to hypoxia.

Flow manipulations in the spine and in the spinal cord itself are similar. The principles outlined in Vol. 2, Chap. 1 apply to these territories and are illustrated in Vol. 5, Chaps. 1 and 2.

Flow manipulations in the cerebral vasculature can be used for more distal catheterization, to reverse flow in an attempt to cross the anterior or posterior portions of the circle of Willis, to reverse flow at the level of a gyrus, or through leptomeningeal collaterals. Despite such helpful techniques, there is no replacement for anatomical knowledge.

1. Distal Catheterization

In some situations, distal catheterization is not possible either because of the size of a vessel or its tortuousity. Flow in such cases can be augmented by raising the systemic blood pressure or by temporarily occluding a neighborhood or contributing artery, thereby resulting in temporary compensatory vasodilatation. The resultant flow increases in turn facilitate more distal navigation. Although valuable, such techniques are seldom needed. Staged embolization may permit a remaining channel to enlarge for future catheterization.

2. Flow Reversal

Due to the ability of the arterial system and its collaterals and anastomoses to carry flow in either direction, one can artificially modify the flow. Flow modification or reversal is possible and may be used at different levels of the cerebral circulation.

a) Modification at the Circle of Willis

Temporary occlusion at the level of the cervical internal carotid arteries is a simple and very useful technique to redirect flow across the anterior cerebral artery when attempting catheterization of it or of medially originating perforators (Berenstein 1981). The reversal of flow can be accomplished by simple manual compression of the contralateral internal carotid artery at the neck. Inflation of a calibrated leak balloon ipsilaterally during systole assists in propelling the microcatheter forward (synchronization with the EKG and balloon inflation). Occlusion of the contralateral internal carotid artery can alternatively be accomplished either by manual compression or with a single or double lumen balloon catheter placed in the cervical internal carotid artery (Berenstein 1981). The technique is also applied to the cervical vertebral artery(ies) when attempting to enter the posterior communicating artery or one of its branches via catheterization of the internal carotid artery.

b) Flow Modification above the Circle of Willis

Flow modification can be accomplished by temporary distal occlusion of a pedicle, thereby increasing the preferential flow into a side branch. This technique uses flow to overcome unfavorable geometric features of the angioarchitecture. For example, temporary occlusion of the M2 segment may redirect flow to permit flow assisted catheterization of a lateral lenticulostriate artery originating at an acute angle from M1 (Fig. 4.37). Temporary occlusion of the internal carotid artery above the posterior communicating artery or anterior choroidal artery can facilitate flow assisted catheterization of these vessels as well or aid in entering an aneurysm (Vol. 3, Chap. 3, Fig. 3.7). This technique has been used in the embolization of midline AVMs with particulate agents such as silicone spheres (Hilal and Michelsen 1975). With variable stiffness microcatheters, used without a balloon and assisted by steerable microguide wires, flow guidance is less important. Such flow modification is seldom necessary for simple catheterization.

Flow modification can also enhance acrylic deposition in a lesion. Temporary flow arrest of a collateral feeder to the AVM is done with a balloon, while embolic liquid is injected through another pedicle. The temporary occlusion produces a local diminution of pressure at the nidus, resulting in better penetration (Fig. 4.14). Proximal occlusion at the M1 segment can reverse the flow in distal cortical territories enabling more selective flow of embolic materials (Apsimon, unpublished).

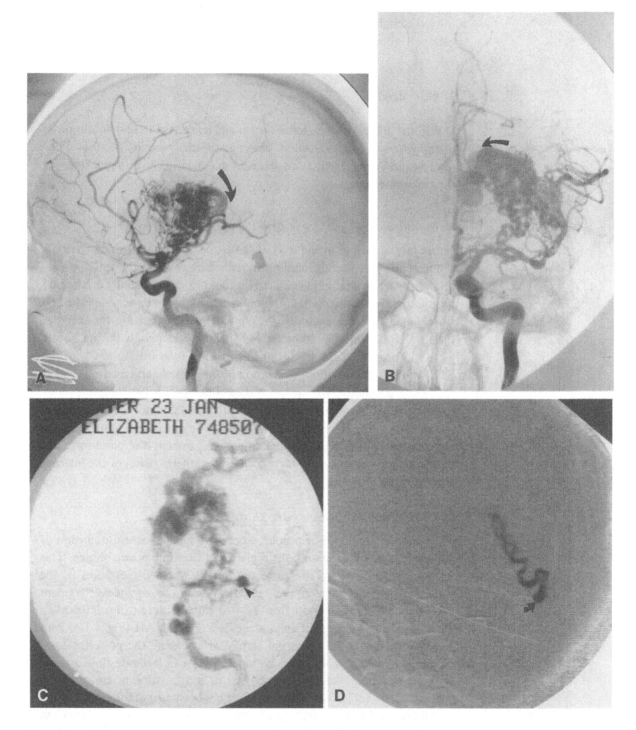

Fig. 4.37 A–E. Basal ganglionic arteriovenous malformation supplied by lateral lenticulostriate arteries, double catheter techniques. **A** Lateral and **B** frontal views of the left internal carotid artery demonstrate the basal ganglionic malformation with supply from the lenticulostriate arteries and draining into the deep venous system (*curved arrow*). **C** Occlusive balloon in the middle cerebral artery distal to the lenticulostriate artery (*arrowhead*). **D** Second microballoon catheter enters the lateral lenticulostriate artery (*curved arrow*). **E** Postembolization lateral view shows significant diminution in the nidus of the malformation with its venous drainage (*curved arrow*). This size malformation is suitable for radiosurgery

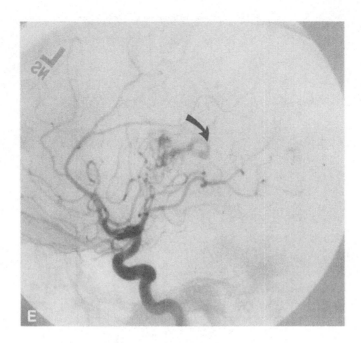

c) Modification at the Cortical Level

Flow reversal to protect a normal vessel distal to the nidus can be accomplished with proximal control at the intracranial carotid bifurcation. Acrylic is delivered selectively into the nidus with preservation of the distal (normal) artery.

d) Modification at the Level of the Leptomeningeal and/or Watershed Area

When superselectivity cannot clear a normal branch and distal penetration is needed, flow reversal can be accomplished using a calibrated leak microballoon placed in a relatively proximal position to obtain flow arrest. Balloon inflation will then produce a reversal in blood flow at the leptomeningeal collaterals (Fig. 4.38) or long anastomotic arteries. If the balloon remains inflated and slow gentle hand injection of contrast material is monitored fluoroscopically, one can clearly see the dilution of the contrast material column, as nonopacified blood (which has reversed its flow secondary to balloon occlusion of the natural afferent direction) displaces the contrast material towards the desired territory (Fig. 4.38 C). If a more forceful injection is done or the balloon is deflated, the distal runoff will be towards both the lesion and the normal pedicle that is to be preserved (Fig. 4.38 D). The demonstration of such viable collateral flow is of major significance. It provides indirect evidence that if the particular pedicle is blocked proximally, there will be no ischemic consequences (Fig. 4.38 G). However, it also illustrates a potential source for reperfusion of a territory if particulate emboli are used or if proximal occlusion occurs.

The necessary force and rate of injection to accomplish flow reversal is mastered by the repeated injections of contrast material under fluoroscopic monitoring prior to liquid acrylic embolization which is done in a similar manner (Fig. 4.38 E – G). One must nonetheless be aware that once the first

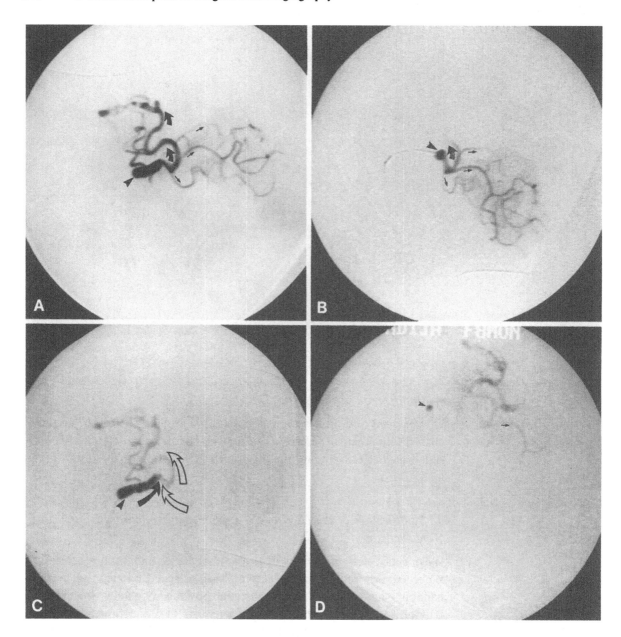

Fig. 4.38 A – G. Flow reversal at the gyra level. **A** Lateral digital subtraction angiogram (DSA) of the P3 segment using an occlusive balloon (*arrowhead*). Note filling of the posterior medial choroidal artery supplying a choroidal malformation (*curved arrows*) and filling of normal distal vessels (*small arrows*). **B** Superselective catheterization of the choroidal artery (*curved arrow*) proved impossible with inability to clear the normal vessel (*small arrows*). **C** Flow reversal is obtained by inflating the balloon (*arrowhead*), obtaining flow control at the proximal segment (*curved arrow*). Nonopacified flow (*open curved arrows*) has been reversed in the normal leptomeningeal circulation by the balloon occlusion and dilutes the contrast material in the choroidal artery. **D** Deflation of the balloon (*arrowhead*) produces

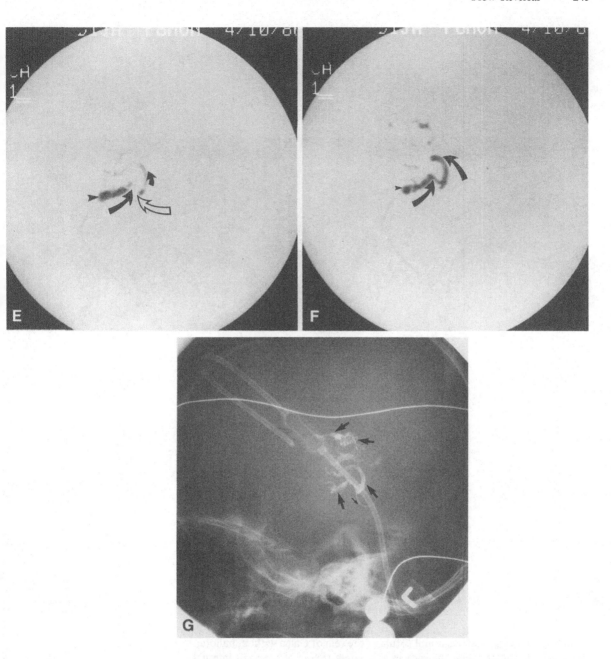

antegrade flow towards the normal branch (*small arrow*). **E** DSA image obtained during the injection of IBCA with flow reversal produced by the inflated balloon (*arrowhead*). The continuous column of acrylic is seen (*curved arrow*) until the nonopacified blood which is reversed (*curved open arrow*) displaces the acrylic towards the choroidal circulation (*curved arrow*). **F** Now the continuous column of acrylic is permeating the choroidal artery and malformation (*curved arrows*), and the balloon (*arrowhead*) is being deflated. **G** Cast obtained of the very distal penetration into the malformation (*arrows*). A proximal segment of the normal branch has been occluded (*small arrow*) without clinical consequence, as the distal territory is perfused by the leptomeningeal collaterals

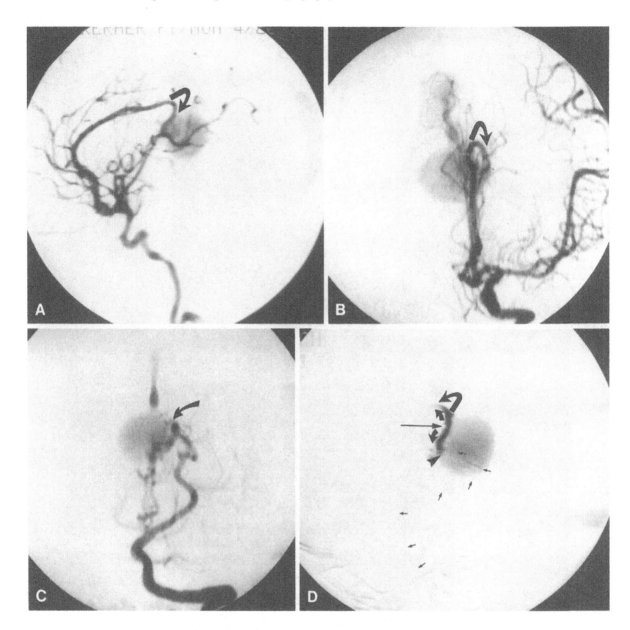

Fig. 4.39 A – G. Flow reversal in a mural fistula of the vein of Galen without balloon. **A** Lateral and **B** frontal digital subtraction angiogram (DSA) of the right internal carotid artery demonstrating the choroidal branch of the anterior cerebral artery (*bent arrow*) supplying a mural fistula. **C** Frontal view of the left vertebral artery injection demonstrates the posterior medial choroidal supply to the same fistula (*curved arrow*). **D** Lateral DSA of the superselective catheterization of the posterior medial choroidal artery on the left with a Tracker microcatheter (*small arrows*) without balloon. With sufficient pressure of injection at the tip of the catheter (*long arrow*) there is antegrade flow towards the fistula (*curved arrow*) and retrograde flow into the anterior cerebral artery (*bent arrow*). **E** Lateral coned down plain film

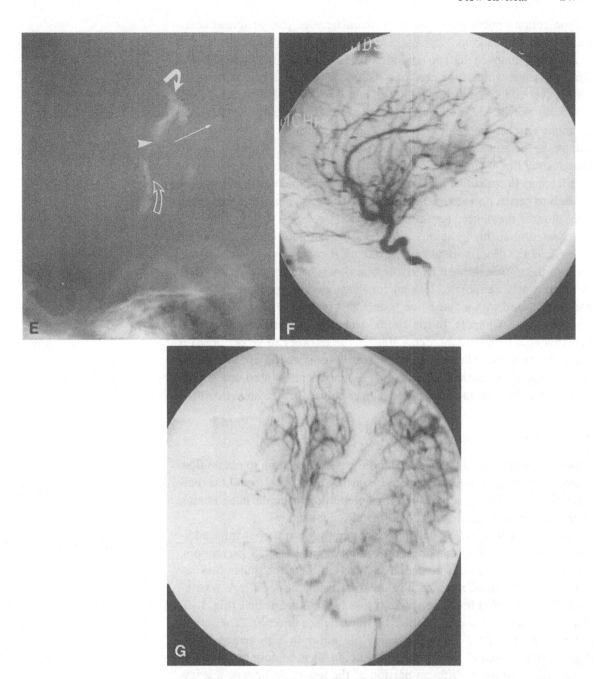

demonstrates the occlusion of the fistula (*arrowhead*) with some acrylic in the vein (*arrow*). Note the retrograde occlusion of the choroidal branch of the anterior cerebral artery (*bent arrow*). Additional embolization in a second choroidal artery is also seen (*open curved arrow*). **F** Lateral and **G** frontal DSAs in late arterial phase of the left internal carotid artery after the embolization via the posterior route; there is not filling of the fistula. The anterior cerebral artery was never catheterized or embolized directly acrylic column polymerizes the flow characteristics change immediately, unlike contrast material.

A fistula supplied by two anastomotic sources can be occluded in a similar manner without the need of a balloon (Fig. 4.39). Of importance to note is that contrast material will travel and wash out, whereas acrylic will eventually polymerize, stop, and then be redirected; however, the technique is simple and can be easily monitored fluoroscopically. If proper control cannot be accomplished one may perform the acrylic injection in two movements, first by injecting a small amount of embolic agent, observing it as it enters the proximal part of the normal vessel, and waiting for several seconds to permit polymerization. Additional embolic liquid can then travel only towards the desired territory.

A variation in this technique is useful when, in addition to attempting to preserve the distal normal runoff, one must preserve the proximal segment of the pedicle through which the injection is being made. In this case, flow arrest with a calibrated leak microballoon obtains reversal of the flow and is combined with a "push" or "sandwich" technique of acrylic deposition (see Vol. 2, Chap. 1). In the "push" technique a small volume of embolic material (0.05–0.2 ml, depending on the territory to be occluded) is placed in the microcatheter and a controlled bolus injection of 5% distilled water is made to push the acrylic into the lesion. We rarely used this "push" technique in brain embolization but it may be used in the spinal cord.

3. Flow Arrest

Flow arrest may be used, as discussed in the previous section, to obtain flow reversal. However, flow arrest is more frequently used to better fill the malformation or pathological territory, thus preventing or diminishing mixing of the acrylic with autologous blood (see Recanalization).

The use of calibrated leak balloons to obtain flow arrest gives some additional flexibility during embolization of, for example, small perforators, where distal penetration is needed. The injection is started under flow arrest, with the 5% distilled water solution first rinsing the pedicle. A relatively small volume of radiopaque acrylic is injected into the pedicle (Fig. 4.40) and the balloon is allowed to deflate by stopping the injection. The acrylic will then be propelled forward towards the nidus by nonopaque blood (Fig. 4.39D). A second injection of acrylic can then be done to close the vessel or to permeate a different portion of the lesion. As always, it is important that the vessel to be occluded does not supply any functional area, a fact determined either by anatomical analysis or by preceding the embolization with a provocative amobarbital test (see Provocative Testing). Flow arrest by a wedged catheter (Moret, unpublished data) may be of assistance to better fill the nidus.

4. Systemic Hypotension

Manipulation of the systemic blood pressure is another means to alter the flow in the malformation and surrounding brain. It can permit better filling of the nidus as the malformation is directly dependent on the systemic blood pressure, whereas normal brain is dependent on autoregulation. Controlled lowering of the systemic blood pressure will produce vasodilatation

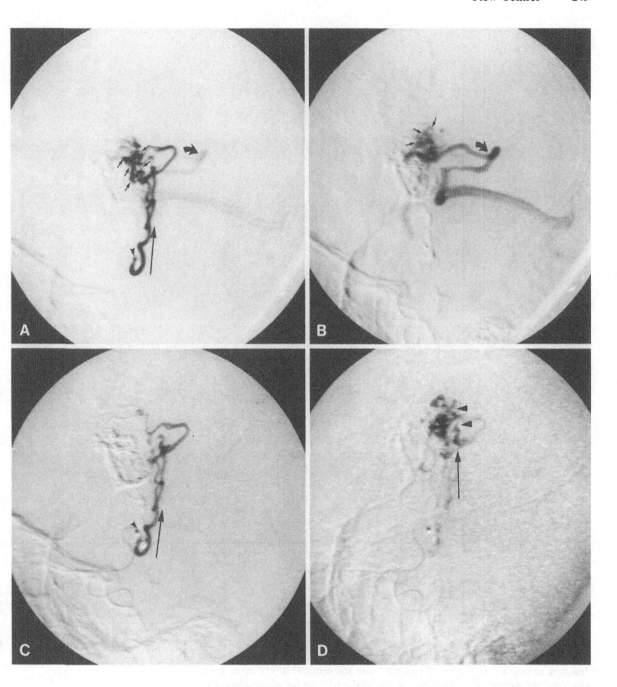

Fig. 4.40 A–D. Flow arrest variation; acrylic embolization with a calibrated leak balloon. **A** Lateral digital subtraction angiogram (DSA) of a lateral lenticulostriate artery catheterized with a calibrated leak microballoon in arterial phase. Note flow arrest by the balloon (*arrowhead*), filling of the lenticulostriate artery (*long arrow*), the nidus (*small arrows*) and draining vein (*curved arrow*). **B** As the balloon is deflated, contrast material rapidly advances passing through the nidus (*small arrows*), and fills the venous drainage (*curved arrow*). **C** IBCA injection with flow arrest by the microballoon (*arrowhead*). The pedicle is filled with the radiopaque acrylic (*arrow*) until the beginning of the nidus. Note the subtracted IBCA from previous depositions. **D** The balloon is deflated; nonopacified blood forwardly displaces the radiopaque acrylic column (*long arrow*) towards the nidus of the malformation (*arrowheads*). Same patient as in Fig. 3.13

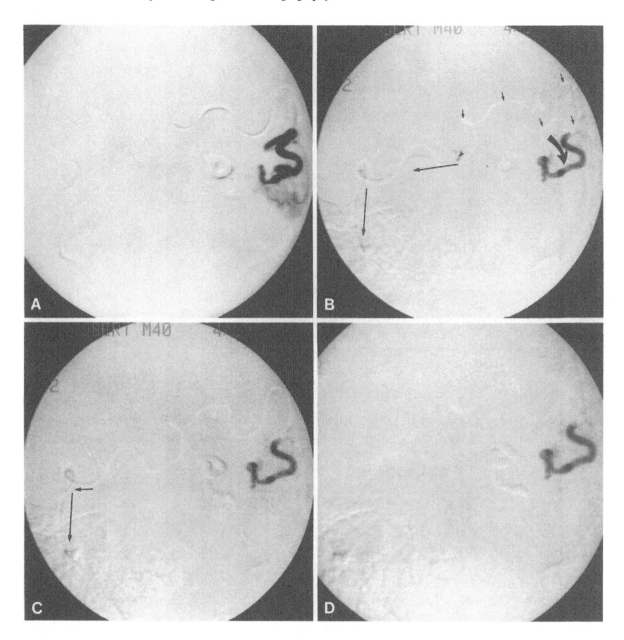

Fig. 4.41 A – D. Catheter withdrawal. Same patient as in Fig. 4.13. **A** Lateral digital subtraction angiogram (DSA) of the distal posterior cerebral artery after acrylic deposition. Negative pressure is applied to deflate the balloon (or non-balloon catheter) to retrieve back any excess acrylic into the microcatheter prior to withdrawal. The negative pressure is maintained as the microcatheter and/or introducer are being withdrawn. **B** Lateral DSA after the acrylic deposition (*curved arrow*). Note the tip of the microcatheter with the balloon deflated (*arrowhead*) and withdrawal of the radiopaque IBCA filled catheter (*arrows*). The white line of the original catheter position can be seen from the original mask (*small arrows*). If a balloon is used, the introducer catheter must be withdrawn to prevent accidental acrylic spillage when the microcatheter enters the introducer. **C** Further withdrawal of the catheter (*arrows*). **D** Final cast

of the normal brain, while diverting flow away from the malformation and slowing flow through the nidus. The slowing of flow in the nidus is clearly seen on fluoroscopy with better opacification of the AVM (Fig. 4.1). If hypotension is used, the catheter should be close to the malformation with no normal vessels between the catheter tip and the nidus. In such cases the security point (Fig. 4.2) is brought forward, and, if a normal vessel exists within the location, it will dilate and can be easily penetrated by the liquid emboli.

5. Catheter Withdrawal

Prior to the acrylic injection one must check that no proximal leaks exist in the system. The microcatheter and introducer are then checked and all excess catheter removed before embolization to insure proper response when withdrawing the microcatheter and/or introducer. The balloon is deflated or suction is applied to the catheter at the end of injection of acrylic (with or without balloon, Fig. 4.41).

Prior to embolization, one must determine the "security point" of venous occlusion, defined as the point in the venous system past which no acrylic should penetrate. In general, this point is proximal to the opening of the first normal vein. The best example is in VGAM, in which the outflow to the fistula is specifically occluded to "trap" the fistula (Fig. 4.7).

VIII. Postoperative Care

1. Cerebral AVMs

The postoperative care of patients with cerebral vascular malformations after embolization by the endovascular route is minimal. The principles previously discussed as to blood pressure monitoring, fluid restriction, anticonvulsants, corticosteroids, etc., have been reviewed. In general, it is best to avoid abrupt raises of systolic blood pressure in the postoperative period, bed rest is primarily related to the puncture site and ambulation is resumed the following day.

2. Aneurysm

The care of patients with aneurysms is similar to that of patients with other types of aneurysms or major vessel occlusion (internal carotid artery, vertebral artery, etc.) treated by other modalities. Bed rest in a flat position for the first 24–48 h with gradual elevation over 2 days, is warrented. It permits stagnant blood clots to become more stable and avoids abrupt orthostatic changes while the circulation adapts to the new arrangement (Vol. 2, Chap. 7 and Vol. 5, Chap. 3, Fig. 3.15).

3. Spinal AVMs

After spinal cord AVM embolization, bed rest for the first 24 h is followed by progressive elevation of the head in patients with cervical lesions. In those with thoracolumbar malformations, the legs should be above the heart level to assist in drainage. In patients with spinal dural AVMs with stagnant flow, a period of heparinization postoperatively may be warranted (see Vol. 5, Chap. 1).

IX. Complications of Cerebral Embolization

Major complications of cerebral embolization include ischemic episodes, which may be either temporary or permanent. Distal migration of embolic material into normal territory (stroke), embolization of the venous side or pulmonary circulation, and hemorrhage (subarachnoid and/or intracerebral) are also possible and may present either during the procedure or in the immediate postoperative period. Gluing of a microcatheter is less common but still possible. In the treatment of patients with aneurysms, stenoses, or occlusions of the parent vessel, embolic complications and vasospasm (usually secondary to previous subarachnoid hemorrhage) may occur.

1. Medical Therapy for Acute Stroke

One of the most important complications that may occur during endovascular procedures in the CNS is acute ischemia and stroke. Potential etiologies are multiple. Ischemia may follow an embolic complication from autologous clot secondary to endovascular manipulation or result from traumatic dissection of a major cerebral artery or from the iatrogenic introduction of an air bubble or other foreign material. Perhaps the most grave complication is that of the injection of embolic agent into an undesired location. Therapy for this complication is limited, due to the high sensitivity to hypoxia and ischemia of the CNS. Therefore, immediate aggressive therapy is pursued in the hope of salvaging areas of partial ischemia or a "penumbra" prior to the development of tissue death. The aim of therapy in such instances is preserving maximal brain tissue viability to maximize neurological recovery. It is a fact that infarcted brain tissue cannot be revived, but it is also recognized that functionally impaired brain tissue with critically reduced blood flow may not undergo irreversible ischemic damage if sufficient blood flow is maintained or restored. Therefore, the main goal of therapy is to preserve as much as possible of the "ischemic penumbra area," which represents tissue that is dysfunctional from ischemia but not irreversibly damaged.

The clinical management of stroke is based on a presumed pathophysiology of arterial occlusion; little experimental data exists on venous infarctions. In the complications that follow BAVM embolization, a significant, if not the most frequent, cause of postoperative symptoms are probably related to venous dysfunction. The following discussion, although based on experimental and clinical work relating to arterial occlusion, applies to improving the microcirculation at the venular level as well.

Acute ischemic stroke therapy is geared toward six major elements of potential therapeutic intervention: (1) immediate recanalization; (2) the microcirculation; (3) platelet antiaggregation drugs; (4) anticoagulation; (5) biorheologic factors; and (6) antiedema agents and pharmacological protection (Yatsu et al. 1987).

a) Recanalization

If autologous blood clot occludes a normal artery during the procedure resulting in a neurological deficit, reperfusion can usually be accomplished by the direct injection of urokinase or tissue plasminogen activator (TPA) into the clot itself. Urokinase appears best for intra-arterial injection; a starting bolus of 30000–50000 units is required, followed by infusion of up to 300000 units in 2×3 h. Caution is needed in postoperative patients, those with a previous hemorrhage, and in those in whom the lesion is still patent. Longer experience is needed to fully assess the true value of this procedure, but it may be of great assistance.

The value of tissue reperfusion, using antifibrinolytic agents, in preventing tissue damage remains unproven. Current studies, under experimental conditions, are now being carried out as to the value of antifibrinolytic therapy in association with Ca^{2+} channel blockers and free radical inhibitors. For our interest, the use of TPA or urokinase may be something to consider in an acute situation in which the embolic material is fresh and iatrogenic blood clot emboli exist. The obvious cautions are to be taken in patients with previous subarachnoid or intracerebral hemorrhagic events, in whom the TPA may dissolve autologous clot and produce cerebral hemorrhage. In addition close observation at the arteriotomy site is needed. Significant investigation is still required prior to recommending the use of TPA (see Pharmacological Protection).

If, in addition, mechanical obstacles to flow exist (balloon, stenosis), reocclusion will result and a dilatation may be needed (Fig. 4.42).

b) Microcirculation Agents

No clear-cut agent is effective in the protection of the microcirculation; however, naloxone, an opiate antagonist is potentially useful. Although no solid evidence exists as to its value, some investigators feel justified in using naloxone in view of its harmless and inexpensive nature. Furthermore, a report by Hosobuchi in 1982 suggested a beneficial effect. The recommended dose of naloxone is 0.4–1.2 mg IV and is given in the acute period (Yatsu 1987).

Vasopressure agents may carry the risk of causing intracerebral hemorrhage; they may be used occasionally to carefully elevate the diastolic pressure and initiate improvement. Vasodilators such as prostacyclins show no clear benefit. They may, in fact, produce an intracerebral reversal of flow or so called "Robin Hood" effect by "stealing" blood from the poor or ischemic tissue and diverting blood towards normal brain.

c) Platelet Antiaggregation Drugs

Platelet hyperaggregability may occur within ischemic tissue, immediately after the acute ischemic event; therefore, the use of an antiplatelet agent in

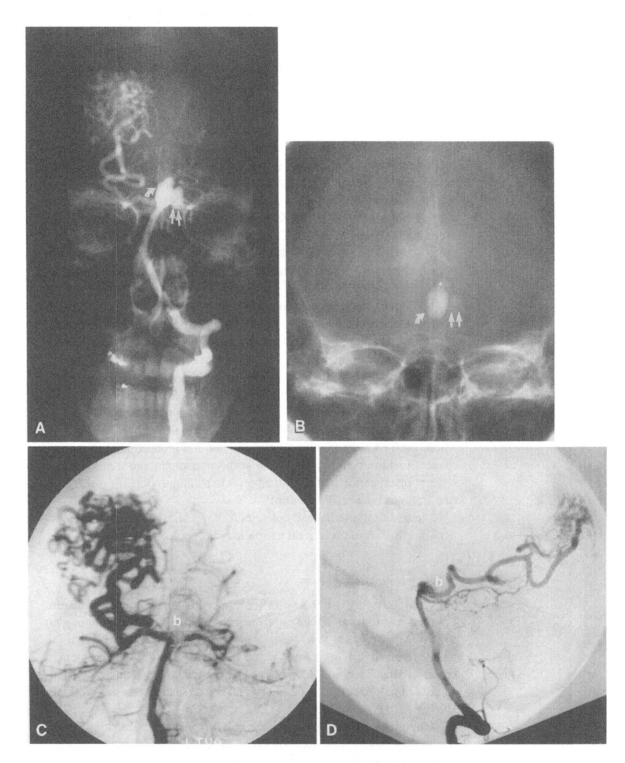

Fig. 4.42 A–H. Recanalization and angioplasty. **A** Frontal view of the left vertebral artery injection shows a basilar aneurysm (*curved arrow*) with a second dome (*double arrow*) proximal to an arteriovenous malformation (AVM). The patient presented with compression of the left pons by the aneurysm. **B** A #9 Debrun balloon filled with HEMA (Hydroxy-ethymethacrylate) has been detached in the

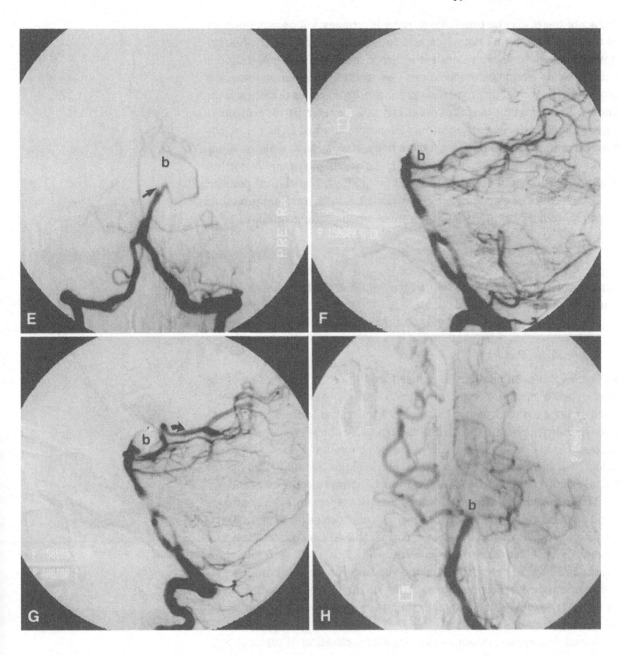

proximal dome (*curved arrow*). Note the stagnation of contrast material on the second dome (*double arrow*). **C** Frontal and **D** lateral angiograms of the left vertebral artery after balloon (*b*) detachment. There is complete exclusion of the aneurysm and preservation of all normal branches. **E** Some 36 h later the patient became comatose. Frontal digital subtraction angiogram (DSA) of the left vertebral artery 30 min after demonstrates occlusion of the distal basilar artery (*arrow*) with clot. The balloon (*b*) has come down slightly. **F** After immediate intra-arterial infusion of 150 000 units of urokinase (intermittent bolus injections of 5000–20 000 units at a time), the basilar tip has been repermeated. However, there is no filling of the right posterior cerebral artery occluded by the balloon. **G** After angioplasty to reposition the balloon, the posterior cerebral artery on the right (*curved arrow*) has been repermeated. **H** After a second angioplasty there is filling of both posterior cerebral arteries; *b*, balloon. A significant portion of the AVM was also embolized the acute stages may be beneficial to prevent propagation or augmentation of thrombosis. Aspirin or dipyridamole can reduce the recurrence of infarctions seen in patients with transient ischemic attacks. Their exact value in treating acute ischemic complications due to interventional endovascular procedures or their ability to prevent propagation of venous occlusion is unknown. Platelet antiaggregation drugs can thus be reserved for patients in whom there is evidence of repeat and/or propagation of ischemic or embolic phenomena secondary to a foreign body, stagnation in a major vessel, or the unwanted remnant of a device in the vascular system. In our experience this has only been a theoretical possibility, as in clinical practice, even when endovascular catheters have been left "glued" in a major cerebral artery, there has been no delayed thromboembolic complication.

d) Anticoagulation

Anticoagulation agents such as heparin are of limited value unless a cardiac source of emboli is identified.

e) Biorheologic Factors

Biorheological manipulations to reduce blood viscosity may be one of the most valuable measures in the treatment of stroke. Blood viscosity is primarily related to the hematocrit, fibrinogen concentration, and the erythrocyte flexibility; these are the various factors to be considered in improving regional blood flow in the areas of "ischemic penumbra" (Wood 1987). Sufficient evidence exists to recommend biorheologic manipulation in the management of some acute complications of iatrogenic embolization.

The understanding of hemorheology may be important in the management of the acute complications of endovascular occlusion of normal territories. In regions of focal cerebral ischemia, blood flow slows distal to a narrow or occluded cerebral artery segment. This slowing results in a vicious circle wherein elevation of blood viscosity further compromises perfusion and ischemia deepens. Reversibility of the neuronal insult depends on the severity of ischemia and on the ability to provide sufficient collateral circulation to maintain viability.

Animal studies have demonstrated significant elevation of regional cerebral blood flow in focally ischemic brain following hypervolemic infusion of autologous plasma or low molecular weight dextran (Wood and Fleischer 1982). Wood's group has also demonstrated that the volume of hemispheric infarction could be decreased by as much as 60% in animals which received two serial infusions of low molecular weight dextran, each equal to 20% of the total blood volume. The effect of hypervolemic hemodilution on brain perfusion is greater in regions of low blood flow and may be related to infusion-induced alterations in blood viscosity.

Although reduction of hematocrit results in a decrease in blood oxygen content, an actual increase in oxygen delivery to tissue occurs as the hematocrit is lowered to approximately 30%. In clinical practice Wood and coworkers evaluated low molecular weight dextran or 5% serum albumin solutions in patients with ischemic stroke; an improvement in regional cerebral blood flow and in electroencephalographic changes occurred. In addition, the induced augmentation of regional cerebral perfusion correlated inversely with hematocrit. Strand, in Sweden (Strand et al. 1984), confirmed the beneficial effect of hemodilution but suggested that isovolemia may decrease the possibility of edema or fluid overload. An acute reduction in hematocrit using phlebotomy and the use of low molecular weight dextrane infusions to produce an isovolemic hemodilution were recommended. In patients with acute cerebral ischemia of less than 48 h duration, an improvement in neurological scoring in the first 10 days occurred in 85% of those treated with isovolemic hemodilution, whereas only 64% of the control group showed improvement. At 3 months follow-up, both groups had similar mortality rates. In the surviving group of hemodiluted patients, however, the final outcome was significantly better. There were three times more patients able to walk than in the surviving control group. Thus, hemodilution therapy improved the overall clinical outcome of these patients.

Our own experience supports the beneficial use of isovolemic hemodilution in the treatment of acute complications of vessel occlusion during endovascular procedures. In four instances, dramatic reversal of the neurological deficits occurred within less than 48 h in all patients treated with isovolemic hemodilution immediately after appearance of symptoms.

Possibilities for the future may include the use of pentoxifylline, an inhibitor of fibrinogen synthesis, with significant decrease in blood viscosity and plasma fibrinogen concentration. In addition improved platelet deaggregation and erythrocyte filterability improved in patients with cerebral vascular disease as reported by Ott in 1983. He treated patients for 6 weeks with pentoxyifylline claiming that these patients experienced significantly fewer ischemic episodes than did control patients. Similar regimens may also be used in patients with severe stenosis and ischemic manifestations.

Wood also noted the type of patient in whom hemorheologic manipulation will not be beneficial. These include patients with intracerebral hemorrhage and increased intracranial pressure and patients with brainstem lacunar infarction.

It appears that the best regimen is the one recommended by Strand et al. (1984), i.e., isovolemic hemodilution by phlebotomy and simultaneous infusion of osmotically active agent. This regimen resulted in a reduced mean hematocrit, from 43% to 30% – 37%. Treatment should be administered in an intensive care unit, using a central venous line for monitoring of volume status and blood osmolality to prevent complications including acute tubular necrosis. More caution must be exerted in older patients. Properly monitored, this regime is safe and offers a rational means to immediately improve blood flow in the area of "ischemic penumbra." The duration of therapy will vary from a minimum of 72 h to a maximum that depends on the ability to taper the infusion while maintaining the level of improvement obtained during the course of treatment.

Other regimens of hemodilution involve continuous infusion of mannitol (Jafar et al. 1986). This has been used in patients with vasospasm secondary to subarachnoid hemorrhage. Mannitol is a diuretic and therefore a large volume of replacement fluid is needed to prevent nephrotoxicity (acute tubular necrosis). The use of pentyoxyphiline or perfluorocarbons to accomplish viscosity reduction remains to be proven.

f) Antiedema and Pharmacological Protection Agents

Brain edema due to ischemia or infarction may compromise autoregulation, produce mass effect, and further decrease tissue perfusion. The various antiedema agents include mannitol or furosemide and may be of use as temporary measures to avert herniation syndromes. As noted above, continuous infusion of mannitol has been used in some patients with vasospasm with apparently promising results (Jafar et al. 1986), primarily as a biorheologic agent. Steroids which can reduce vasogenic edema, seen primarily in tumors, have no effect on the cytotoxic edema customarily accompanying stroke and are therefore of no value in the management of stroke.

The brain has an exquisite vulnerability to ischemia or anoxia due to its high demands for metabolic substrate. The reduction in these metabolic demands will theoretically avert or minimize brain injury but this tenet is still unproven. The use of barbiturates has not proven to be of benefit for ischemic tissue, although they may be used to obtain a decrease in internal cerebral pressure. Ca^{2+} channel blockers offer a potential means of averting the reversible ischemic damage triggered by cellular influx of Ca^{2+}. In addition Ca^{2+} channel blockers may produce vasodilatation in the microcirculation. At present there is no good evidence supporting their effectiveness but they may be useful prophylactically.

g) Additional Measures

The obvious measures of general medical care to maintain proper cardiovascular competence and other medical needs in the acute stage of stroke must be considered.

Revascularization may be useful in very specific instances in which an intracranial approach to bypass or reopening of an iatrogenically occluded vessel may be warranted. This has been true for patients with prematurely detached balloons in whom immediate surgical intervention and removal of the foreign body may be life saving (Chalif 1987).

2. Hemorrhage

Hemorrhagic complications of endovascular embolizations include both subarachnoid and intracerebral hemorrhage; differentiation is important because the treatment may differ significantly. Angiography may be helpful in differentiation but an immediate CT is of more value in planning surgical treatment, as it will clearly determine if a hematoma is present, its size, location, effect on the surrounding brain, whether there is extension into the ventricular system, etc.

The availability of a properly trained and multidisciplinary team that is familiar with the acute care of patients with these types of emergencies and the need for endotracheal intubation and other types of resuscitation measures can be the key factor in the final outcome.

The hemorrhagic complications of embolization can be divided into those that occur during the procedure and those that occur after the procedure.

Bleeding that occurs during the procedure may be related to rupture of a cerebral artery during catheterization (Berenstein 1980c; Khangure and

Apsimon 1989), rupture of an aneurysm, or to rupture of the AVM itself. In the first instance, the most common cause is balloon overdistention and occurs mainly with the older model balloons, such as the silicone Kerber calibrated leak balloon. With the newer, smaller, softer, latex balloons, with a large enough leak and good memory, vessel rupture can be prevented (see Chap. 4). To avoid rupture of a small vessel, the first injection of contrast material is done very gently without balloon inflation; if the tip of the balloon is in a small branch, one will clearly see the contrast material as it exits the catheter. If the tip is in a larger branch, either rapid washout of the contrast material is noted or no contrast material can be seen fluoroscopically, as the fast flow washes it out. At this point it is safe to inflate the balloon. If one sees inflation of the balloon first, the possibility of distal occlusion or malfunction of the balloon exists and the catheter should be withdrawn to prevent overinflation.

There may be a short delay between the occurrence of the hemorrhage and its clinical manifestation. Thus, immediate recognition of extravasation fluoroscopically can be life saving. Fluoroscopically, various findings should alert one to the possibility that a vessel has been damaged. If the balloon shape changes, if no washout occurs when contrast material is injected, if contrast appearance does not conform to the expected vessel shape, or if frank extravasation is seen (contrast material taking the appearance of a sulcus or cistern; Fig. 4.43), one must be ready to immediately seal off the vessel (Berenstein 1980c). The catheter is left in place as the fastest means to accomplish hemostasis. The microcatheter itself may be tamponading the leak, and if withdrawn further bleeding can occur as the vessel may not be able to retract. Catheter flushing is stopped to avoid additional extravasation.

In view of this potential complication, we routinely have the various materials for acrylic embolization ready, including tantalum, and syringes filled with nonionic 5% distilled water. The acrylic (without iophendylate) is immediately opened and mixed with the tantalum. (In general, if the acrylic is open and exposed to air for a relatively long period of time, it may polymerize at the table or prematurely). The hub of the microcatheter is immediately rinsed with the 5% distilled water solution. Only 0.1 ml of this solution is used to rinse the microcatheter shaft, to avoid excessive additional extravasation. The acrylic-tantalum mixture is then gently injected to produce hemostasis, without balloon inflation. Simultaneous with closing the ruptured vessel, reversal of heparinization is accomplished. The patient's neurological and clinical status are checked, and the appropriate measures are taken. Immediately after stabilization, a control low volume angiogram is done and a CT is performed which will further guide management. The CT appearance of subarachnoid hemorrhage cannot differentiate blood from extravasated contrast material. The purpose of CT is to determine if a surgical lesion exists (Fig. 4.44). If using a Tracker or similar microcatheter, and extravasation is noted, a coil can be used to seal the hole; as the coil is advanced the microcatheter is withdrawn (Halbach 1990, unpublished data).

An additional cause of intraoperative hemorrhage is a small remnant of malformation or a very small branch that remains at or near the embolized pedicle (Fig. 4.45) after occlusion. This situation can be avoided by completely sealing the pedicle at time of acrylic deposition.

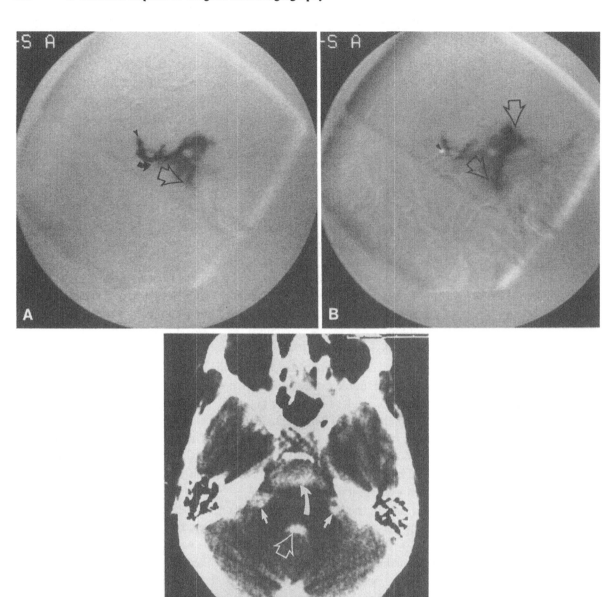

Fig. 4.43 A – C. Extravasation of contrast material. **A** Early and **B** later phases of the superselective injection in a posterior thalamo-perforating artery with a small, occlusive, calibrated leak balloon (*arrowhead*); oblique view. Note the vessel filling (*curved arrow*) and the extravasation into the prepontine cistern (*open arrowhead*). **B** The microcatheter was removed (*arrowhead*) and there is further extravasation (*open arrowheads*). Note the appearance of the contrast material delineating the prepontine cistern. **C** Axial CT demonstrates extravasation into the fourth ventricle (*open arrowhead*), prepontine cistern (*curved arrow*), and cerebellopontine cisterns (*arrows*)

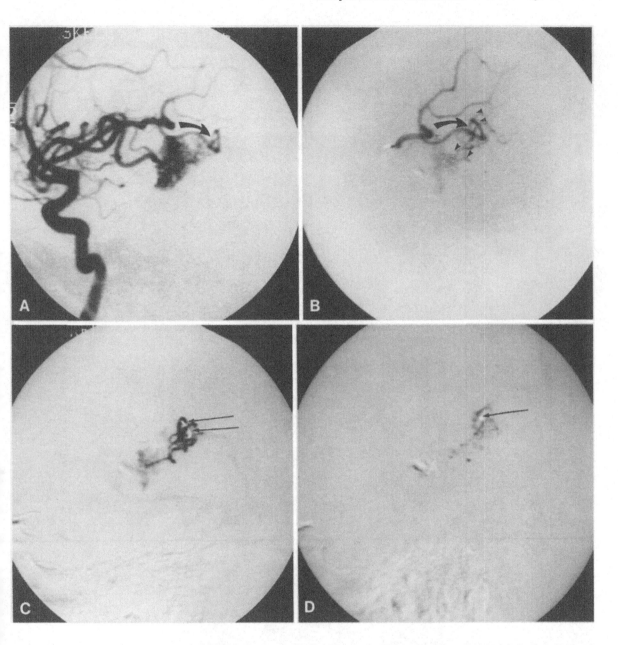

Fig. 4.44 A–G. Postembolization hemorrhage. **A** Lateral view of the left internal carotid artery midarterial phase demonstrates the remaining middle cerebral supply (*curved arrow*) to a temporal vascular malformation in the midtemporal gyrus. **B** Last vessel to be embolized (*curved arrow*) shows small distal vessels going towards the malformation "en passage" (*arrowheads*). **C** Catheterization of the remaining supply (*arrows*). There is no normal vessel filling. **D** Digital subtraction angiogram (DSA) image from the acrylic deposition which is radiopaque. The tip of the catheter has been removed (*arrow*)

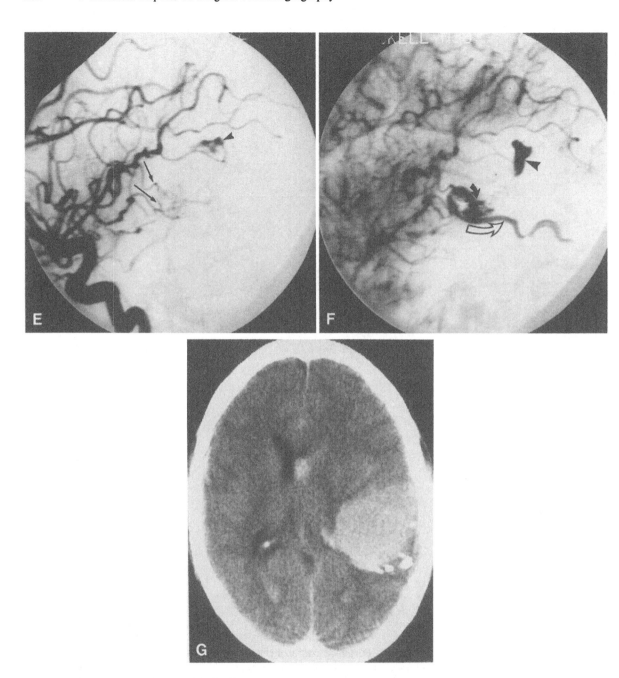

Fig. 4.44. E Immediate postembolization angiogram demonstrates extravasation at the site of occlusion (*arrowheads*). A small contribution to the malformation remains (*arrows*). **F** Midphase of the same injection shows additional extravasation (*arrowhead*), associated with increase in mass effect and small amount of filling of the malformation (*curved arrow*) and draining vein (*open curved arrow*). **G** Immediate CT scan demonstrates the large mass effect with hemorrhage extending into the ventricular system

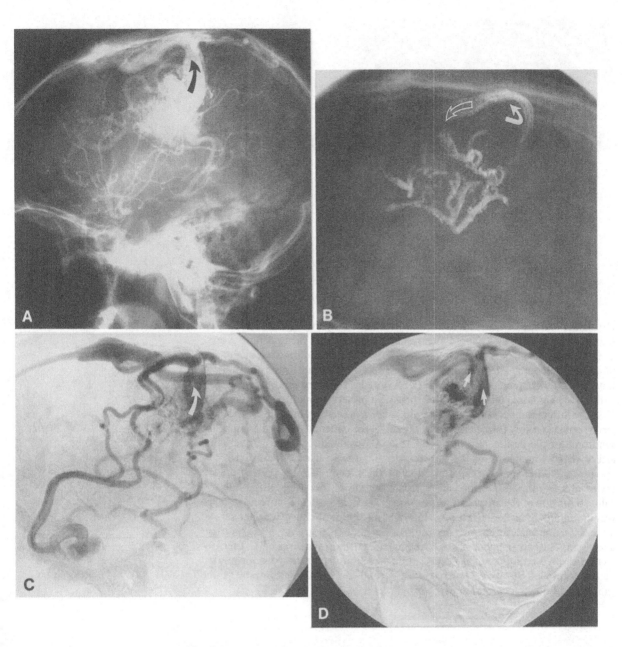

Fig. 4.45 A–D. Low thrombogenicity of the cyanoacrylate. **A** Late phase of the left internal carotid artery demonstrates an arteriovenous malformation with drainage through a hypertrophied cortical parietal vein (*curved arrow*). **B** Plain film of the skull after NBCA embolization. Note the migration of the radiopaque acrylic through the vein (*broken white arrow*) and the dilution of the cyanoacrylate layering against the vessel wall by nonopaque blood. **C** Immediate postembolization control angiogram in the late phase demonstrates contrast material passing around the cyanoacrylate (*white curved arrow*). **D** A 6 month follow-up angiogram demonstrates patency of the same vein. There is no delay thrombosis to the intraluminal cyanoacrylate

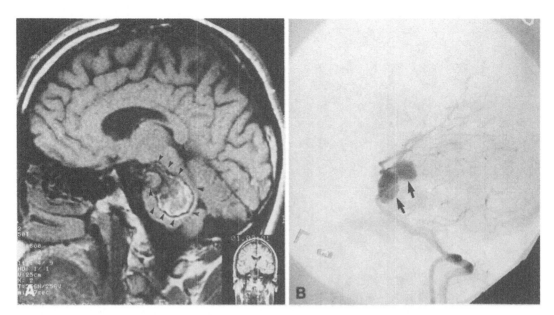

Fig. 4.46 A–F. Use of intravenous tissue plasminogen activator (TPA); midbasilar multilobule partially thrombosed aneurysm. **A** Sagittal MRI demonstrates a large aneurysm of the midbasilar region (*arrowheads*). **B** Lateral subtraction angiogram of the left vertebral artery demonstrates two lobes of the aneurysm (*arrows*). **C** Lateral digital subtraction angiogram (DSA) of the right vertebral artery after a balloon (*b*) has been placed in the first lobe, with preservation of the basilar artery. Note the inflow and outflow (*curved arrows*). There is small amount of contrast material seen posteriorly (*small arrow*). **D** After 72 h the patient developed an ischemic syndrome of the basilar territory. Frontal DSA examination of the left vertebral artery shows thrombosis of the basilar artery at the level of the aneurysm (*arrowhead*). **E** After systemic heparinization and intravenous TPA, a DSA of the left vertebral artery injection demonstrates recanalization of the distal basilar but also filling a portion of the aneurysm (*arrowhead*). The neurological syndrome resolved within minutes after the intravenous TPA administration. **F** Right internal carotid artery injection while attempting occlusion of the midbasilar artery for the recurrent aneurysm. The patient had a massive subarachnoid hemorrhage. Vertebral artery injection showed no intracranial flow. Carotid injection demonstrated extravasation in the region of the clivus (*curved open arrow*) and significant spasm of the supraclinoid internal carotid artery (*arrow*)

Intraoperative hemorrhage is also caused by occlusion of the venous outflow, without occluding the inflow. Some venous embolization occurs frequently without clinical consequences. Venous migration manifests itself fluoroscopically as the column flow is changed in diameter or the diameter of the acrylic column abruptly increases (Fig. 4.5 D). This change in column diameter represents filling of the fistulization site, with flow from other sources washing or "spreading" the polymerizing acrylic column into the periphery of the vein (Fig. 4.45). When radiopaque acrylic is seen to enter the venous side, the injection of additional NBCA should not be discontinued but should actually be speeded up to seal off the shunt and prevent further migration of glue (see Chap. 5, Vein of Galen Aneurysmal Malformation). Alternatively, the injection is resumed 1–2 s later to permit polymerization of the portion that has reached the fistula.

Migration of embolic material into a major sinus structure, such as the straight sinus, is potentially dangerous. In most cases, however, as the un-

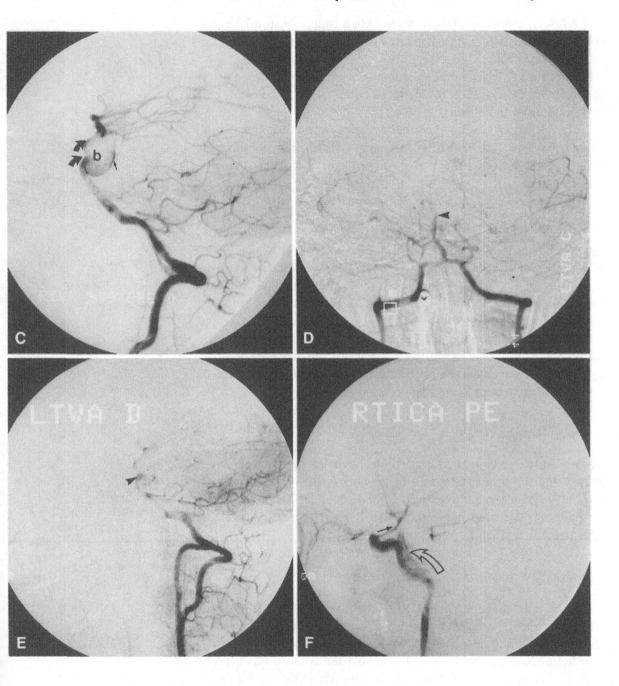

polymerized acrylic reaches a large venous structure it will either fragment or layer against one of the vessel walls without occluding it either acutely or later (Fig. 4.45 D). This lack of occlusion testifies to the mechanical nature of cyanoacrylate occlusion with no or minimal delayed thrombosis.

Migration of embolic material into the pulmonary circulation is usually asymptomatic, even with relatively large amounts in adults (Capan et al. 1983). However, in newborns or infants with a compromised cardiopulmonary system even small amounts of embolic material escaping into the lungs can result in death (Berenstein 1980c).

In infants with high-flow lesions, one can avoid distal migration of acrylic material by using pure acrylic-tantalum mixture injected against the vessel wall, first very slowly and then rapidly to create a "mushroom" (see

Figs. 4.7, 4.11, and Chap. 5). Flow arrest with a balloon that inflates prior to leaking is also useful as is hypotension (Fig. 4.22) or using coils as a buffer (Figs. 4.31, 4.32).

If at the time of injection the balloon is seen to inflate more than before, no further acrylic is injected; the increased distal resistance represents polymerization or no more nidus.

On rare occasions a hemorrhage has occurred some hours after embolization (from 2 to 24 h). The cause is usually difficult to establish and its management is that of other causes of hemorrhage. We have seen this occur in three patients.

3. Distal Embolization

Distal embolization may occur into a normal artery and is handled like other causes of ischemic complications (see Medical Therapy for Acute Stroke). Blood clot formation can be treated with thrombolytic therapy (Fig. 4.46) (see Vol. 5, Chap. 3). It may also occur into the venous or pulmonary circulations.

Embolic material reaching the venous side of an AVM is not an infrequent occurrence. It is usually of no consequence and may even be advantageous as it may promote complete thrombosis of the lesion, provided the nidus and afferent pedicle are also occluded (see Chap. 3).

4. Arterial Stenosis

Stenosis of a cerebral artery can follow balloon detachment (Vol. 4, Chap. 3, Fig. 3.7) or may be caused by the neck of the balloon (Fig. 4.42). Angioplasty of the stenotic segment at the level of the balloon is usually possible using a second nondetachable balloon (Hieshima, unpublished data) (see Vol. 5, Chap. 3, Aneurysm).

5. Vasospasm

Cerebral vasospasm during navigation is infrequent. We have seen it almost exclusively when treating patients in the acute stage after hemorrhage. Therefore, embolization of cerebral AVMs is usually delayed 6–8 weeks after hemorrhage, as the risk of rebleed from the AVM in this period is minimal. The use of Ca^{2+} channel blockers has been advocated as a prophylactic measure to prevent vasospasm during cerebral navigation (Merland, unpublished data) and should be given 24 h prior to the procedure. We have not had the need to use it. Spasm can occur at the level of the internal carotid artery when the introducer catheter is wedged, is at a sharp curve, or is frequently moved. For the most part, slight proximal withdrawal of the introducer will be sufficient to relieve the spasm and Ca^{2+} channel blockers have not been of major help in the acute stages (personal experience). In the few patients with hyperreactive vessels, preoperative Ca^{2+} channel blockers may be useful. If severe spasm is a problem the procedure can be stopped and repeated after Ca^{2+} channel blockers have been given. It is important to recognize this spasm to avoid inadvertent "steal" from the opposite side or from the posterior circulation (see Vol. 2, Chap. 8, CCF).

CHAPTER 5

Arteriovenous Fistulas of the Brain

I. Introduction

In a certain group of patients the angioarchitectural abnormality is a direct arteriovenous fistula(s) (AVFs), without an intervening angiomatous complex (see Chap. 1) (Fig. 5.1). This type of lesion represented 15% of our referred patients (138/900) and 20% of the patients embolized (116/560). Other lesions incorporating direct fistulas are described elsewhere, including in Vol. 2, and Chap. 8, Dural AVFs and in Chap. 3, this volume.

Since most AVFs of the brain are observed in the pediatric population, we believe that they deserve a special section. Two major groups of lesions can be distinguished: (1) Fistulas associated with dilatation of the vein of Galen precursor – the vein of Galen aneurysmal malformations (VGAMs); these are located in the subarachnoid space. (2) Direct AVFs between cerebral arteries and pial veins (brain AVFs); these are located subpially.

VGAMs represented 12.2% of the arteriovenous malformations (AVMs) in patients referred to both centers (New York and Bicêtre, Surgical Neuro-angiography Sections) and 16.9% of those in embolized patients. Pial AVFs are much less common; they were seen in 3.1% of referrals and 3.75% of treated patients.

Patients in these two groups have some similarities in clinical presentation, primarily as a result of the systemic effects of the high-flow fistula. Significant clinical differences do exist, mainly in the neurological consequences of the lesion. Hemorrhage, for example, in a genuine VGAM is a distinct rarity.

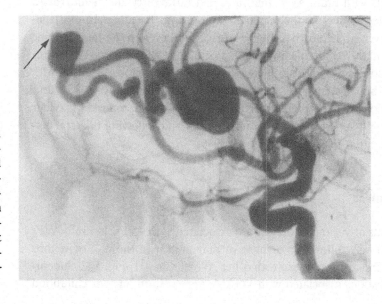

Fig. 5.1. Right internal carotid artery injection in lateral projection. Typical aspect of a pial arteriovenous fistula. The arteriovenous shunt (*arrow*) is easily recognized by the change in vessel caliber. Additional venous changes distal to the shunt can be appreciated by the narrowing and more distal dilatation

II. Systemic and Neurological Manifestations in AVFs

1. Congestive Heart Failure

The abrupt onset of congestive heart failure (CHF) in AVF patients at or shortly after birth has been attributed to the fact that arteriovenous shunting occurs independently of pulmonary vascular resistance. The shunt results from loss of the low resistance placenta with an associated rise of systemic vascular resistance at birth (Rudolph 1970; Ross et al. 1986). In addition to increased preload, the newborn's heart may not be able to adjust cardiac output appropriately in the face of severe changes in preload and afterload (Nelson 1984). In autopsies of newborns with high-flow AVMs, the heart is usually enlarged, but otherwise normal. The causes for the fatal cardiomegaly and events leading to cardiac decomposition are not fully understood.

2. Failure to Thrive

Failure to thrive is a frequent finding in children with AVFs, the cause of which is not always clear. It may represent a combination of factors that lead to decreased tissue perfusion. The main feature appears to be CHF with poor caloric intake and increased metabolic demands in the face of poor tissue perfusion. Arterial "steal" through the arteriovenous shunt as a cause of symptoms is not a satisfactory explanation (Grossman et al. 1984).

3. Prominence of CSF Spaces

Prominence of CSF spaces and hydrocephalus are a well known finding in children with AVFs (Figs. 5.2, 5.3). In many patients presenting with ventricular enlargement or prominent CSF spaces, there is no evidence of mechanical obstruction to CSF flow.

In patients with brain AVFs that have had intraventricular hemorrhage, ventriculomegaly may be the result of the previous bleeding. In most patients, however, no hemorrhage has occurred, and even in the face of some mass effect in the region of the aqueduct or other CSF pathway, the hydrodynamic disorder results from increased intracranial venous pressure, with consequent impairment of CSF reabsorption (Zerah et al. 1992). Hydrocephalus secondary to venous hypertension has also been reported to occur in patients with superior vena cava obstruction and following bilateral cervical vein ligation in dogs (Ross et al. 1986).

4. Calcifications

Calcifications of various etiologies are associated with AVFs. In brain AVFs calcification may follow hemorrhage or may appear in the wall of venous structures, similar to that seen with other AVMs (Chap. 1, Fig. 3.1). Subcortical calcifications associated with VGAMs appear in infancy or childhood

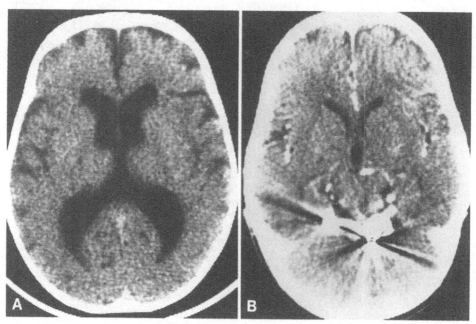

Fig. 5.2 A, B. Decrease in CSF spaces. Axial MRI cuts. **A** CT scans before and **B** 24 h after partial embolization of a choroidal VGAM. Note the decreased ventricular si and reexpansion of the cortical mantle after embolization

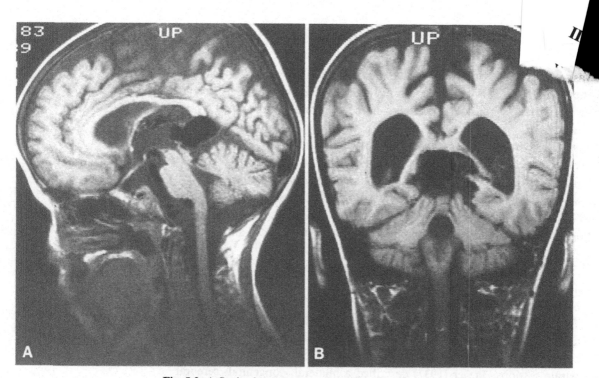

Fig. 5.3. A Sagittal and **B** coronal MRI in a patient presenting with a vein of Galen aneurysmal malformation. Note the large subarachnoid spaces and the patency of the aqueduct of the mesencephalon

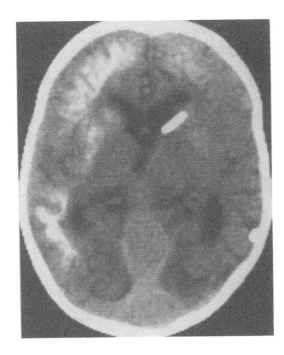

Fig. 5.4. Significant subcortical calcifications. The patient was previously shunted for hydrocephalus

but are not seen in neonates (Fig. 5.4). They have a characteristic appearance and correspond to decreased tissue perfusion at the level of the medullary veins-venous watershed. Their appearance may be precipitated by ventricular shunting (Zerah et al. 1992). They may precede localized atrophy (Fig. 5.5) similar to what is seen in Sturge-Weber syndrome.

II. Arteriovenous Shunts Involving the Vein of Galen

Vascular malformations that involve the vein of Galen region and that are characterized by variable dilatation of the great cerebral vein or its precursor have received considerable interest in the literature. Unfortunately, various types of lesions harboring vastly differing pathologies are often grouped together. In addition, the term "vein of Galen aneurysm" is an ill-suited use of the word "aneurysm" to describe the venous dilatation or ectasia present in such lesions. This imprecise and misleading terminology causes confusion with regard to the cause and classification of these lesions (Lunsden 1947; Wolfe and France 1949; French and Peyton 1954; Thomson 1959; Poppen 1960; Hirano 1960; Gagnon and Boileau 1960; Russell and Newton 1964; Gold et al. 1964; Lorber 1967).

Steinheil (1895) described the postmortem finding in a 49 year old man who had both a VGAM and a separate frontal AVM. This lesion was obviously a cerebral AVM with drainage through an ectatic vein of Galen.

The first attempt at treatment was probably that of Blance (1905), as cited by Pool (1968). The patient, an 11 month old girl with a history of intracranial hypertension, underwent ligation of both carotid arteries at separate sessions. Jaeger (1937) described a bilateral, congenital, cerebral arteriovenous communication into an aneurysm of the vein of Galen. The pathology was reviewed by Padget (1948). Boldrey and Miller (1949) report-

Fig. 5.5. Significant brain atrophy in an 8 month old infant with a nontreated pial arteriovenous fistula who presented with convulsions since birth. Note the atrophy in the left hemisphere adjacent to the fistula

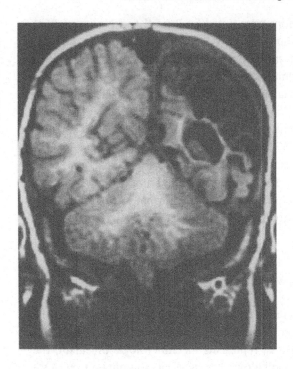

ed on two patients also treated by ligation. Both had what appeared to be a true fistula into an aneurysmally dilated great cerebral vein of Galen, diagnosed for the first time with angiography. Recognition of this type of malformation as the cause of congestive cardiac failure during the neonatal period was reported by Pollock and Laslett (1958) and Claireaux and Newman (1960). Corrin (1959) and Glatt and Rowe (1960) reported additional cases of CHF in newborns or infants which were associated with similar cerebrovascular malformations.

From these early reports, the supposed link between the arteriovenous lesions, hydrocephalus, abnormal collateral circulation, epistaxis, and subarachnoid hemorrhage was postulated. In 1960 Litvak gave the first anatomical definition of these vascular malformations, allowing a clearer distinction to be made between AVFs with dilation of the vein of Galen and other midline AVMs with drainage via a dilated vein of Galen. Litvak referred to these lesions as primary and secondary aneurysms of the vein of Galen, respectively. In 1964 Gold reviewed 34 patients described in the literature and correlated age at presentation, clinical syndromes, and pathophysiology. He established three groups based on clinical grounds which he felt were characteristic: (1) neonates with severe congestive heart failure CHF; (2) infants and young children with hydrocephalus or convulsions; and (3) older children or adults with headaches and/or subarachnoid hemorrhage. Amacher et al. (1979) modified this classification by adding a fourth group of neonates and young infants with mild CHF and macrocephaly. More recently, the clinical descriptions have become more precise.

Following Litvak et al. (1960), Clarisse et al. (1978) suggested that true and false vein of Galen AVMs should be distinguished; however, both authors failed to establish clear-cut definitions for the two groups.

Thomson (1959) commented on the lack of opacification of the straight and transverse sinuses on angiography in patients with "vein of Galen aneurysms". Similar observations were noted by Russell and Newton (1964), Clarisse et al. (1978). Lasjaunias et al. (1987) drew attention to the dural sinus anomalies observed in most vein of Galen aneurysms. Since absence of the straight sinus is extremely rare, the high frequency of these findings in association with vein of Galen aneurysms is remarkable. Often, a falcine sinus drains the aneurysmal sac towards the posterior third of the superior sagittal sinus. Such a pattern has been previously recognized (Glatt and Rowe 1960; Clarisse et al. 1978) and is frequently apparent in the illustrations of many authors (Gomez et al. 1963; Lehman et al. 1966; Agee et al. 1969; O'Brien and Schechter 1970; Montoya 1970; Long et al. 1974; Bartal 1975 and others). This venous configuration is normal in the human embryo (Okudera 1984) and is occasionally observed after birth (Huang 1984).

1. Embryology

A major advance in the understanding of this group of lesions was the recognition by Raybaud et al. (1989) that the dilated midline vein cannot be the vein of Galen but instead represents its embryologic precursor, the median vein of the prosencephalon. The arterial anatomy in VGAMs indicates that the event leading to the defect occurs after the stage of 21−23 mm embryo, prior to the development of the vein of Galen and straight sinus (Raybaud et al. 1989, see Vol. 3, Chap. 7). The transient median vein of the prosencephalon normally disappears before the 50 mm stage. During the period between 21−23 mm (6 weeks) and 50 mm (11 weeks), the pallium itself is only beginning to grow and its intrinsic vascularization is not yet established.

As vascularity in the region develops, an adaptation to the particular condition created by the "parasitic" fistula shunting the pericerebral blood away should occur. Dilated veins may also be related to redirection of blood from the fistula or to compensation in the drainage of the normal brain. When redirection of the normal venous flow is present, it routes to the cavernous sinus through the deep and superficial middle cerebral veins and then to the ophthalmic veins and/or the pterygoid venous plexus. These collateral pathways explain the prominent facial and scalp veins in these patients and the reported cases of epistaxis (Litvak et al. 1960; Hoffman et al. 1982; Johnston et al. 1987) (Figs. 5.22−5.24). The enlarged veins may eventually disappear if complete obliteration of the fistula is accomplished (Fig. 5.23) but may persist as the only outflow of the normal cerebral circulation (Fig. 5.24).

These are therefore fundamental differences between lesions which we term VGAM in which the vein of Galen is absent (malformed) and those in which the vein of Galen is present but is aneurysmally dilated. The latter arise secondary to a deep-seated AVM draining into a true vein of Galen with compromised venous outflow resulting in aneurysmal venous dilatation (Lasjaunias et al. 1987). Based on these significant angioarchitectural differences, various groups of patients can be recognized. These are described below.

Fig. 5.6. A vein of Galen malformation demonstrating the different arterial feeders opening either directly into the ectatic venous pouch or into choroidal venous afferents (*asterisks*). *1*, anterior choroidal artery; *2*, posterolateral choroidal artery; *3*, medial choroidal artery; *4*, circumferential artery; *5*, subependymal channel; *6*, subfornical artery. (Reprinted from Lasjaunias et al. 1989a)

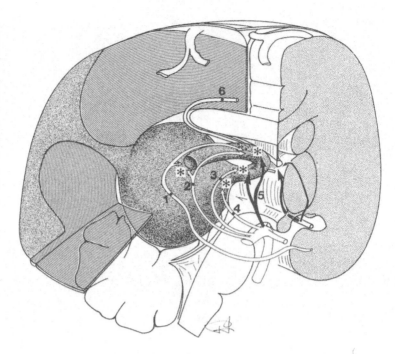

2. Vein of Galen Aneurysmal Malformation

a) Architecture

In this type of lesion there is a true malformation in the development of the vein of Galen (Fig. 5.6). The lesion is an arteriovenous shunt(s) involving the embryologic precursor to the vein of Galen, the median vein of the prosencephalon. The vein of Galen as a confluence of normal cerebral venous tributaries does not exist. It is "replaced" by the persistence of an

Fig. 5.7. Superolateral view of the choroid fissure demonstrating the deep cerebral venous pathways in a vein of Galen aneurysmal malformation. *1*, septal vein; *2*, internal cerebral vein; *3*, thalamostriate vein; *4*, longitudinal caudate vein; *5*, atrial vein; *6*, ventral diencephalic vein; *7*, anterior pontomesencephalic vein; *8*, inferior choroidal vein; *9*, tentorial sinus; *10*, subtemporal vein; *11*, interstriate anastomosis; *12*, basal vein; *13*, media/parietal vein. (Reprinted from Lasjaunias et al. 1991a)

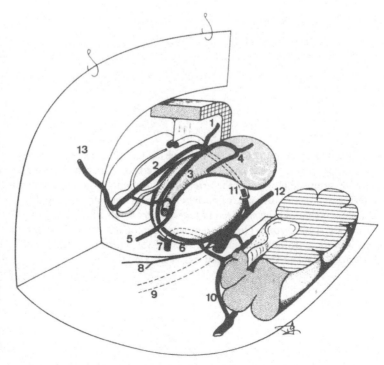

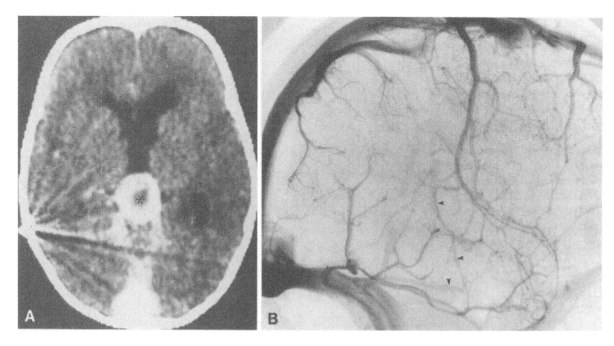

Fig. 5.8. A Axial CT and **B** late venous phase of the internal carotid artery injection in a patient with spontaneous closure of a vein of Galen aneurysmal malformation diagnosed 6 months following ventricular shunting for hydrocephalus. Note the typical shape of the deep venous drainage (*arrowheads*) opening into a tentorial sinus. (Reprinted from Lasjaunias et al. 1987)

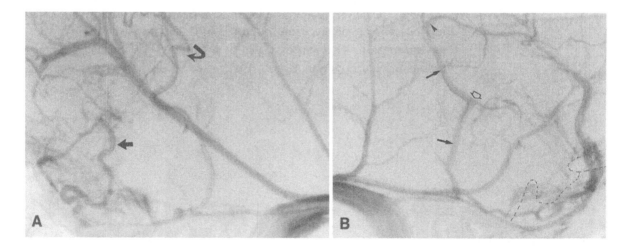

Fig. 5.9. A Left and **B** right venous phases of the internal carotid injection, lateral projections, in a patient with a previously embolized vein of Galen aneurysmal malformation, with complete closure of the arteriovenous shunt. Note the typical embryonic pattern in the venous drainage of both hemispheres opening into subtemporal veins. On the left side (**A**) the striate vein (*curved arrow*) also drains into the deep sylvian venous system (*arrow*). On the right side, the thalamostriate vein (*arrowhead*) opens into the retrothalamic and subtemporal veins (*arrows*); basal vein junction, *open arrow*. (Reprinted from Lasjaunias et al. 1991)

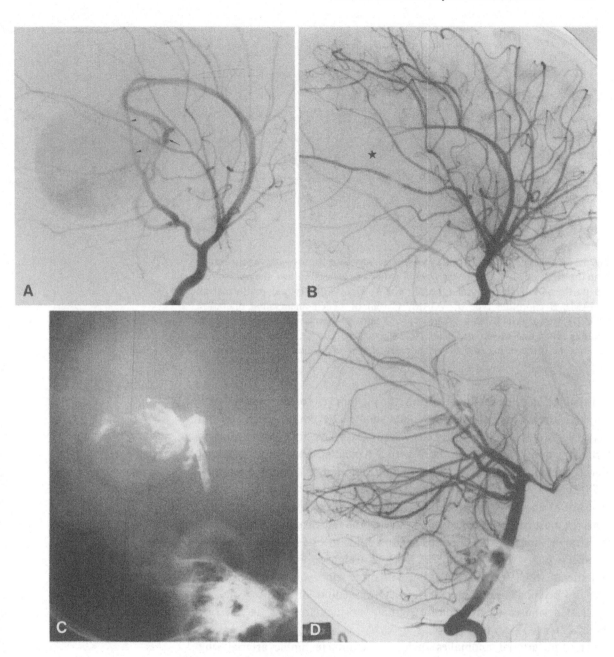

Fig. 5.10. Right internal carotid angiogram **A** before and **B** after embolization with NBCA. **C** Plain skull film and **D** left vertebral angiography in lateral projection after embolization. **A** Mural type of vein of Galen aneurysmal malformation (*arrow*). Note the persistant limbic arterial ring (*arrowheads*). **B** Following complete closure of the lesion there is a complete spontaneous regression of the limbic system (*star*). In the vertebral artery injection (**D**) note the compensatory supply to the singular gyrus territory taken over by the posterior cerebral artery

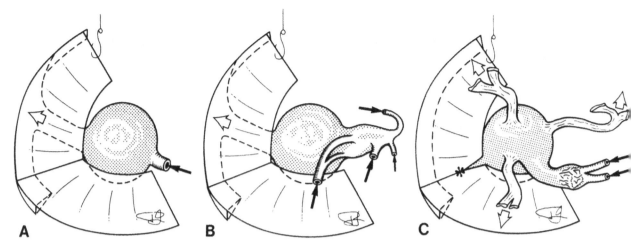

Fig. 5.11A–C. The three different types of arteriovenous shunts with venous ectasias in the pineal region. The *solid arrows* illustrate the arterial inflow, the *open arrow* the outflow. **A** Typical mural type of vein of Galen aneurysmal malformation (VGAM); **B** choroidal type of VGAM; **C** vein of Galen aneurysmal dilatation (VGAD) with arterial afferents (*arrows*) to a cerebral arteriovenous malformation draining into a dilated vein of Galen. Note the distal occlusion of the straight sinus (*asterisk*) and the reflux into the usual cerebral venous afferents (*open arrows*)

embryologic midline venous structure (the median vein of the prosencephalon) that drains only the arteriovenous shunt. The normal deep cerebral structures drain through alternate venous pathways that correspond to "frozen" embryonic configurations with a typical epsilon shape on lateral view (Lasjaunias et al. 1991; Mayberg and Zimmerman 1988; Yokota et al. 1978) (Figs. 5.7–5.10). This drainage is through dural sinuses that present anatomical anomalies representing persistence of embryologic configurations. In most cases drainage occurs through the falcine sinus (precursor of the straight sinus) to the superior sagittal sinus in one or more than one channel (Chap. 4, Fig. 4.31 and Fig. 5.11). A straight sinus is seldom present in patients with VGAMs. Persistence of other embryologic dispositions, such as occipital and marginal sinuses, or venous anomalies, such as duplicated sinuses or hypoplastic sigmoid or jugular veins, is not rare (Fig. 5.22).

Persisting arterial anomalies such as a complete limbic arterial ring (Vol. 3, Chap. 3, Figs. 3.10, 3.14, 5.10) further illustrate the embryonic onset of the VGAM. Following partial or complete occlusion of the arteriovenous shunt, maturation of both the cortical venous system and the embryonic arterial ring disposition can be observed (Fig. 5.10).

The AVF in VGAM may be single or multiple. If single it may be either a single pedicle or multiple pedicles which converge into the same fistula site (Chap. 4, Fig. 4.39). According to the location of the fistula two different subtypes of VGAM can be distinguished, choroidal and mural (Fig. 5.11).

Choroidal VGAMs

In the choroidal VGAM multiple fistulas are located in the cistern of the velum interposition anywhere within the tela choroidea. The shunt is extracerebral, subarachnoid, and communicates with the anterior aspect of

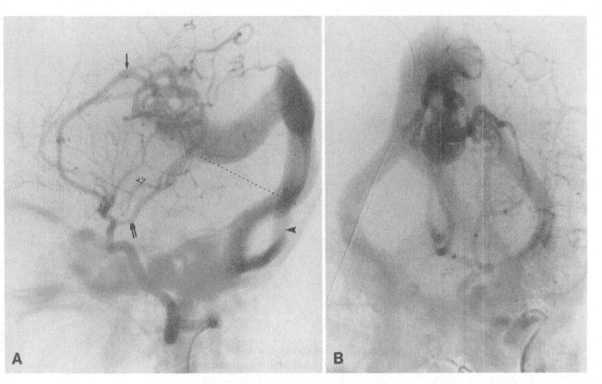

Fig. 5.12 A, B. Typical aspects of the choroidal type of vein of Galen aneurysmal malformation (VGAM) in a neonate. **A** Internal carotid artery injection in lateral and **B** frontal projections. Multiple arterial feeders can be recognized on frontal views (*asterisks*). The straight sinus is outlined by the *interrupted line*. Note the anterior choroidal supply (*open arrow*), the subfornical contribution (*arrow*), the posterior cerebral artery branches (*double arrows*), and the medial occipital sinus (*arrowhead*)

the median vein of the prosencephalon. The arterial feeders are usually bilateral and correspond to the normal choroidal arteries, subfornical branch, or pericallosal artery or subependymal branches of the thalamo-perforators. This type of VGAM usually causes heart failure in newborns and can be recognized by its complex arterial network (Figs. 5.11B, 5.12, Chap. 4, Fig. 4.32).

Mural VGAMs

In the mural type of VGAM, the fistula is in the wall of the median pros-encephalic vein, usually in its inferolateral margin and is also extracerebral and subarachnoid. The vessels supplying the shunt are usually the collicular and/or the posterior choroidal arteries and may be unilateral or bilateral. Clinically, the mural types of VGAMs present later in infants with macrocephaly or failure to thrive and may be associated with mild cardiac failure or asymptomatic cardiomegaly (Figs. 5.11A, 5.13).

b) Clinical Manifestations

The clinical manifestations are grossly characteristic of each age group (Fig. 5.14). In neonates cardiac failure is usually the most prominent clinical feature, while in older infants macrocephaly or neurological symptoms are

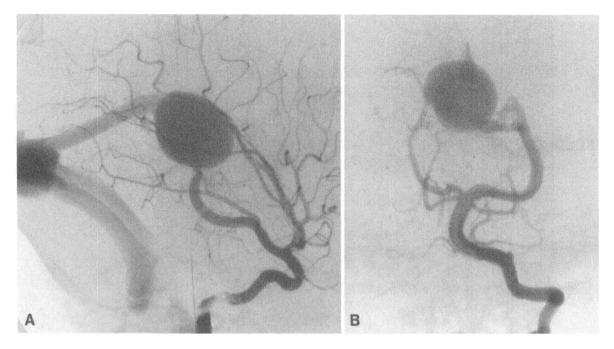

Fig. 5.13. Internal carotid angiogram in lateral projection (**A**) and vertebral artery in frontal projection (**B**) in a mural vein of Galen aneurysmal malformation in an infant. Note the normal development of the straight sinus in this patient with a single-hole fistula

more frequent. Incidental discovery of a VGAM is only possible when secondary complications occur, as will be discussed below. Different angioarchitectural groups of lesions will often present in patients at different ages. The natural history also differs significantly (Table 5.1) (Conqvist et al. 1972; Cumming 1980; Levine et al. 1962; Ross et al. 1986; Al Watban and Banna 1987).

Cardiac Manifestations

These are mostly seen in the neonate group. The degree of cardiac symptomatology is extremely variable, spanning a broad range from asymptomatic cardiomegaly to multiple organ failure resistant to all medical the-

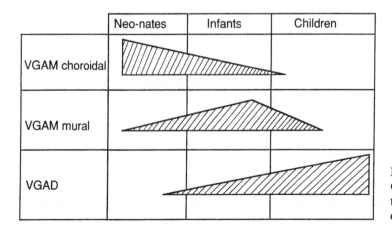

Fig. 5.14. Frequency of vein of Galen aneurysmal malformation (VGAM) and aneurysmal dilatation per age group

Table 5.1. Differential characteristics between vein of Galen aneurysmal malformation (VGAM) vein of Galen aneurysmal dilatation (VGAD)

	VGAM		VGAD
	Choroidal	Mural	
Vein of Galen afferents	No	No	Yes
Dorsal vein of the prosencephalon	Yes	Yes	No
Falcine sinus	Frequent	Possible	Rare
Communication with cerebral veins	No	No	Yes
Most frequent age of onset	Newborns	Infants	Children
CHF	Almost constant	Frequent	Rare
CSF disorders	Frequent	Frequent	Rare
Failure to thrive	Yes	Possible	Possible
Expected rate of cure per type with embolization	High	Very high	Low
Natural history	Unknown	Unknown	Same as deep-seated AVM with an already existing venous stenosis
Risk of future hemorrhage	If distal, dural spinal thrombosis[a]	If distal, dural spinal thrombosis[a]	Very high
Risk of future focal neurological symptoms	If ventricular shunting or calcification[b]	If ventricular shunting of calcification[b]	Very high

[a] Reflux of the arteriovenous shunt previous dural drainage into the cerebral vein.
[b] Mechanical and or hemodynamic impairment of transcerebral venous drainage and unfavorable anatomical disposition.

rapy. The reasons for this wide spectrum of cardiac manifestations are still poorly understood. The size of the shunt, the type of venous drainage, the degree of outflow restriction, the complexity of arterial supply, and the response of the host must be considered, although the exact role of each of these factors is neither conclusive nor sufficiently proven. In our series, major cardiac failure, when present, was always diagnosed before 2 weeks of age, none appeared later. Failure often evolves during the first 5 days of life before responding to medical management (Garcia-Monaco et al. 1991).

Patients with choroidal types of VGAMs usually present with heart failure and therefore are diagnosed earlier than those with the mural form. Mural VAGMs seldom produce severe cardiac symptoms and patients present later with macrocephaly. Occasionally, cyanosis may be associated with the heart failure; a right to left shunt or a persistent fetal type of circulation are the features usually responsible for the cyanosis. An atrial communication may be present when right atrial pressure overload hinders the closure of the foramen ovale. Patent ductus arteriosus in these patients should not be regarded as a true associated cardiac malformation but as an adaptive response to flow and oxygen pressure changes. Patent ductus, however, oc-

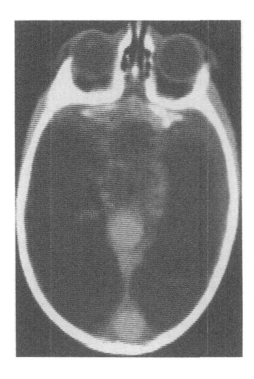

Fig. 5.15. Axial CT in a neonate with a vein of Galen aneurysmal malformation. Bilateral diffuse encephalomalacia is clearly demonstrated

casionally worsens the clinical condition, requiring cardiac surgery (Hernandez et al. 1956; Crawford et al. 1990). Prenatal diagnosis of cardiac overload has been made in a few patients, each time reflecting an aggressive lesion which almost invariably produces major neonatal cerebral ischemia and encephalomalacia (Fig. 5.15) (Norman and Becker 1974).

CSF and Neurological Disorders

CSF and neurological disorders have been recognized as being associated with VGAM for many years (Dandy 1919; Bedford 1934; Schlesinger 1940). Neurological dysfunction from VGAM rarely presents in newborns and when such dysfunction exists it is always secondary to severe heart failure. Only the most severe deficits will be diagnosed in the neonatal age group. Early brain ischemia or encephalomalacia can be demonstrated by transfontanel ultrasound (US), computerized tomography (CT), or magnetic resonance imaging (MRI) (Fig. 5.15). Minor neurological symptoms with normal US and CT are difficult to evaluate and diagnosis is even more difficult in the presence of heart failure.

In infants the presenting symptoms of VGAM are usually a macrocephaly or hydrocephalus (Russell and Nevin 1940; Askenasy et al. 1953; Milhorat et al. 1970; Hammock et al. 1971; Rosman and Shands 1978; Pribil et al. 1983; Rosenfeld and Fabinyi 1984). Although cardiac manifestations may be present they are well tolerated or discovered incidentally (cardiomegaly in X-ray chest film) (Fig. 5.16). Hydrocephalus occurs secondary to impaired CSF resorption due to venous hypertension (Hooper 1961; Kinal 1962; Stroobandt et al. 1986; Lamas et al. 1977; Johnston 1973; Janny et al. 1981; Young 1979; Yi and KeWei 1985; Sainte-Rose et al. 1984; de Lange and de Vlieger 1970). Although compression of the aqueduct of Sylvius by

Fig. 5.16. Chest X-ray in a neonate with a vein of Galen aneurysmal malformation with major cardial failure; significant cardial involvement. There was a good response to medical treatment. Artificial ventilation was not needed and endovascular management could be delayed

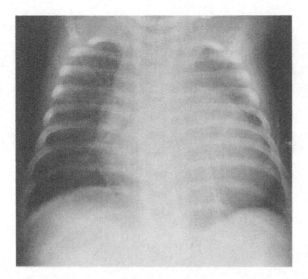

the aneurysm may be present, obstructive hydrocephalus is rare (Figs. 5.17, 5.18). The existence of hydrocephalus is therefore not an absolute indication for ventricular shunting. Although technically simple, shunting is not innocuous and in our experience almost all shunted children have had some neurological impairment at the time of referral (Zerah et al. 1992) (Fig. 5.19) (Tables 5.2, 5.3). Ventricular shunting interferes with water balance between the extracellular and intravascular compartments and may favor brain edema and cortico-subcortical ischemia.

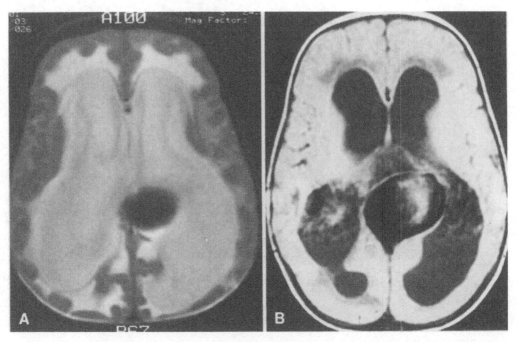

Fig. 5.17. Progressive active hydrocephalus in patient presenting with a vein of Galen aneurysmal malformation as demonstrated on axial MRI cuts (**A, B**) with abnormal signals around the frontal and occipital horns of the lateral ventricle. (Reprinted from Zerah et al. 1992)

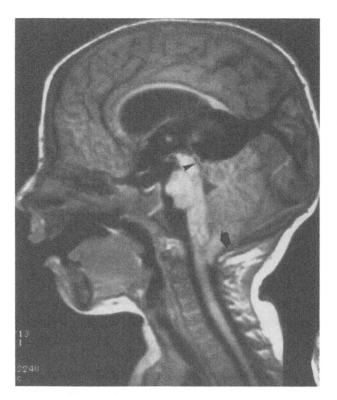

Fig. 5.18. Sagittal MRI study in an infant presenting with a macrocephaly associated with vein of Galen aneurysmal malformation. Note the patency of the mesencephalic aqueduct (*arrowhead*) and the existence of a Chiari malformation (*arrow*)

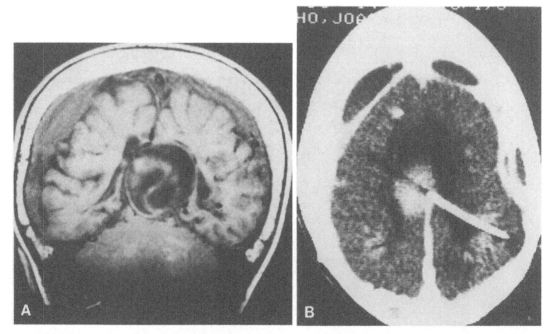

Fig. 5.19. A Coronal MRI and **B** axial CT sections in an 8 year old child with bilateral subdural hematoma, following ventricular shunting. At this stage, in spite of complete occlusion of the arteriovenous shunt by embolization, no improvement was noted. (Reprinted from Zerah et al. 1992)

Table 5.2. Size of ventricle and subarachnoid spaces in VGAM (from Zerah 1992) ($n = 43$)

	Ventricular dilatation		
	Absent	Mild	Significant
Aqueduct stenosis	1/9	1/12	0/2
No stenosis	8/9	11/12	2/2
Normal subarachnoid spaces	3/9	1/15	1/4
Enlarged subarachnoid spaces	6/9	14/15	3/4

The aqueduct in 20 cases and the subarachnoid space in 15 could not be assessed with sufficient reliability.

Table 5.3. Complications of ventricular shunt[a] (from Zerah 1992) ($n = 43$)

Complication	n
Enlargement of the vein of Galen	7
Continuous seizure	3
Infections	1
Mechanical problems	3
Subdural hematomas	6
Slit ventricles	1

[a] There was a total of 17 patients with VP (Ventriculo Peritoneal Shunt) shunt (only 1 without any problem).

Embolization of a VGAM is the treatment of choice and should be the first line therapy to manage CSF disorders. Reduction of venous hypertension will immediately improve CSF circulation and reabsorption (Figs. 5.2 and 5.20). Acute hydrocephalus is rare in VGAM but if present represents an indication for urgent embolization. If embolization fails to relieve the ventricular enlargement sufficiently, the decrease in blood flow should make surgical shunting safer.

Cerebral venous hypertension is the cause of most VGAM-associated neurological symptoms in the neonate. The drainage of the arteriovenous shunt increases the pressure in the torcular or superior sagittal sinus thereby creating a hemodynamic obstacle to the normal cortical and deep venous drainage of the brain. Distal venous stenosis or secondary venous occlusion will further alter this venous drainage (Figs. 5.21 – 5.23). Thus, cerebral venous circulation is often reversed and rerouted towards the cavernous sinus and ophthalmic veins (producing dilatation of facial veins or epistaxis) (Fig. 5.21) or to the basisphenoid sinus and pterygoid veins (Figs. 5.24, 5.25). If these alternative pathways of venous drainage are not yet well developed, cerebral venous congestion leading to brain edema, hypoxia, and hydrocephalus will develop, worsening the neurological prognosis (Andeweg 1989). Psychoneurological retardation and axial hypotony may be the clinical correlates of these hemodynamic alterations.

Mental retardation is part of the clinical history of patients with VGAM regardless of the type of lesion. Its presence is often associated with the hydrodynamic disorders (Tardien 1990; Zerah et al. 1992). Moderate delay (<20% of chronological age) will be reversed by proper therapeutic

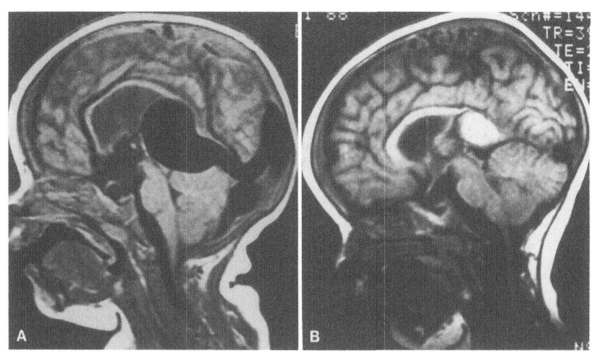

Fig. 5.20. Sagittal MRIs **A** before and **B** 6 months after embolization. Note that despite the dramatic shrinkage of the vein, there is no significant change in the patency of the mesencephalic aqueduct. Clinically, the child has grown normally without requiring shunting. (Reprinted from Zerah et al. 1992)

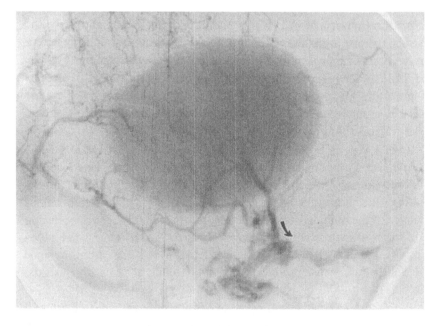

Fig. 5.21. Venous phase of a right internal carotid angiogram, lateral view, in a large dilatation of the median vein of the prosencephalon in an infant. Note the satisfactory opening of the cerebral venous drainage into the cavernous sinus and its drainage through the superior ophthalmic vein (*curved arrow*)

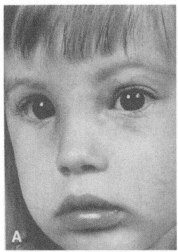

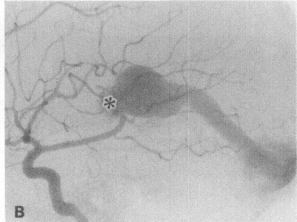

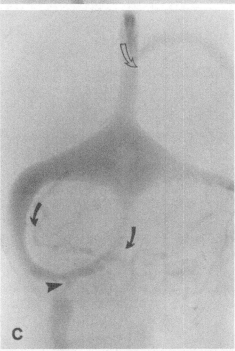

Fig. 5.22 A–C. A 7 year old child presenting with enlargement of the facial vein (**A**) related to retrograde drainage of both vein of Galen malformation (*asterisk*) into the sagittal sinus and to a cortical vein (*open curved arrow* in **C**) before reaching the cavernous sinus and the ophthalmic vein. **B** Left internal carotid angiogram in lateral and **C** frontal view. Note the distal jugular stenosis (*arrowhead*) and the insufficient drainage through the right sigmoid and lateral sinus and medial occipital sinus (*curved arrows*). (Reprinted from Lasjaunias et al. 1987)

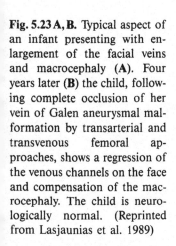

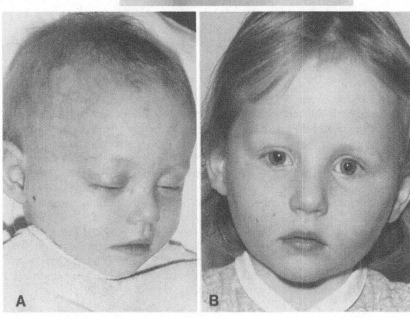

Fig. 5.23 A, B. Typical aspect of an infant presenting with enlargement of the facial veins and macrocephaly (**A**). Four years later (**B**) the child, following complete occlusion of her vein of Galen aneurysmal malformation by transarterial and transvenous femoral approaches, shows a regression of the venous channels on the face and compensation of the macrocephaly. The child is neurologically normal. (Reprinted from Lasjaunias et al. 1989)

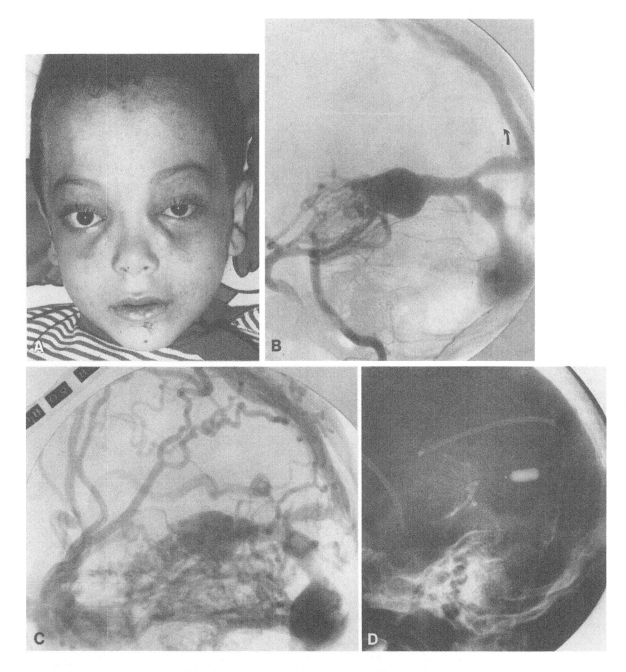

Fig. 5.24 A–G. An 8 year old child presenting with enlargement of the facial veins
(A) draining both the vein of Galen aneurysmal malformation and the normal
brain. On the vertebral angiography in lateral projection (B) early and (C) late
phases, complete occlusion of the posterior fossa sinuses is demonstrated. The entire venous blood flow is rerouted (*curved arrow* in B) towards the cavernous sinus
and the facial veins. Following several transarterial embolizations, significant reduction of the arteriovenous shunt was obtained; however, persistent reflux into the
cerebral veins led us to seek complete exclusion of the lesion. **D** Transvenous deposition of detachable gold valve balloon into the common portion of the falcine sinus
was performed. Control angiogram of the vertebral artery in lateral projection (E)
and in early (F) and late (G) phases of the left internal carotid artery shows complete
closure of the malformation. Only the normal brain drains into the facial veins.
Some 2 h after the venous approach, the patient developed a cerebral hemorrhage
that resulted in hemiparesis. (Reprinted from Lasjaunias et al. 1991)

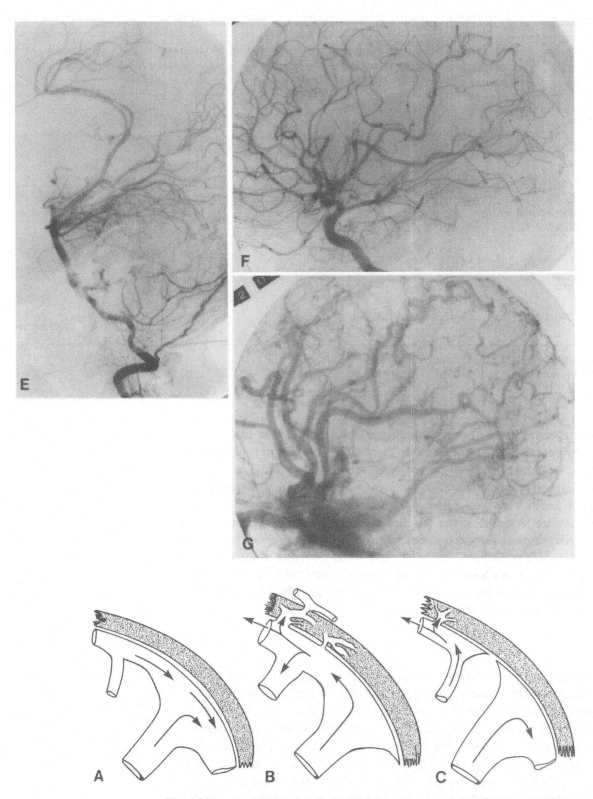

Fig. 5.25 A–C. Different types of drainage in vein of Galen aneurysmal malformation (VGAM). **A** Common drainage of the brain and of the VGAM anterograde into the sagittal sinus and towards the posterior fossa sinuses. **B** Common drainage of the VGAM and normal brain after closure of the posterior fossa sinuses resulting in retrograde flow into the cerebral and diploic veins. **C** Separate drainage of the VGAM into the posterior fossa sinuses, whereas the cerebral venous system opens into the diploic vein and towards the cavernous sinus anteriorly. (Reprinted from Lasjaunias et al. 1989)

Table 5.4. Comparison of clinical outcome in patients shunted or not shunted (from Zerah 1992)

	n	Complete exclusion	Clinically normal	Mild symptoms[a] neurologically normal	Moderate mental retardation (<20%) or focal symptoms	Significant retardation (>20%)	Death
Embolized patients							
With VP shunt	13	10	4	0	6	2	1
		77%	31%	–	46%	15%	8%
Without VP shunt	21	6	7	7	5	1	1
		29%	33%	33%	24%	5%	5%
Total	34	16	11	7	11	3	2
		47%	32%	21%	32%	9%	6%
Non-embolized patients							
With VP shunt	4	2	1	0	1	0	2
		50%	25%		25%		50%
Without VP shunt		0	1	0	0	0	4
	5		20%		–	–	80%
Total		2	2	0	1	0	6
	9	22%	22%		11%		67%
All patients	43	18	13	7	12	3	8
		42%	30%	16%	28%	7%	19%

Death in neonates, 27.8%; death in infants and children 12%.
[a] Moderate cardiac overload or residual macrocephaly (<2 SD).

management leading to either amelioration of retardation or to neurologically normal children (all VGAMs together in all age groups) (Table 5.4) (Fig. 5.23).

Cerebral calcifications, always located in the transcerebral venous watershed area between the superficial and deep venous system, present objective anatomical evidence of the presence of venous hypoxic disorder and its hydrodynamic consequences. Calcification is often associated with brain atrophy and secondarily may produce seizures, testifying to cerebral damage (Fig. 5.4). We have not, however, seen seizures or focal neurological deficit in VGAM patients unless a ventricular shunt had been placed or spontaneous venous changes or calcifications have occurred.

Risks of Hemorrhage

We have not observed intracranial hemorrhage in patients with genuine VGAM. As the arteriovenous shunt drains into the median vein of the prosencephalon, which may be viewed as a subarachnoid extension of a dural sinus and not as a true cerebral vein, the chances of bleeding are minimal (Lasjaunias et al. 1986, 1987). Many reports in the literature state that hemorrhage in late childhood or adulthood is a feature of the natural history of VGAMs. This erroneous statement reflects the failure to recognize the different types of "vein of Galen" and the acquired changes that modify its early drainage pattern (Seljeskog et al. 1968; Stehbens et al. 1973; Castaigne et al. 1972; Ventureyra et al. 1980; Kalyanaraman et al. 1971). In fact, most of the reported cases of hemorrhage belong to vein of Galen aneurysmal dilatation (VGAD) (parenchymatous AVMs).

Hemorrhage is possible in VGAM patients if venous stenosis or the venous drainage of the arteriovenous shunt is rerouted into pial veins

(Figs. 5.24, 5.25). Such rerouting may occur secondary to venous stenosis or to thrombosis of distal sinus outlets. These congested veins may then rupture, a situation similar to any dural AVM with retrograde cortical venous drainage or to any cerebral AVM. Other types of bleeding such as hemorrhagic infarction, intraventricular hemorrhage, or subdural hematomas may occur following ventricular shunting (Fig. 5.18) or after transvenous embolization (Fig. 5.24).

Spontaneous thrombosis of the venous pouch and/or of its outlet(s) have been observed by many (Gigson 1959; Rodesch et al. 1988; Lazar 1974; Olin et al. 1982; Oscherwitz and Davidoff 1947; Sartor 1978; Siqueira and Murray 1972; Wilson and Roy 1964; Zampella et al. 1988; Bots 1971; Heinz et al. 1968) (Figs. 5.26, 5.27). Although it has been said to be a favorable and desirable outcome, it may also be associated with increased intracranial pressure and/or venous ischemic episodes, thus illustrating how anatomical and clinical cure are not necessarily linked together in neonates and infants.

The occurrence of partial or total thrombosis in a given patient is hardly predictable (Figs. 5.8, 5.28). Retrospective analysis of the venous pattern suggests that these "spontaneous cures" seem to occur most often in patients with the mural type of VGAM.

c) Incidence and Epidemiology

As we have seen, the various groups of vascular lesions referred to as "vein of Galen malformations" in the literature are actually a heterogeneous group of lesions which are often inappropriately grouped together. It is therefore difficult to establish useful figures for the incidence of these lesions in relation to the number of births or other standard reference figures. In the cooperative study on subarachnoid hemorrhages, "vein of Galen malformation" represented less than 1% of all AVMs (Sahs 1969) and the various groups were not recognized.

Knudson (1979) studied all cases of neonatal cardiac failure due to an AVM collected by the U.S. Armed Forces Institute of Pathology. Intracranial AVMs accounted for 81 (52%) of 156 patients. Of these, 52 (64%) were labeled as having vein of Galen malformations, a somewhat surprising number, as in our experience other types of cerebral vascular malformations producing CHF are rare (see Vol. 2, Chap. 8, and AVFs of the Brain, this chapter).

In Hoffman's review (Hoffman et al. 1982) of 128 patients, 45 (35%) were neonates. Of these 43 (96%) presented with CHF, a group probably representing patients with VGAM. In the older infant group, only 2 (6%) of 36 infants presented with CHF, and 33 infants (92%) presented with hydrocephalus or neurological deficit, probably representing patients with VGAMs of the mural type, with most having VGADs.

Johnston et al. (1987) reported on 13 patients with malformations involving the vein of Galen out of 34 with intracranial AVMs presenting to his pediatric service over a 10 year period. Of these 13, 10 presented with CHF in the first months of life. In his review of 245 patients, there were 80 (33% of all) neonates; 78 (98% of neonates) of which presented with CHF and only 5 with CSF obstruction, 3 with seizures, and 1 with focal signs. (In his description of vascular anatomy most neonates with severe CHF had choroidal fistulas and belong to the group of patients with VGAMs.) In

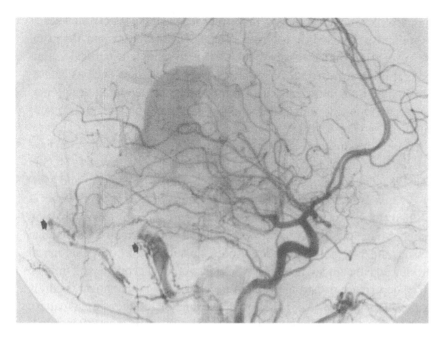

Fig. 5.26. Right common carotid angiogram. Same patient as in Fig. 5.19. Bilateral spontaneous occlusion of the proximal sigmoid sinuses that produced a slow-flow dural shunt draining into a more distal patent portion of the sigmoid sinuses (*arrows*)

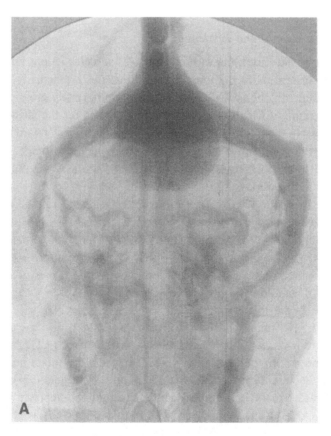

A

Fig. 5.27. Late phase of the left vertebral artery injection **A** before, **B** after partial embolization, and **C** over a 3 month period. Same patient as in Fig. 5.18. Note the progressive thrombosis of the right sigmoid sinus (*star*) and the significant narrowing of the left one (*solid arrow*). The relative shrinkage of the venous pouch and the absence of increase in the superior sagittal sinus system led us to believe that the arteriovenous shunt outflow was the only one to preserve the patency of the distal sinuses. Progressive reduction of the shunt produced a spontaneous adaptation of the outlets and therefore thrombosis. No symptoms followed this observation. The lesion was completely occluded in two sessions; the patient is clinically normal

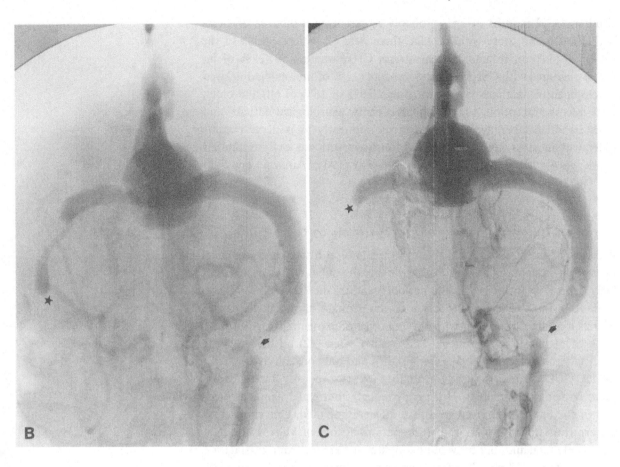

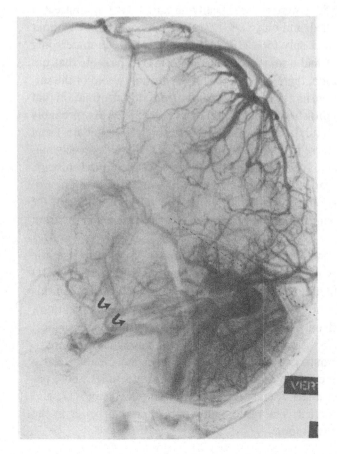

Fig. 5.28. Left vertebral angiogram in lateral projection in a patient with a spontaneous thrombosis of a calcified vein of Galen aneurysmal malformation. Note the choroidal vein opening into the lateral mesencephalic vein and secondarily into the petrous vein bilaterally (*bent arrow*). The straight sinus is not demonstrated (*interrupted line*). (Reprinted from Lasjaunias et al. 1987)

children 1–12 months of age (probably representing a mixture of those with VGAM and those with VGAD), there were 82 patients (33% of the total); 28 (34% of infants) presented with CHF, whereas 58 (71% of infants) presented with CSF obstruction and 10 (12% of infants) had delayed development. In patients 1–5 years of age (39% or 16% of all) and older, CHF was the exception, whereas macrocephaly, neurological deficits, and intracerebral hemorrhage were seen more frequently as patients became older, with most having VGADs; this is consistent with our analysis. Similar incidences are found in the reports by Gold et al. (1964), Amacher and Shillito (1973), and Long et al. (1974).

d) Natural History and Results of Previous Treatments

A review of the literature, as it relates to the natural history and results of previous treatment in both groups, shows that the outcome has been singularly depressing (primarily in the newborn and infant ages).

In Johnston's review of 245 cases, in the neonatal group there was an overall mortality of 91.4%, with the majority of patients dying within 1 week of diagnosis or treatment. Those not treated (12) all died. Of the medically treated patients, 95% (38/40) died and only one survivor had no deficit. Of 17 patients surgically treated, 14 (82%) died; only 2 were reported to be without deficit. In Hoffman's report, nontreated neonates died, and of the few that survived treatment all were impaired. One can clearly discern from this information that the natural history of VGAM is almost universally fatal and that conventional treatments are far from satisfactory.

In patients 1–12 months of age there was an overall mortality of 48%, and of the survivors 50% were neurologically impaired. Of the nontreated infants, 73% (8/11) died, and only 18% (2/11) were reported to be without deficit. Of those treated only for CHF, 33% died (2/6); those undergoing only shunt placement had a mortality of 64% (7/11). In patients that underwent direct operation, there was a 32% (13/41) mortality, and of the survivors 66% (27/41) were impaired. One can infer from this information that this group of cases consists of patients with less severe VGAMs (probably representing simpler mural fistulas and the best surgical candidates) and that the majority of these patients harbored a VGAD with a "parenchymatous" nidus and were poor surgical candidates. The natural history, therefore, of VGAD patients is a very high mortality and significant neurological deficits, with only a very small group of "normal" children. Of those treated, direct surgery had better results, but these were still far from satisfactory.

In Johnston's review of cases involving children 1–5 years of age, the overall mortality was 42% (13/31); of those that survived, 65% (11/31) were impaired. Of interest to note is that, of the untreated patients in this group (which should correspond to those with VGAD in our classification), 67% (4/6) died and only one was reported to be without neurological deficit. This testifies to the poor outcome in this group and that in comparison to the VGAM group, patients may survive longer but eventually also have a dismal outcome. In the treated group in Johnston's series, those patients that underwent direct operation had a mortality of 35% (6/17) and 53% (10/17) had a deficit. The results, although somewhat better in the older age group, are still poor.

In patients older than 6 years of age, the exact type of lesion is difficult to evaluate, as it includes midline malformations draining into the deep venous system, which is a completely separate group of lesions.

e) Treatment of VGAMs

A major breakthrough in treatment began in the early 1980s with the use of endovascular embolization in the management of patients with VGAMs (Berenstein 1982, 1985), with the first, reported, complete, transarterial occlusion and cure reported by Lasjaunias et al. in 1989. Mickle and Quisling (1986) and Quisling and Mickle (1989) introduced the neurosurgical transtorcular venous approach to control severe CHF. By 1987, the technical capability existed to reach the aneurysmally dilated vein by anterograde catheterization from the femoral artery or by retrograde catheterization of the feeding pedicle to the fistula from the femoral vein, permitting complete obliteration of choroidal fistulas (Chap. 4, Fig. 4.31) (Kendall 1986, unpublished data; Dowd et al. 1990; Mickle and Quisling 1986; Quisling and Mickle 1989; O'Donnabhain and Duff 1989; Circillo et al. 1990; Wisoff et al. 1990; Lasjaunias et al. 1986, 1987, 1989, 1991).

Before undertaking treatment one should evaluate as objectively as possible the chances that the child may develop normally. Depending on the age, type, onset, and dominant symptoms, the objectives of treatment will vary and the tools should be chosen accordingly. Various methods of treatment, medical, surgical, and/or endovascular, are used, either alone or combined.

The primary goal in neonates is obliteration of the major portion of the fistula to allow resolution of the CHF. Since these patients cannot tolerate a significant volume load and usually have borderline renal function, the extent of angiographic evaluation must be limited. The clinical history of severe CHF in a newborn gives a high degree of suspicion that the lesion is probably choroidal and less likely a mural VGAM (Fig. 5.14); the CT and MRI will add information as to which types is involved and what are the main contributing pedicles; the eccentricity of the aneurysmal vein will suggest the site of the larger fistulization (Fig. 5.29). Thus, all noninvasively obtained information to aid analysis of the most likely anatomy prior to embolization is crucial. Such information may minimize the amount of angiography required.

In general, the left (or right) vertebral artery injection in frontal projection (if biplanar equipment is not available) is preferred to identify the largest fistula, the obliteration of which should be the first goal in treatment. All additional injections and projections, if needed, will be derived from the result of that series. The total amount of contrast material used varies in relation to the weight of the baby. Between 4 and 8 ml/kg body weight of contrast material (nonionic or low osmolarity) are tolerated in most neonates, with the total amount in an individual patient dependent on the total time of the procedure and the urinary output. In both children and adults, the goal is to obtain appropriate and complete preliminary angiographic studies. If the patient is older, there is less problem of CHF and fluid overload. In older infants clinical problems are usually not an emergency, therefore appropriate work-up can be done, as in adults with AVMs. Staging the procedure in neonates over consecutive days, leaving the vascular access in situ, has been done by one of us (AB). Once the limits

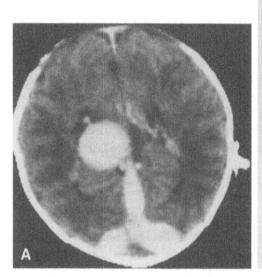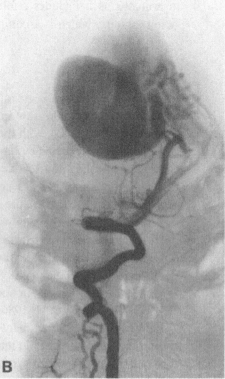

Fig. 5.29. A Enhanced axial CT and **B** right vertebral artery injection in frontal view in a neonate with a left sided choroidal type of vein of Galen aneurysmal malformation. Note the lateralization of the ectasia corresponding to the choroidal venous tributary and the maximum jet of the fistula region

for contrast material or fluid have been reached for the day, the procedure is stopped. The introducer sheath at the puncture site is fixed in place, the infant is kept intubated, and if the systemic symptoms do not improve in the intervening 12–24 h, additional embolization is performed.

I. Medical Treatment

Palliative medical treatment including support measures are performed while awaiting the best timing for the definitive treatment, that is, closure of the arteriovenous shunt by embolization.

The management of cardiac manifestations by the use of diuretics, pressors, or assisted ventilation is determined by the severity of the cardiac failure. The indications for digitalis are uncertain in the newborn period, since in most of the patients cardiac symptoms are related to volume overload and not to an impaired systolic function. In some patients, when despite medical treatment the cardiac status is unstable, careful search for associated cardiac manifestations should be undertaken. Embolization is indicated in newborns in the absence of brain damage, and even partial embolization of the arteriovenous shunt offers rewarding results with rapid clinical improvement (Berenstein 1982; Garcia-Monaco et al. 1991).

Table 5.5. Mortality in VGAM patients

	n	Nontreated (%)	n	Treated (%)[a]
Newborns	12	100	56	93
Infants	11	72	57	38
Children below 5 years	6	66	25	36

From Johnston's review (Neurosurgery 1987) of 167 patients.
[a] Embolization was not used as part of treatment.

II. Surgical Treatment

Surgical correction of VGAM (Gibson et al. 1959; Verdura and Shafron 1969; Amacher et al. 1979; Menezes et al. 1981; Smith and Donat 1981; Weir et al. 1968; Alvarez-Garijo et al. 1980; Hoffman et al. 1982; de Marais and Lemos 1982; Yasargil et al. 1976) is no longer indicated as a primary form of treatment since its results are uniformly poor (Table 5.5). A surgical craniotomy to allow transtorcular embolization might be indicated on some occasions when an arterial or venous femoral approach are not possible. We have used this approach only in a few patients of our series. Ventricular shunting should not be performed in patients with hydrocephalus, unless proper endovascular management cannot be rapidly instituted. As discussed above, shunting prior to closure of the arteriovenous shunt may aggravate the neurological conditions and worsen outcome (Tables 5.3, 5.4) (Zerah et al. 1992).

III. Endovascular Treatment

Endovascular embolization of VGAMs is the present treatment of choice, if properly timed and performed by a well trained group in pediatric interventional neuroradiology. The technical goal is to occlude the arteriovenous shunt, disconnecting the pathological arteries and aneurysmal vein from the brain circulation. This may be accomplished by occlusion of the shunt and vein via the arterial route (arterial embolization) or by occluding the ectatic vein from the venous route (venous embolization). Whenever possible, the transarterial route is tried first and only if unsuccessful do we try a venous approach. The risk of immediate or delayed hemorrhagic complications has been significantly less with transarterial embolizations. To accomplish satisfactory results, proper patient selection is mandatory. If the venous route is to be used, one must be absolutely certain that the aneurysmal vein is not connected to other cerebral veins (Table 5.1).

There are no indications for endovascular therapy of VGAM (or even angiography) in the neonatal age in a patient without severe heart failure (e.g., incidental finding or mild and controlled symptoms) in view of the technical limitations of embolization at this age (Fig. 5.30). Endovascular therapy may be postponed if strict periodical monitoring assures that growth, neurological development, and brain parenchyma (as evaluated by CT and MRI) remain normal. At 6 months of age technical conditions are optimal and both morphological and clinical results are dramatically enhanced (Fig. 5.31).

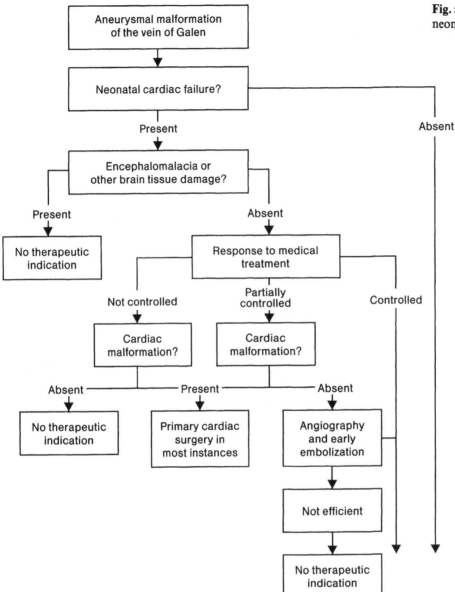

Fig. 5.30. Decision tree in the neonatal period

Neurological damage, assessed by CT, US, or MRI, is a contraindication for endovascular therapy since, despite an anatomical cure, clinical results are not satisfactory (Wisoff et al. 1990) (Tables 5.6, 5.7; Fig. 5.32). However, hydrodynamic disorders, failure to thrive, or delayed neurological development clinically may represent rapid indications for embolization at the infant age. The conjunction of neonatal macrocephaly or moderate hydrocephalus with CHF that is not life threatening is not a mandatory indication for urgent treatment. Both symptoms arise from different unrelated mechanisms.

Embolization should be postponed if ventricular shunting has been done recently, since occlusion of the shunt produces a shrinkage of the mass effect from the ectatic vein (Figs. 5.33, 5.34). The combination of rapid volume modifications in a relatively short (few days) interval may create a sig-

Fig. 5.31. Decision tree based on the infant's age

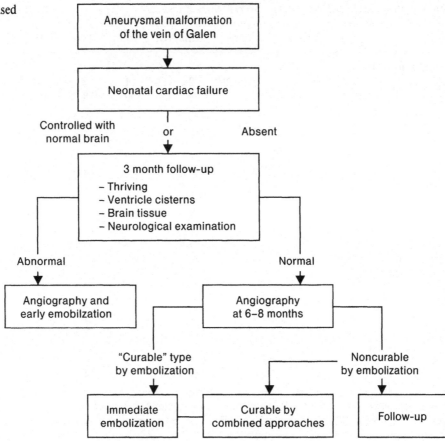

nificant and acute decrease of supratentorial pressure leading to ascending cerebellar herniation. Following shunting alone, an increase in the size of the venous pouch is noted in almost half the patients (Fig. 5.33 and Chap. 3, Fig. 3.35).

Technique of Embolization

We favor the transarterial route since it has shown the best clinical and morphological results with lowest risks. Comparative series of patients treated with the venous approach, based on different architectural analyses and objectives, have shown very high morbidity with unrewarding clinical results

Table 5.6. Bicêtre series (1984 – 1990): recruitment profile

	Neonate	Infant	Children	Adult	Total
Age of onset (*n*)	31	14	7	0	52
Age of referral (*n*)	21	17	13	1	52
Age of first embolization (*n*)	5	19	13	1	38

Two spontaneous occlusions, five patients yet to be admitted, one normal child refused treatment, and six patients rejected treatment.

Table 5.7. Bicêtre series (1984 – 1990): overall clinical results

	Neonate	Infants	Children	Adults	Total
Clinically normal					
n	4	5 (+2)	2 (+1)	1	12 (+3)
%	19	41.2	23.1	100	28.8
Neurologically normal but with mild manifestations[a]					
n	2 (+1)	4 (+1)	6	0	12 (+2)
%	14.3	29.4	46.1		26.9
Mild neurological symptoms or mental retardation <20%					
n	6 (+1)	3	2	0	11 (+1)
%	33.3	17.6	15.4		23.1
Significant neurological deficit or mental retardation >20%					
n	2	0	1	0	3
%	9.6		7.7		5.8
Death					
n	5	2	1	0	8
%	23.8	11.8	7.7		15.4

Complete occlusion: 19 patients (41%) and 10 yet to come (63%). There have been 88 sessions, 2.3 per child. More than 130 arteries have been embolized, including 4 venous approaches (3 torcular, 1 femoral).

[a] Stable macrocephaly and/or asymptomatic increase in cardiothoracic index.
(+n) Children, to be admitted for endovascular management.
% have been calculated by age group. Neonates 21; Infants 17; Children 13; Adults 1.

Fig. 5.32 A – C. Young infant presenting with a choroidal type of vein of Galen ▶ aneurysmal malformation. Born as a premature baby (1.8 kg), during the first 3 months the child survived under medical treatment and gained weight. This led to an infant presenting with macrocephaly and at that time retardation difficult to assess. In view of the unusual survival of the child, an angiogram was performed which demonstrated significant dysplastic changes with a moyamoya type network on the right side (**A**) and intense arterial irregularities on both the anterior (**B**) and posterior circulations (**C**). At present this pattern represents a contraindication to treatment

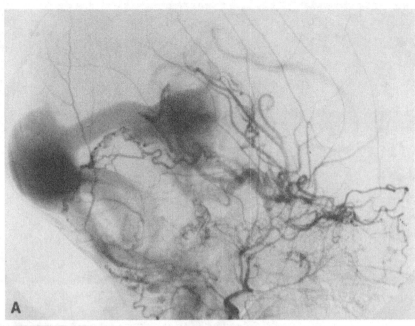

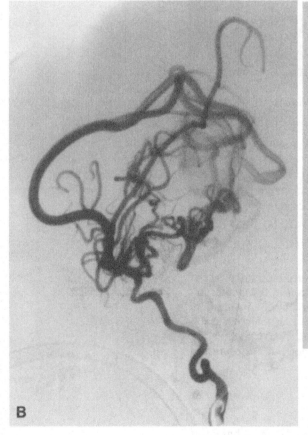

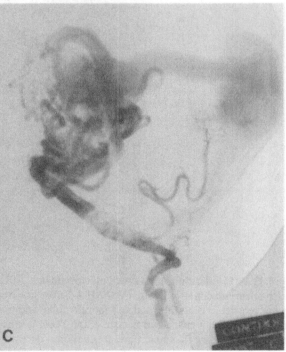

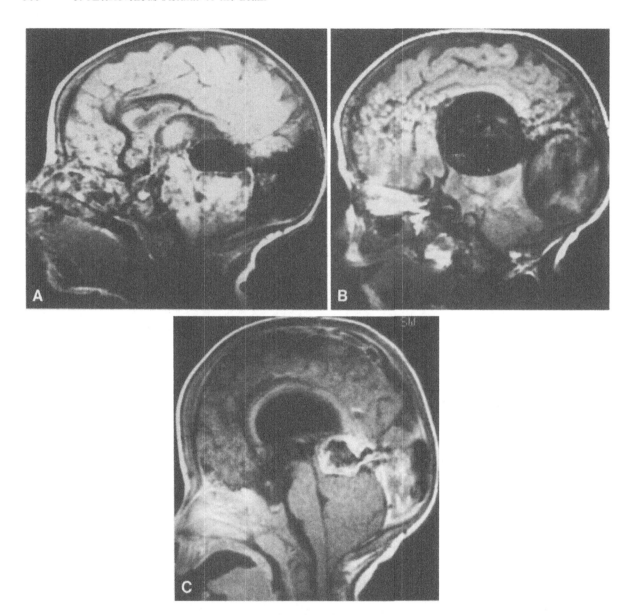

Fig. 5.33 A–C. Infant presenting with macrocephalus. MRI demonstrates a vein of Galen aneurysmal malformation (VGAM) **A** before any treatment, **B** 2 months following ventricular shunting, and **C** 3 months following transarterial embolization. Note the significant changes in the size of the VGAM, the torcular following shunting, and their return to a more normal situation after embolization. Chiari malformation was not clearly demonstrated on the early examination but was confirmed later on. (Reprinted from Zerah et al. 1992)

(Figs. 5.24, 5.35) (Circillo et al. 1990; Dowd et al. 1990; O'Donnabhain and Duff 1989). We have used the technique of transtorcular or transfemoral venous approach in a few instances with variable results. In these patients the venous approach was chosen because of the impossibility of achieving a safe, distal, arterial catheterization to occlude the arteriovenous shunts (Figs. 5.24, 5.35 and Chap. 4, Fig. 4.31). In all other patients we used transarterial embolization by the femoral approach after percutaneous puncture. The technique employed by one of us (Lasjaunias) will be detailed since

Fig. 5.34. Usual head circumference curve as seen in an infant after embolization following our protocol and without ventricular shunting. Satisfactory interruption of the abnormal curve is observed shortly following partial and then complete occlusion of the vein of Galen aneurysmal malformation. Same patient as in Figs. 5.2 and 5.20

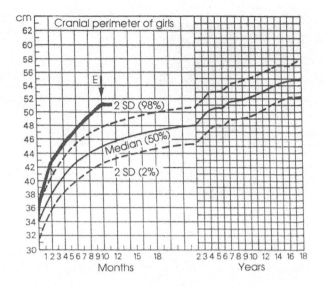

management by the other (Berenstein), although not fundamentally different, was presented in Chap. 4.

Since 1984, percutaneous catheterization of the femoral artery can be accomplished without the need of a cutdown, even in newborns. A 4F femoral sheath is used at the arteriotomy site. Pretherapeutic angiography is done with a 4F catheter and low osmolarity (Hexabrix) or nonionic contrast material. In the same session a variable stiffness microcatheter, such as the Mini-Torquer (Chap. 4, Fig. 4.6) (NYCOMED Ingenor, Paris, France) is used from the femoral route without the need of a coaxial system. The Mini-Torquer can be used either with or without a guide wire (Chap. 4, Figs. 4.7, 4.8) (Garcia-Monaco 1990) to catheterize the afferent artery of the

Fig. 5.35. Right internal carotid artery injection in an infant previously embolized transarterially and transtorcularly at the neonatal age, with coils to control major cardiac failure. Note the remaining patency around 80 cm of coils introduced by transtorcular approach. The neonate came out of failure; however, mental retardation >25% led us to perform a second transtorcular embolization. Following this procedure the lesion was completely excluded, but the patient had a lethal hemorrhage a few hours after the procedure

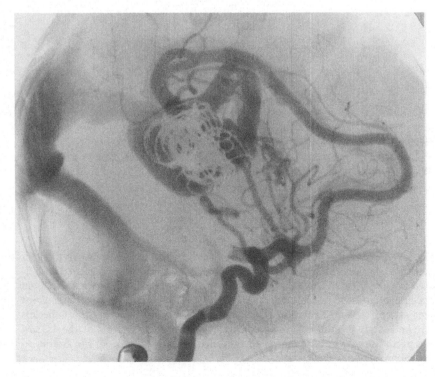

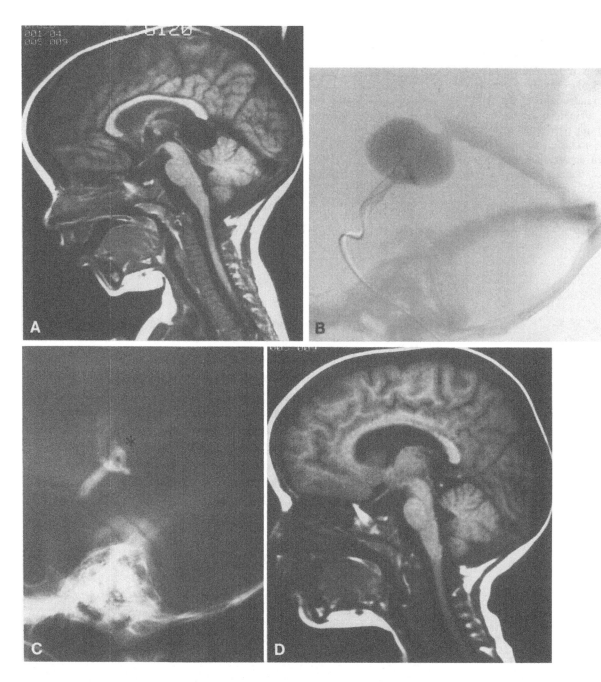

Fig. 5.36. A Sagittal MRI in a young child presenting with a mural vein of Galen aneurysmal malformation. Transarterial embolization was performed with IBCA (**B** and **C**). Note the rapid shrinkage of the dilated vein in a few weeks (**D**) as demonstrated on MRI. (Reprinted from Lasjaunias et al. 1989)

Fig. 5.37A–C. Mural vein of Galen aneurysmal malformation (VGAM) in an infant. **A** Plain skull film after the more prominent feeder has been occluded with liquid acrylic. **B** Left vertebral artery injection immediately after **A** shows residual opacification of the pouch with stagnation of contrast material. The patient was kept asleep for 24 h. Evolution was uneventful. **C** Control angiogram of the left vertebral artery 3 months later demonstrates complete thrombosis of the VGAM and partial shrinkage of the mass, with normal opacification of all the arteries to the region

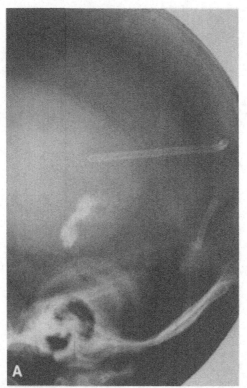

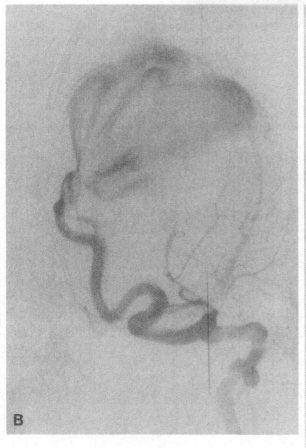

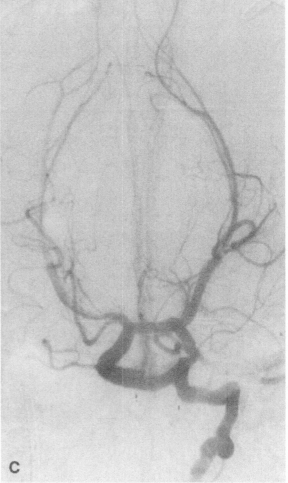

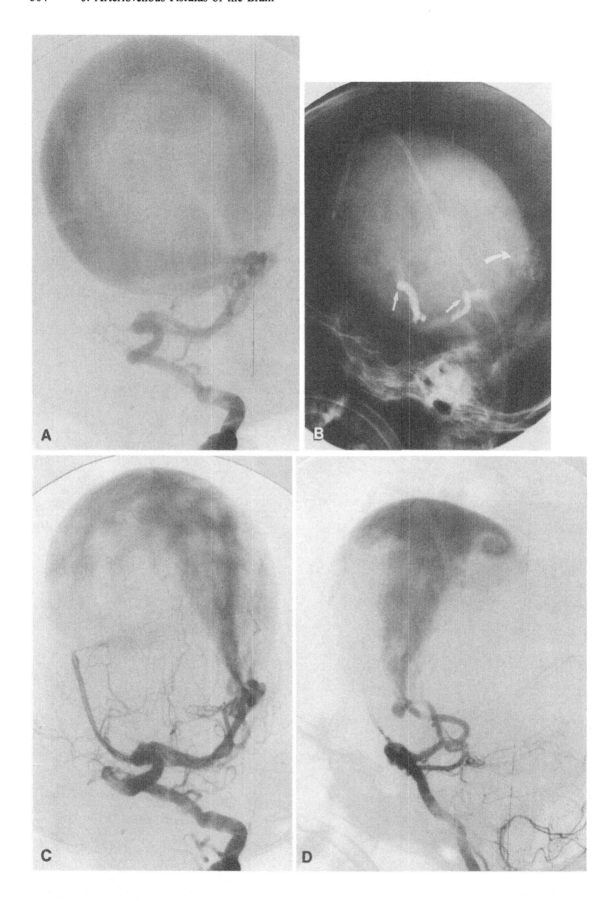

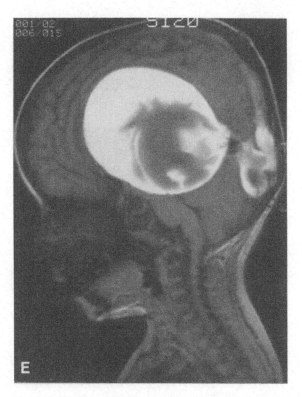

Fig. 5.38 A–E. Multiple feeders to a mural type of vein of Galen aneurysmal malformation embolized in one session. **A** Left vertebral angiography in frontal view. **B** Skull X-ray demonstrates the position of the glue in the two most prominent feeders (*arrows*) and the radiopaque acrylic at the exit of the dilated pouch (*curved arrow*). **C** Frontal and **D** lateral views of the left vertebral artery injection immediately after the embolization of the two most prominent feeders embolized on the right side. On the left, additional filling remains through small contributors that were not embolized. **E** Sagittal MRI performed a few days after the embolization demonstrates the complete occlusion of the lesion extending into the torcular, as the normal brain had adapted to the fistula and was draining into the cavernous sinus

shunt (Chap. 4, Figs. 4.7, 4.8 and 5.36). No balloon is used at the tip of the catheter. Embolization in these high-flow lesions is usually accomplished using NBCA-tantalum, without iophendylate (Chap. 4, Figs. 4.7, 4.8 and Figs. 5.37–5.39). The goal is to occlude both the segment of the supplying artery beyond the last normal branch and the exit of the ectatic vein (Chap. 4, Figs. 4.36 and 5.35, 5.36). If there is a closed stenosis at the distal end of the dilated vein, this technique can be performed with relative safety. When the vein is widely open, however, it represents a more difficult situation that requires considerable experience in the use of glue for embolization (Fig. 5.39).

Immediately after proper embolization with NBCA, the blood stagnates in the venous aneurysm, resulting in gradual thrombosis (Chap. 3, Fig. 3.32, Chap. 4, Fig. 4.7, and Fig. 5.38). A few weeks later, CT or MRI usually shows shrinkage of the ectatic vein (Figs. 5.20, 5.33, 5.36).

On some occasions complete closure of the shunt is accomplished in one session, particularly in patients with mural types of VGAM. In such cases

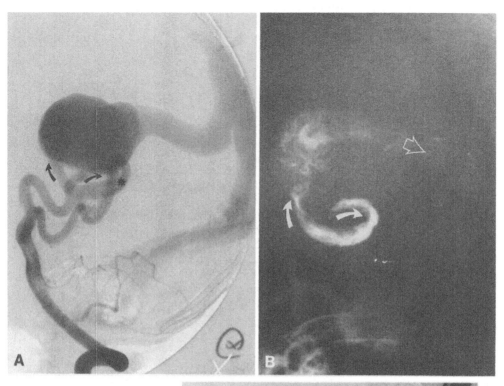

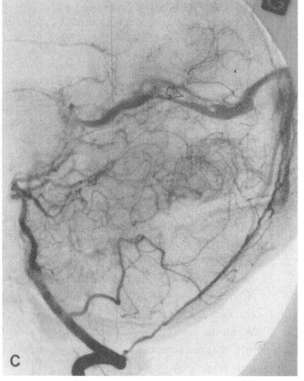

one of us (PL) keeps the infant or newborn intubated under general anesthesia for approximately 36 h following the procedure. Blood pressure is kept at normal levels; we have not had any perfursion pressure breakthrough phenomena in our series nor have we observed secondary cerebral venous thrombosis. One of us (AB) does not keep the patient intubated or under anesthesia and has also not seen perfusion pressure breakdown or secondary venous thrombosis.

In other instances, particularly in patients with choroidal VGAMs, embolization should be staged, because total occlusion is seldom achieved in one session due to the complex arterial supply. Clinical symptoms usually improve even after partial embolization; however we try to accomplish an anatomical cure every time, if possible (Chap. 4, Fig. 4.31). The procedure is done under general anesthesia without hypotension. Heparin is not needed if no coaxial system is used in children under 3 years of age. The average duration of the procedure is 90 min (60–180, PL). For one of us (AB), the procedure may be prolonged (3–5 h) to permit excretion of some contrast material and thereby accomplish more embolization in one session.

Children are followed neuroradiologically (CT and/or MRI are performed some days after and a control angiography 3 months after) and clinically by both ourselves and the pediatric neurologist. Morbidity and mortality using this protocol have been very low so far and almost exclusively observed following venous approaches: two deaths in the embolized group, two patients with neurological deficits following venous approaches (Lasjaunias et al. 1991). In rare cases secondary occlusion of the venous outlet has occurred, as if the flow from the arteriovenous shunt was necessary for patency (Figs. 5.27, 5.39). None has led to significant manifestations. In four patients, ventricular shunting followed embolization with complete occlusion of the shunt. In all patients, despite correction of the hemodynamic disorder, it was felt that irreversible dysfunction of CSF resorption was present. None of the patients had any permanent deficit. Two children experienced one or two seizure episodes a few months after the shunt. Except for these rate situations, our experience shows that,

◀ **Fig. 5.39 A–C.** Embolization of a mural type of vein of Galen aneurysmal malformation without outflow restriction at the sinus. **A** Left vertebral angiogram in lateral projection. Note the absence of restriction at the level of the falcine sinus. The embolization was carried on into one of the prominent feeders (*curved arrows*). Note the arterial-arterial anastomosis (*star*). **B** Plain skull X-ray of the cast. Due to the lack of outflow restriction in the venous side, the acrylic injection is preformed more proximally, against the vessel wall, and in a rapid injection (*curved arrows*). Note the glue in the proximal part of the sinus (*open arrow*). **C** Left vertebral angiogram in lateral projection 1 year after embolization. There is only minimal filling of the vein, with the subtracted acrylic (*open arrow*). The postoperative course was uneventful, and the lesion went onto complete thrombosis

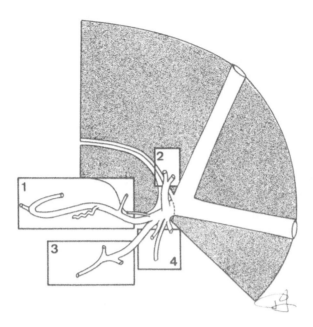

Fig. 5.40. The cortical and deep territories drained by the great cerebral vein (vein of Galen). *1*, deep nuclei territory; *2*, medial parietal and occipital territory; *3*, medial temporal territory; *4*, infratentorial territory. (Reprinted from Lasjaunias et al. 1989)

both for direct treatment of the primary lesion and for control of resulting the hydrodynamic disorders, the endovascular approach must be considered first and surgery used only after failure of the former technique.

3. Vein of Galen Aneurysmal Dilatation

In this group of lesions the ectatic venous structure is, in contrast to the situation in VGAM, the great cerebral vein (vein of Galen). In such cases, although it drains the AVM, the vein of Galen receives drainage from normal brain veins as well (Figs. 5.40, 5.41). Two types of lesions can be distinguished: parenchymatous (Fig. 5.42) and dural (see Vol. 2, Chap. 8).

a) Parenchymatous AVM

In the parenchymatous AVMs with VGAD there is a subpial AVM which drains into a tributary of the vein of Galen and thereby into the deep cerebral venous drainage (pial veins) (Fig. 5.42 C). Aneurysmal dilatation of the vein is secondary to an outflow obstruction (see Chap. 1). Due to this outflow constraint the vein of Galen dilates and blood flow refluxes into other normal cerebral veins (internal cerebral, vermian, hippocampal, basal vein, medial ventricular, parietal, occipital, or other normal tributaries of the vein of Galen) (Fig. 5.43).

Clinically this type of VGAD usually presents in childhood or young adulthood and shares clinical manifestations with other deep-seated AVMs: intracerebral hemorrhage, focal neurological deficit, seizures, etc. The venous outflow restriction is an added weakness in this angioarchitecture and can explain the early onset of symptoms in this group of patients as compared to those with other deep-seated brain AVMs without outflow restrictions.

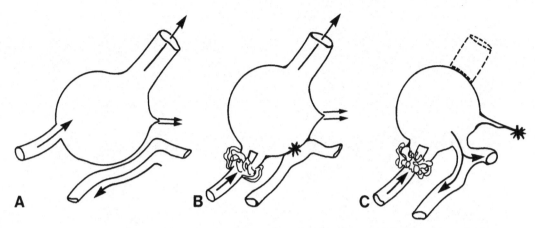

Fig. 5.41 A – C. The possible communications between the normal cerebral venous system and the venous ectasia. **A** Absence of communication with the cerebral veins. The straight sinus is not patent (*double arrow*). The drainage occurs through an embryonic sinus (*arrow*). The cerebral veins have already bypassed the shunting zone and do not communicate with it. This type corresponds to most mural and choroidal type of vein of Galen aneurysmal malformation (VGAM). **B** Similar situation in which a network of more or less enlarged, abnormal, choroidal capillaries is demonstrated at the entrance to the dilated vein (*arrow*). Here, the communication with the venous territory of the brain may be secondarily occluded and not visualized during the procedure (*asterisk*). This theoretical type may correspond to intermediate forms in which the medial vein of the prosencephalon (MVP) has regressed incompletely and some communications have occurred with the pouch via choroidal veins. The straight sinus is not patent (*double arrow*). **C** Vein of Galen aneurysmal dilatation (VGAD) following acquired thrombosis of the straight sinus (*asterisk*). The nidus is located on an afferent vein to the vein of Galen (VG). Reflux into the other afferents to the VG and therefore into the cerebral tissue is demonstrated (*curved arrows*). (Reprinted from Lasjaunias et al. 1989)

Angiographic recognition of VGAD is simple and is based on proper analysis of the venous drainage of the lesion. The venous outflow of the AVM will include the cerebral vein. The deep venous system does not show the bilateral "epsilon shape" that is encountered in VGAM (Figs. 5.8, 5.9) (Lasjaunias et al. 1991). Differentiation between a VGAM and a tectal AVM based only on angiography can sometimes be difficult, but demonstration of transmesencephalic vessels by MRI (Chap. 1, Fig. 1.21) confirms a tectal location and therefore confirms the VGAD (Lasjaunias et al. 1988). Management of VGAD is the same as with any deep-seated lesion; the venous approach is *contraindicated* since it may produce extensive venous thrombosis in deep cerebral veins. The VGAD may, however, mimic closely VGAM with which it should not be confused (Fig. 5.43).

b) Dural Shunts into a Dilated Vein of Galen

Dural arteriovenous shunt with VGAD corresponds to an acquired lesion in which there is an arteriovenous shunt located in the wall of the vein of Galen itself: the dilatation is secondary to a straight sinus obstruction (stenosis or thrombosis). Reflux is always noted into afferent cerebral veins to the vein of Galen (Fig. 5.44). The clinical presentation shares characteristics of other dural AVMs draining into cerebral veins. Although the number of

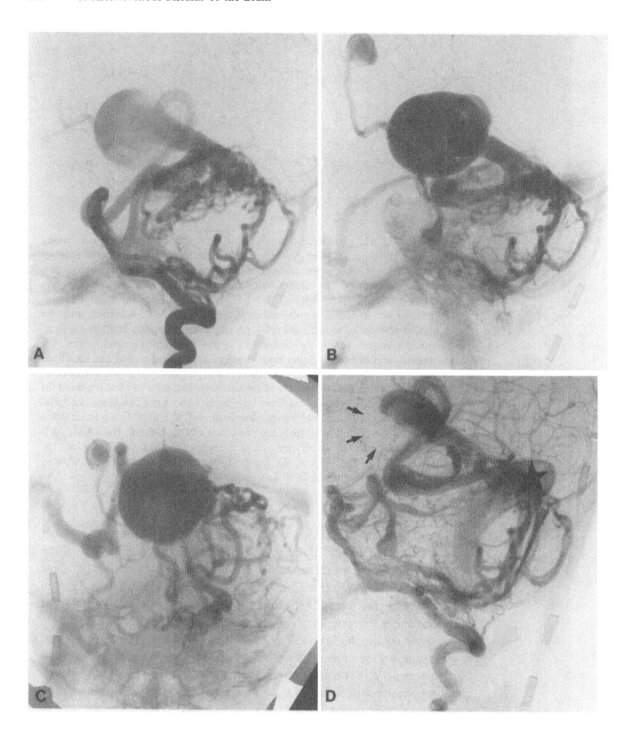

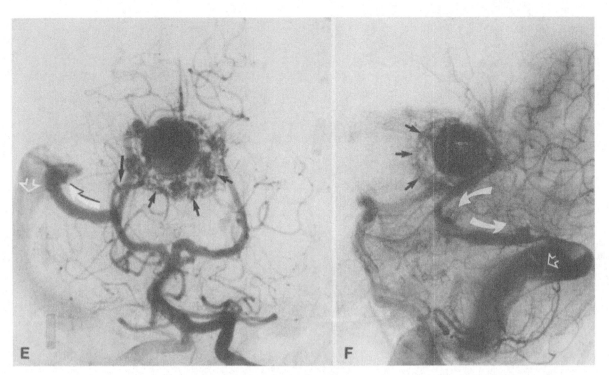

Fig. 5.42 A–F. A 7 year old child presenting with a posterior fossa vermian arterio-venous malformation (AVM) draining into the superior vermian vein, and reaching an aneurysmally dilated vein of Galen-straight sinus. Left vertebral artery angiogram in lateral projection **A** early and **B** late phases. **C** Frontal projection early phase. Note the reflux into cerebral veins and in particular into the right subtemporal veins. **D** Following partial embolization the shunt is significantly reduced (*star*) and the venous dilatation of the VG has partially thrombosed (*arrows*). Residual channels drain the small remaining part from the AVM. In view of the remaining AVM, surgical intervention was elected. Following surgery, the nidus was removed, leaving the VG untouched. **E** Frontal and **F** lateral control angiograms of the left vertebral artery following surgery demonstrated a capillary network (*arrows*) at the level of the previously, partially thrombosed portion of the ectasia and draining into the previous venous outlet of the lesion (*curved arrows*). These unusual findings were interpreted as an acquired angiogenesis and/or recanalization within the clot via the vasa vasorum which originated from the P2 segment of the posterior bilaterally; similar pathogenesis as dural AVMs. The sigmoid sinus (*open arrow*) is now draining the shunt (*curved arrows*). (Reprinted from Fournier et al. 1991)

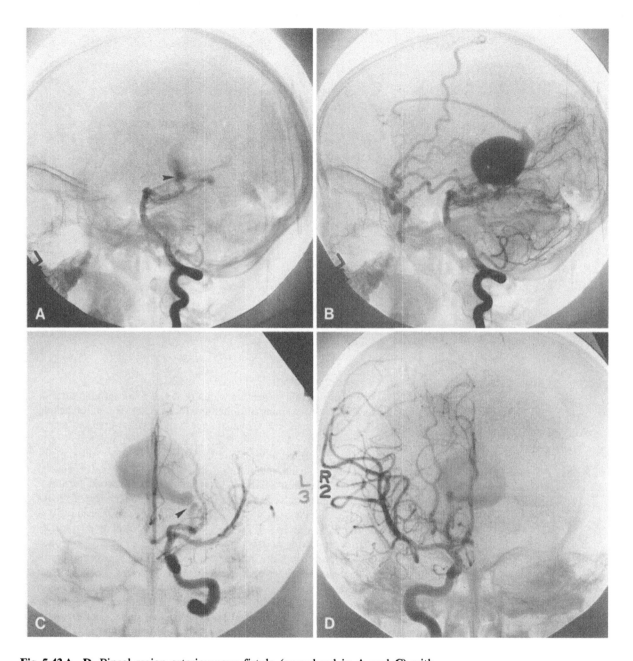

Fig. 5.43 A–D. Pineal region arteriovenous fistula (arrowhead in **A** and **C**) with dilatation of the vein of Galen. **A** Early and **B** late phases of the vertebral artery angiogram in lateral projection. **C** Left and **D** right frontal projection of both internal carotid arteries. In this particular case, the ectasia does not correspond to the medial vein of the prosencephalon but to the vein of Galen itself that is dilated because of an outflow restriction. Note the confluence of the deep venous system has already been established; and there is reflux towards the inferior sagittal sinus, the sylvian and superior sagittal sinuses are demonstrated

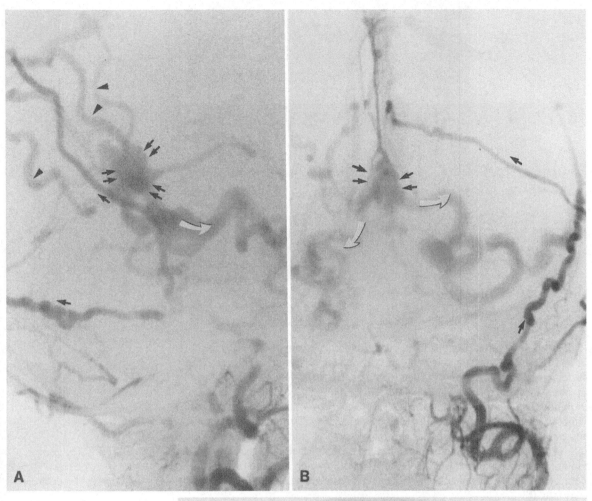

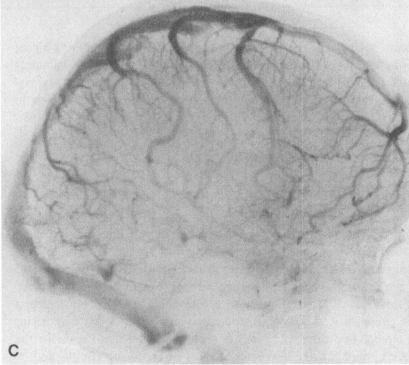

Fig. 5.44 A–C. Dural shunt at the level of the vein of Galen. **A** Right external carotid artery in lateral projection. **B** Left external carotid artery in frontal projection. **C** Late phase of the internal carotid angiogram on the right side. These studies demonstrate dural arteries with middle meningeal feeders (*arrows*) supplying a typical dural shunt at the level of the vein of Galen (*double arrows*). Note the absence of the straight sinus and the reflux into the afferents of the basal vein of Rosenthal (*curved arrow*) and internal cerebral vein. Medial veins are also demonstrated (*arrowhead*). The late phase of the carotid angiography (**C**) shows the absence of visualization of any deep venous system. (Reprinted from Fournier et al. 1991)

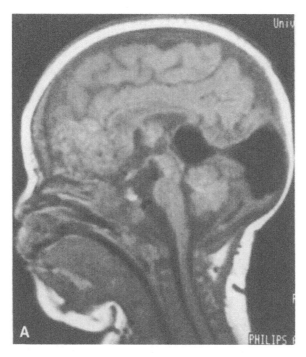

Fig. 5.45 A – E. Brain arteriovenous fistula draining into the vein of Galen. **A** Sagittal, **B** and **C** axial MRI cuts in a neonate presenting with a convulsive episode. The scans demonstrates a large vein of Galen with a dilated atrial vein proximally from a narrowed junction (arrows in **C**). Note the fistulous site of what is a direct arteriovenous fistula at the mesencephalic level (*double arrow* in **B**). The patient was not embolized at that time; 2 months later nonenhanced CT (not shown) demonstrated early calcifications. **D** MRI showed major cerebral damage bilaterally, with venous hemorrhagic infarct predominantly on the right side (see Chap. 4, Fig. 4.32). The infant was successfully treated from her fistula; however, at 6 months, except for control of seizures, there has been irreversible cerebral damage with bilateral diffuse atrophy (**E**)

patients is small, the risk of progressive dementia in this group is higher than in patients with other DAVMs. The arterial supply is predominantly dural originating from falcotentorial arteries of the carotid or vertebral system and from the vasa vasorum to the wall of the vein of Galen which, in turn, arise from pial arteries (see Vol. 3, Chap. 7) (Figs. 5.42, 5.44) (Fournier et al. 1991).

IV. AVFs of the Brain

Brain AVFs are superficial lesions in which a direct communication exists between a pial artery and a pial vein. The effects are similar to those associated with VGAM and include systemic manifestations (high output CHF) and cerebral venous hypertension that can produce atrophy, hydrocephalus, or calcifications. However, because of the direct shunting into cerebral veins, complications analogous to conventional brain AVMs may occur, e.g., cerebral hemorrhage, seizures, or neurological deficits. The earlier the onset of symptoms, the higher the chances of producing atrophy and irreversible brain damage (Figs. 5.5, 5.45). The closer to the midline (or in the

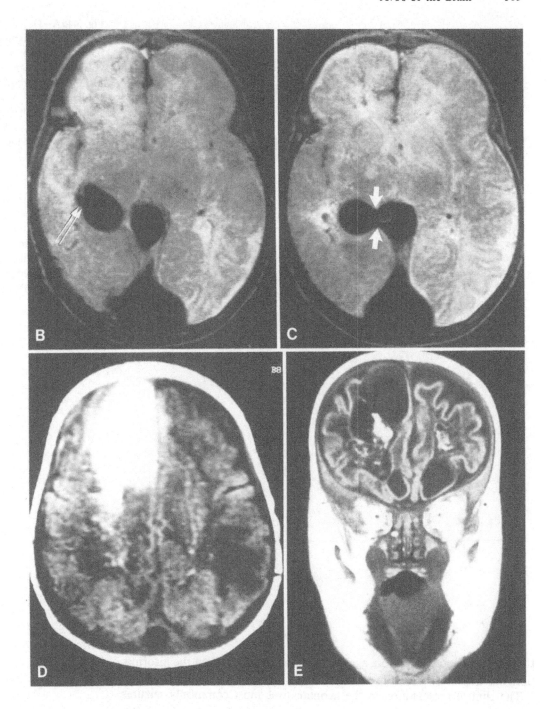

face of bilateral venous drainage), the more extensive the cerebral impairment (Fig. 5.45). In the literature, no specific mention of these type of lesions exists; they are usually included with other vascular malformations. We found 30 cases in the literature in which an appropriate diagnosis could be inferred from available angiograms or autopsy descriptions (Niimi 1990). From over 900 patients referred to us for consultation, we found 28 patients with direct AVFs of cerebral artery(ies) to cerebral vein(s) (four times less than VGAM). There was a slight female predominance. The age of presentation ranged from the neonatal period to 40 years old. Presentation was earlier than in patients with other brain AVMs; 30% were diagnosed before

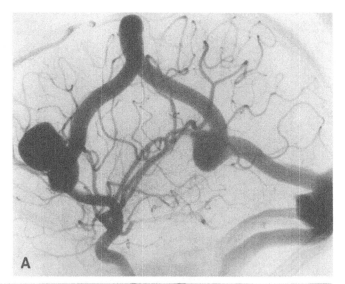

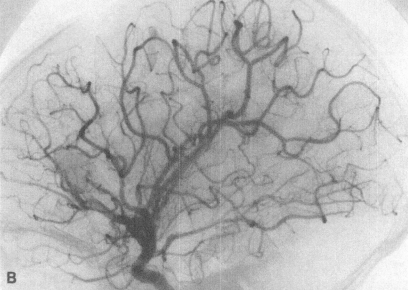

Fig. 5.46 A–D. Single-hole arteriovenous fistula in an infant presenting with a convulsive episode. Following two sessions of embolization, the fistula could be completely excluded. **A** Internal carotid angiogram in lateral projection; **B** control following the second attempt. Complete occlusion was confirmed 1 year later. **C** Chest X-rays before embolization demonstrate an enlarged cardiothoracic index. **D** The cardiothoracic index has normalized 6 months following complete occlusion of the shunt. (Reprinted from Garcia-Monaco et al. 1991)

the age of 10 and 67% before age 20. In all patients in whom the information was available, a loud bruit could be heard during auscultation.

The clinical presentation in the neonates was most commonly seizures (Fig. 5.45) or CHF. In infants, cardiomegaly was most frequent (Fig. 5.46). The presence of seizures, not seen in association with VGAM, should immediately suggest a true brain AVM. An additional symptom of brain AVM included failure to thrive in 39% of children. Hemorrhage as the initial presentation was seen in 30% of patients; in 28% of them the hemorrhage was lethal and only one patient who bled had no sequelae. Some 13% of the patients presented with seizures. When seen as a group, only 30% of patients with brain AVMs were neurologically normal at the time of diagnosis (Niimi 1990).

CT and/or MRI are the preliminary screening modalities, but angiography is the most sensitive and important diagnostic test to analyze the lesions and from which to plan treatment. The arterial supply to the fistula

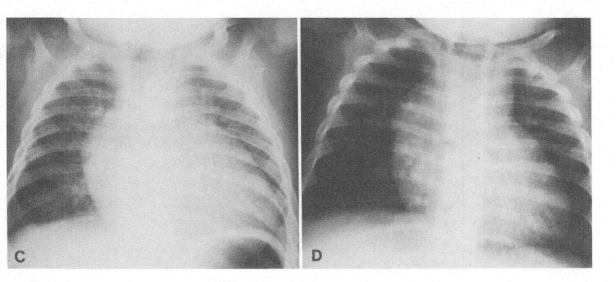

may be single (Fig. 5.46), but is frequently multiple (Chap. 3, Fig. 3.9) (57% of patients). The lesions are primarily supratentorial (85% of patients). Multiple (multifocal) fistulas are not infrequent, particularly in children (Chap. 3, Fig. 3.4). There may be multiple fistulas entering the same venous structure. Alternatively, sites of fistulization may be multifocal with separate venous outlets with or without Rendu-Osler-Weber disease (Chap. 1, Figs. 1.6, 1.62). Only neonates present with any significant CHF in association with these lesions.

Brain AVFs have a relatively high potential for partial or complete spontaneous thrombosis (Chap. 1, Fig. 1.62). In 23% of our patients there was evidence of direct lesional thrombosis, which eventually led to complete occlusion in half of them. The symptoms worsened, leaving permanent sequelae in some patients (Chap. 1, Fig. 1.6). Thus, although spontaneous thrombosis is often perceived as a favorable outcome and sometimes expected in spite of mild symptoms, it is not necessarily a benign process. Conversely, thrombosis resulting from embolization does not produce the same complication, and only temporary deficit occurred in one patient, related to progressive venous thrombosis after embolization.

1. Treatment of Brain AVFs

The therapeutic goal in brain AVFs can safely be accomplished by occlusion of the arterial feeder distal to the last arterial branch and proximal to the first normal venous tributary. Regardless of the method, the fistula can be excluded by either arterial or venous closure. Management and techniques presented for VGAMs in neonates and infants applies also to BAVFs. The various techniques are reviewed in Chap. 4.

Treatment is best accomplished in a hemodynamically stable child and can usually be done when the child weighs 5–6 kg; however intervention may be mandatory at an earlier age. The fact that only 30% of brain AVF patients are neurologically normal points to the need for early treatment.

References

Agee OF, Musella R, Tweed CG (1969) Aneurysm of the great vein of Galen. Report of two cases. J Neurosurg 31:346−350

Al Watban J, Banna M (1987) Infantile cardiomegaly as a complication of vascular malformations of the brain: report of 2 cases. Ann Saudi Med 8:373−376

Alvarez F, Roda J (1986) Experimental model for induction of cerebral aneurysms in rats. J Neurosurg 675:398−400

Alvarez-Garijo JA, Mengual MV, Gomial DT, Martin AA (1980) Giant arteriovenous fistula of the vein of Galen in early infancy treated successfully with surgery: case report. J Neurosurg 53:703−806

Amacher AL, Shillito J (1973) The syndromes and surgical treatment of aneurysms of great vein of Galen. J Neurosurg 39:89−98

Amacher AL, Drake CG, Hovind L (1979) The results of operating upon cerebral aneurysms and angiomas in children and adolescents. Child's brain 5:166−173

Ambrosetto P, Albrosetto G, Michelucci R, Bacci A (1983) Sturge-Weber syndrome without port-wine facial nevus. Report of 2 cases studied by CT. Childs Brain 10:387−392

Ancri D, Pertuiset B (1985) Instantaneous measurements of flow velocity in internal carotid arteries by pulsed doppler in cerebral arteriovenous malformations. Neurochirurgie 31:1−6

Anderson RM, Blackwood W (1959) The association of arteriovenous angioma and saccular aneurysm of the arteries of the brain. J Pathol Bacteriol 77:101−110

Andeweg J (1989) Intracranial venous pressure, hydrocephalus and effects of cerebrospinal fluid shunts. Childs Nerv Syst 5:318−323

Aoki N, Mizutani H (1985) Arteriovenous malformation in the territory of the occluded middle cerebral artery with massive intraoperative brain swelling: case report. Neurosurgery 16(5):660−662

Askenasy HM, Herzberger EE, Wijsenbeek HS (1953) Hydrocephalus with vascular malformations of the brain: a preliminary report. Neurology (NY) 3:213−220

Auer LM, McKenzie ET (1984) Physiology of the cerebral venous system. In: Kapp JP, Schimdek HH (eds) The cerebral venous system and its disorders. Grune & Stratton, New York

Avanzo RC, Chierego G, Marchetti C, Pozza F, Colombo F et al. (1984) L'irradiazone stereotassica con acceleratore lineare. Radiol Med (Torino) 70:124−129

Barnett GH, Little JR, Ebrahim ZY, Jones SC, Friel HT (1987) Cerebral circulation during arteriovenous malformation operation. Neurosurgery 20(6):836−842

Barre RG, Suter GG, Rosenblum WI (1978) Familial vascular malformation or chance occurrence: case report of two affected family members. Neurology 28:98−100

Bartal AD (1975) Classification of aneurysm of the great vein of Galen (letter to the editor). J Neurosurg 42:617−619

Bartynski WS, O'Reilly GV, Forrest MD (1987) In vitro arteriovenous malformation model for simulated intravascular embolization procedures (a). AJNR 8:969

Batjer H, Suss RA, Samson D (1986) Intracranial arteriovenous malformations associated with aneurysms. Neurosurgery 18(1):29−35

Batjer H, Mickey B, Samson D (1987) Enlargement and rupture of distal basilar artery aneurysm after iatrogenic carotid occlusion. Neurosurgery 20:624−629

Batjer HH, Devoius MD, Meyer YJ, Purdy PD et al. (1988a) Cerebrovascular hemodynamics in arteriovenous malformation complicated by normal perfusion pressure breakthrough. Neurosurgery 22(3):503−509

Batjer HH, Devous MD, Seibert B, Purdy P et al. (1988b) Intracranial arteriovenous malformations: relationships between clinical and radiographic factors and ipsilateral steal severity. Neurosurgery 23:322–328

Becker DH, Townsend JJ, Kramer RA, Newton TH (1979) Occult cerebrovascular malformations. A series of 18 histologically verified cases with negative angiography. Brain 102:249–287

Bedford THB (1934) The venous system of the velum interpositum of the rhesus monkey and the effect of experimental occlusion of the great vein of Galen. Brain 57:255–265

Belloti C, Medina M, Oliveri G, Barrale S, Ettore F (1985) Cystic cavernous angiomas of the posterior fossa. J Neurosurg 63:797–799

Benati A, Beltramello A, Maschio A, Perini S, Rosta L, Piovan E (1987) Combined embolization of intracranial AVMs with multi-purpose mobile-wing microcatheter system; indications and results in 71 cases. AJNR 8:938

Bentson JR, Wilson GH, Newton TH (1971) Cerebral venous drainage pattern of the Sturge-Weber syndrome. Radiology 101:111–118

Berenstein A (1980a) Flow controlled silicone fluid embolization. AJNR 1:61–77

Berenstein A (1980b) Transvascular fracture and repair of a cerebral artery (a). AJNR 1:358

Berenstein A (1981) Technique for catheterization and embolization of the lenticulostriate arteries. J Neurosurg 54:783–789

Berenstein A, Choi IS (1988) Surgical neuroangiography of intracranial lesions. Imaging in neuroradiology, part II. Radiol Clin North Am 26(5):1143–1151

Berenstein A, Epstein F (1982) Vein of Galen malformations. Combined neurosurgical and neuroradiological intervention. In: McLaurin R, Schut L, Venes J (eds) Pediatric neurosurgery. Grune & Stratton, New York, pp 637–647

Berenstein A, Kricheff II (1978) Therapeutic vascular occlusion. J Dermatol Surg Oncol 4:874–880

Berenstein A, Kricheff II (1980) Treatment of vascular abnormalities of the cerebral artery with detachable balloons (a). AJNR 1:358

Berenstein A, Kricheff II (1979a) A new balloon catheter for coaxial embolization. Neuroradiology 18:239–241

Berenstein A, Kricheff II (1979b) Catheter and material selection for transarterial embolization: technical considerations. I. Catheters. Radiology 132(3):619–630

Berenstein A, Kricheff II (1979c) Catheter and material selection for transarterial embolization: technical considerations. II. Materials. Radiology 132(3):631–639

Berenstein A, Kricheff II (1981) Neuroradiologic interventional procedures. Semin Roentgenol 16:79–94

Berenstein A, Lasjaunias P, Kricheff II (1983) Functional anatomy of facial vasculature in pathologic conditions and its therapeutic application. AJNR 4:149

Berenstein A, Ransohoff J, Kupersmith M et al. (1984a) Transvascular treatment of giant aneurysms of the cavernous carotid and vertebral arteries. Functional investigation and embolization. Surg Neurol 21:3–12

Berenstein A, Young W, Ransohoff J, Benjamin V, Merkin H (1984b) Somatosensory evoked potentials during spinal angiography and therapeutic transvascular embolization. J Neurosurg 60:777–785

Berenstein A, Choi IS, Kupersmith M, Flamm E, Kricheff II, Madrid MM (1989a) Complications of endovascular embolization in 202 patients with cerebral AVMs. AJNR 10:876

Berenstein AB, Krall R, Choi IS (1989b) Embolization with n-butyl-cyanoacrylate in management of CNS lesions (a). AJNR 10:883

Berenstein A, Choi IS, Neophytydes A, Benjamin V (1990) Endovascular treatment of spinal cord arteriovenous malformations (SCAVMs) (a). AJNR 10:898

Bergstrand H, Olivecrona H, Tonnis W (1936) Gefäßmißbildungen und Gefäßgeschwülste des Gehirns. Thieme, Leipzig

Berry RG, Alpers BS, White JC (1966) Angiomas. In: Millikan CH (ed) Cerebrovascular disease. Williams and Wilkins, Baltimore

Bicknell JM, Carlow TJ, Kornfeld M, Stouring J, Turner P (1978) Familial cavernous angiomas. Arch Neurol 35:746–749

Bitoh S, Hasegawa H, Fujiwaram M, Sakurai M (1978) Angiographically occult vascular malformations causing intra cranial hemorrhage. Surg Neurol 17: 35–42

Bitoh S, Hasegawa H, Kato A, Tamura K, Mabuchi E, Kobayashi Y (1987) Meningeal neoplasms associated with cerebral vascular malformations. Surg Neurol 27:469–475

Boldrey E, Miller ER (1949) Arteriovenous fistula (aneurysm) of the great cerebral vein (of Galen) and the circle of Willis. Arch Neurol Psychiatry 62:778–783

Bonnet P, Dechaume J, Blanc E (1937) L'anévrysme cirsoide de la rétine (anévrysme racemeux) ses relations avec l'anévrysme cirsoide de la face et avec l'anévrysme cirsoide du cerveau. J Med Lyon 18:165–178

Bots GAM (1971) Thrombosis of the galenic system veins in adults. Acta Neuropathol (Berl) 17:227–233

Boyd MC, Steinbok P, Paty DW (1985) Familial arteriovenous malformations. Report of four cases in one family. J Neurosurg 62(4):597–599

Boynton RC, Morgan CB (1973) Cerebral arteriovenous fistula with possible hereditary telangiectasia. Am J Dis Child 125:99–101

Brothers MF, Kaufmann JCW, Fox AJ, Deveikis JP (1989) N-butyl-2-cyanoacrylate – substitute for IBCA in interventional neuroradiology: histopathologic and polymerization time studies. AJNR 10:777

Brown RD, Wiebers DO, Forbes G, O'Fallon WM, Piepgras DG, Marsh R, Maciunas RJ (1988) The natural history of unruptured intracranial arteriovenous malformations. J Neurosurg 68:352–357

Bucci MN, Chandler WF, Gebarski SS, McKeever PE (1976) Multiple progressive familial thrombosed arteriovenous malformations. Neurosurgery 19:401–404

Buonaguidi B, Cvanapicci R, Mimassin N, Ferdeghini M (1984) Intrasellar cavernous hemangiomas. Neurosurgery 14:732–734

Capan LM, Labdizabal S, Sinha K, Ashok U et al. (1983) Acute pulmonary embolism during therapeutic arterial embolization with silicone fluids. Anesthesiology 58:569–571

Castaigne P, Rondot P, Escourolle R, Brunet P, Ribadeau Dumas JL (1972) Malformation de la veine de Galien à révélation tardive: étude anatomoclinique. Rev Neurol 126:304–312

Cersoli M, Campanile S, Campanile A, Amore A (1989) Unusual findings in Sturge-Weber syndrome. AJNR 10:S85

Chaudary RR (1987) Sturge Weber syndrome with extensive intracranial calcifications contralateral to the bulk of the facial nevus, normal intelligence, and absent seizure disorder. AJNR 8:736

Choi IS, Berenstein A, Flamm E (1988) Superselective catheterization and embolization of cerebral AVMs. In: Pluchino F, Broggi G (eds) Advanced technology in neurosurgery. Springer, Berlin Heidelberg New York, pp 183–192

Choi IS, Berenstein A, Kagetsu NJ (1990) Irrigation device for neuroangiographic procedures. Radiology 177:580

Chovanes GI, Truex R Jr (1987) Association of a ganglioneuroma with an arteriovenous malformation: case report. Neurosurgery 21:241–243

Circillo SF, Edwards MSB, Schmidt KG, Hieshima GB (1990) Interventional neuroradiological management of vein of Galen in the neonate. Neurosurgery 27:22–28

Claireaux AE, Newman CGH (1960) Arteriovenous aneurysm of the great vein of Galen with heart failure in the neonatal period. Arch Dis Child 35:605–612

Clarisse J, Dobbelaere P, Rey C, D'Hellemes P, Hassan M (1978) Aneurysms of the great vein of Galen. Radiological-anatomical study of 22 cases. J Neuroradiol 5:91–102

Clark JV (1970) Familial occurrence of cavernous angiomata of the brain. J Neurol Neurosurg Psychiatry 33:871–876

Colombo F, Benedetti A, Casentini L, Zanusso M, Pozza F (1987) Linear accelerator radiosurgery of arteriovenous malformations. Appl Neurophysiol 50: 257–261

Colombo F, Benedetti A, Pozza F, Marchetti C, Cherego G (1989) Linear accelerator radiosurgery of cerebral arteriovenous malformations. Neurosurgery 24(6):833–840

Conqvist S, Granholm L, Lundstrom NR (1972) Hydrocephalus and congestive heart failure caused by intracranial arteriovenous malformations in infants. J Neurosurg 36:249–254

Constantino A, Vitners HV (1986) A pathogenic correlate of the "steal" phenomenon in a patient with cerebral arteriovenous malformation. Stroke 17:103–106

Corrin B (1959) Three cases of intracranial vascular malformations in infants. J Clin Pathol 12:412–418

Cosgrove GR, Bertrand G, Fontaine S, Robitaille Y, Melanson D (1988) Cavernous angiomas of the spinal cord. J Neurosurg 68:31–36

Courville CB (1945) Pathology of the nervous system, 2nd edn. Pacific Press, Mountain View

Crawford JV, Russel DS (1956) Cryptic arteriovenous and venous hamartomas of the brain. J Neurol Neurosurg Psychiatry 19:1–11

Crawford PM, West CR, Chadwick DW, Shaw MDM (1986) Arteriovenous malformations of the brain: natural history in unoperated patients. J Neurol Neurosurg Psychiatry 49:1–10

Crawford JM, Rossitch EK, Oakes WJ, Alexander E (1990) Arteriovenous malformation of the great vein of Galen associated with patent ductus arteriosus. Report of 3 cases and review of the literature. Childs Nerv Syst 6:18–22

Cromwell D, Kerber C (1980) Modification of cyanoacrylate for therapeutic embolization: preliminary experience (a). AJNR 1:113

Cromwell LD, Harris AB (1980) Treatment of cerebral arteriovenous malformations. A combined neurosurgical and neuroradiological approach. J Neurosurg 52:705–708

Cronqvist S, Granholm I, Lundstrom NR (1972) Hydrocephalus and congestive heart failure caused by intracranial arteriovenous malformations in infants. J Neurosurg 36:249–254

Cumming GR (1980) Circulation in neonates with intracranial arteriovenous fistula and cardiac failure. Am J Cardiol 45:1019–1024

Dandy WE (1919) Experimental hydrocephalus. Ann Surg 70:129–142

De Lange SA, de Vlieger M (1970) Hydrocephalus associated with raised venous pressure. Dev Med Child Neurol 12 [Suppl]:28–32

De Marais JV, Lemos S (1982) Calcified aneurysm of the vein of Galen. Successful removal. Surg Neurol 17:304–306

Debrun G, Vinuela F, Faox AJ, Drake CG (1982a) Embolization of cerebral arteriovenous malformations with bucrylate: experience with 46 cases. J Neurosurg 56:615–627

Debrun GM, Vinuela FV, Fox AJ, Kan S (1982b) Two different calibrated leak ballons: experimental work and application in humans. AJNR 3:407

Deshpande DH, Vidyasagar C (1980) Histology of the persistent embryonic veins in arteriovenous malformations of brain. Acta Neurochirurgica 53:227–236

Deutsch G (1983) Blood flow changes in arteriovenous malformation during behavioral activation. Ann Neurol 13(1):38–43

Dias MS, Sekhar LN (1990) Intracranial hemorrhage from aneurysms and arteriovenous malformations during pregnancy and the puerperium. Neurosurg 27:855–866

Dion JE, Vinuela FV, Lylyk P, Lufkin R, Bentson J (1988) Ivalon 33% ethanol avitene embolic mixture: clinical experience with neuroradiological endovascular therapy in 40 arteriovenous malformations (a). AJNR 9:1029

Dobbelaere P, Jomin M, Clarisse J, Laine E (1979) Interet pronostique de l'étude du drainage veineux des anévrysmes artérioveineux cérébraux. Neurochirurgie 25:178–184

Dotter CT, Rosch J, Kalin PC (1972) Injectable flow guided coaxial catheterization for selective angiogram and controlled vascular occlusion. Radiology 104:421–423

Dowd CF, Halbach VV, Barnwell SL, Higashida RT, Edwards MS, Hieshima GB (1990) Transfemoral venous embolization of vein of Galen malformations. AJNR 11:643–648

Drake CG (1979) Cerebral arteriovenous malformations: considerations for an experience with surgical treatment in 166 cases. Clin Neurosurg 26:145–208

Duckwiller GR, Dion JE, Vinuela F, Martin N, Jabour B, Bentson J (1989) Intravascular microcatheter pressure monitoring experimental work and early clinical evaluation (a). AJNR 10:876

Dusser A, Boyer-Neumann C, Wolf M (1988) Temporary protein C deficiency associated with cerebral arterial thrombosis in childhood. J Pediatr 113:849–852

Duvernoy HM, Delon S, Vannson JL (1981) Cortical blood vessels of the human brain. Brain Res Bull 7:519–579

Eisenman JI, Alekoubides A, Priba MH (1972) Spontaneous thrombosis of vascular malformations of the brain. Acta Radiol Diagn (Stockh) 13:77–85

El Gohary M, Tomita T, Guitierrez FA, McLone DG (1987) Angiographically occult vascular malformations in childhood. Neurosurgery 20:759–766

Eskridge JM, Hartling RP (1989) Angioplasty of vasospasm. AJNR 10:877

Fabbrikant JI, Lyman JT, Hosobuchi Y (1984) Stereotactic heavy-ion Bragg peak radiosurgery: method for treatment of deep arteriovenous malformations. Br J Radiol 57:479–490

Fabbrikant JI, Frankel KA, Phillips MH, Levy RP (1989) Stereotactic heavy charged particle Bragg peak radiosurgery for intracranial arteriovenous malformations. In: Edwards MSB, Hoffman HJ (eds) Cerebral vascular diseases in children and adolescents. Williams and Wilkins, Baltimore, pp 389–409

Faria MA, Fleischer AS (1980) Dual cerebral and meningeal supply to giant arteriovenous malformations of the posterior cerebral hemisphere. J Neurosurg 52:153–161

Fehlings MG, Tucker WS (1988) Cavernous hemangioma of Meckel's cave. J Neurosurg 68:645–647

Feindel W, Yamamoto Y, Hodge C (1979) Red cerebral veins and the cerebral steal syndrome: evidence from fluoroscein angiography and microregional blood flow by radioisotopes during excision of an angioma. J Neurosurg 35:167–179

Fischer N (1979) Collagen dysplasia in matrix vesicles. Research with the electric microscope into the problem of so called "weakness of the vessel wall". Pathol Res Pract 165:374–391

Fischer WS (1989) Decision analysis: a tool of the future: an application to unruptured arteriovenous malformations. Neurosurgery 24(1):129–136

Folkman J (1986) How is blood vessel growth regulated in normal and neoplastic tissue? GHA Clowes memorial award lecture. Cancer Res 46:467–473

Fontaine S, Melanson D, Cosgrove R, Bertrand G (1988) Cavernous hemangiomas of the spinal cord: MR imaging. Radiology 166:839–841

Forster DMC, Steiner L, Hakanson S (1972) Arteriovenous malformations of the brain. A long-term clinical study. J Neurosurg 37:562–570

Fournier D, Rodesch G, Terbrugge K, Flodmark R, Lasjaunias P (1991) Acquired mural (dural) arteriovenous shunts of the vein of Galen. Report of 4 cases. Neuroradiology 33:52–55

Fox AJ, Lee DH, Pelz DM, Brothers MF, Deveikis JP (1988) Thrombotic mixture as a polymerizing agent (a). AJNR 9:1029

French LA, Peyton WT (1954) Vascular malformations in the region of the great vein of Galen. J Neurosurg 11:488–498

Friedmann D, Berenstein A, Choi I (1991) Neonatal vein of Galen malformations. Experience in developing a multidisciplinary approach using an embolisation treatment protocol. Clin Pediatric (Phila) 30(II):621–627

Gabrielsen TO, Heinz ER (1969) Spontaneous aseptic thrombosis of the superior sagittal and cerebral veins. AJR 107:579–588

Gagnon J, Boileau G (1960) Anatomical study of an arteriovenous malformation drained by the system of Galen. J Neurosurg 17:75–80

Gamache FW, Patterson J (1985) Infratentorial AVMS. In: Fein H, Flammes G (eds) Cerebrovascular surgery, vol 10. Springer, Berlin Heidelberg New York, pp 1117–1132

Garcia JC, Roach S, McLean WT (1981) Recurrent thrombotic deteroration in the Sturge-Weber syndrome. Childs Brain 8:427–433

Garcia-Monaco R, Alvarez H, Goulao Z, Pruvost Ph, Lasjaunias P (1990a) Posterior fossa arteriovenous malformations. Angioarchitecture in relation to their hemorrhagic episodes. Neuroradiology 31:471–475

Garcia-Monaco R, Alvarez H, Lasjaunias P (1990b) Utilization of the mini-torquer in cerebral arteriovenous malformations of the newborn and infant. Diagn Int Radiol 2:123–124

Garcia-Monaco R, De Victor D, Mann C, Hannedouche A, Terbrugge K, Lasjaunias P (1991a) Congestive cardiac manifestations from cerebrocranial arteriovenous shunts. Childs Nerv Syst 7:48–52

Garcia-Monaco R, Rodesch G, Terbrugge K, Burrows P, Lasjaunias P (1991b) Multifocal dural arteriovenous shunts in children. Childs Nerv Syst 7:48–52

Garretson HD (1985) Intracranial arteriovenous malformations. In: Wilkins RH, Rengachary SS (eds) Neurosurgery. McGraw-Hill, New York, pp 1448–1457

Gibson JB, Taylor AR, Richardson AE (1959) Congenital arteriovenous fistula with an aneurysm of the great cerebral vein and hydrocephalus treated surgically. J Neurol Neurosurg Psychiatry 22:224–228

Giombini S, Morello G (1978) Cavernous angiomas of the brain. Account of fourteen personal cases and review of the literature. Acta Neurochir (Wien) 40:61–82

Glatt BS, Rowe RD (1960) Cerebral arteriovenous fistula associated with congestive heart failure in the newborn: report of 2 cases. Pediatrics 26:596–603

Gold AP, Ransohoff J, Carter S (1964) Vein of Galen malformation. Acta Neurol Scand 40:5–31

Gomez MR, Whiteen CF, Nolke A, Bernstein J, Meyer J (1963) Aneurysmal malformation of the great vein of Galen causing heart failure in early infancy: report of 5 cases. Pediatrics 31:400–411

Goodkin R, Zaias B, Michelsen J (1990) Arteriovenous malformation and glioma: coexistent or sequential? J Neurosurg 72:798–805

Graf CJ, Perret GE, Torner JC (1983) Bleeding from cerebral arteriovenous malformations as part of their natural history. J Neurosurg 58:331–337

Graves VB, Partington CR, Rufenacht DA et al. (1989) Platinum coil placement with Tracker 18 catheter. Observation in dog carotid model (a). AJNR 10:876

Grossman RI, Bruce DA, Zimmerman RA, Goldberg HI, Bilaniuk LT (1984) Vascular steal associated with vein of Galen aneurysm. Neuroradiology 26:381–386

Hacke W, Zeumer H, Berg-Dammer E (1983) Monitoring of hemispheric and brainstem functions with neurophysiological methods during interventional neuroradiology. AJNR 4:382–384

Halbach VV, Higashida RT, Hieshima GB et al. (1987) Normal perfusion pressure breakthrough occurring during treatment of carotid and vertebral fistulas. AJNR 8:751–756

Halbach VV, Higashida RT, Hieshima GB, Hardin CW, Dowd CF, Barnwell SL (1989a) Transarterial occlusion of solitary intracerebral arteriovenous fistulas. AJNR 10:747

Halbach VV, Higashida RT, Hieshima GB, Mehringer CM, Hardin CW (1989b) Transvenous embolization of dural fistulas involving transverse and sigmoid sinuses. AJNR 10:385

Hammock MK, Milhorat TH, Earle K, DiChiro G (1971) Vein of Galen ligation in the primate: angiographic, gross and light microscopic evaluation. J Neurosurg 34:77–83

Hanieh A, Blumbergs PC, Carney PG (1981) Arteriovenous malformations associated with soft-tissue vascular malformations: case report. J Neurosurg 54:670–672

Harris GY, Jzkobiec FA (1979) Cavernous hemangiomas of the orbit. J Neurosurg 51:219–228

Hash CJ, Grossman CB, Shenkin HA (1975) Concurrent intracranial and spinal cord arteriovenous malformation: case report. J Neurosurg 43:104–107

Hashima SM, Asakura T, Koichi U, Kadota K, Awa H, Kusumoto K, Yamashita K (1985) Angiographically occult arteriovenous malformations. Surg Neurol 23:431–439

Hashimoto N, Handa H, Nagata I (1980) Experimentally induced cerebral aneurysms in rats, part V. Relations of hemodynamics in the circle of Willis to formation of aneurysms. Surg Neurol 13:41–45

Hassler W (1986) Hemodynamic aspects of cerebral angiomas. Acta Neurochir (Wien) [Suppl] 37:1–6

Hassler W, Steinmetz H (1987) Cerebral hemodynamics in angioma patients: an intraoperative study. J Neurosurg 67:822–831

Hayashi S, Arimoto T, Itakura T, Fujii T, Nishiguchi T, Komai N (1981) The association of intracranial aneurysms and arteriovenous malformations in the brain. Case report. J Neurosurg 55:971–975

Hayman LA, Evans RA, Ferell RE, Fahr LM, Ostrom P, Riccocdi VM (1982) Familial cavernous angiomas. Natural history and genetic study over a 5 year period. Am J Med Genet 11:147–160

Heinz ER, Schwartz RA, Sears RA (1968) Thrombosis in the vein of Galen malformations. Br J Radiol 41:424–428

Hernandez J, Schwartz JF, Goldring D (1956) Cerebral arteriovenous fistulas and congenital heart disease. J Pediatr 66:722–728

Heros RC, Korosue K (1989) Hemodilution for cerebral ischemia. Stroke 20(3):423–427

Hieshima GB, Higashida RT (1987) Aneurysm neck remnant following balloon embolization. J Neurosurg 67:322–323 (letter)

Hieshima GB, Grinnell VS, Mehringer CM (1981) A detachable balloon for therapeutic transcatheter occlusions. Radiology 138:227–228

Hieshima GB, Higishida RT, Wapenski J et al. (1986) Balloon embolization of large distal basilar artery aneurysms. J Neurosurg 65:413–416

Hieshima GB, Higishita RT, Wapenski J et al. (1987) Intravascular balloon embolization of large midbasilar artery aneurysms: case report. J Neurosurg 66:124–127

Hilal SK, Michelson WJ (1975) Therapeutic percutaneous embolization for extraaxial vascular lesions of head, neck and spine. J Neurosurg 43:275–287

Hilal SK, Sane P, Michelson WJ, Kossein A (1978) The embolization of vascular malformations of the spinal cord with low-viscosity silicone rubber. Neuroradiology 16:430–433

Hilal SK, Khandji AG, Chi TL, Stein BM, Bello JA, Silver AJ (1988) Synthetic fiber-coated platinum coils successfully used for endovascular treatment of arteriovenous malformations and direct arteriofistulas of CNS (a). AJNR 9:1030

Hirano A, Solomon S (1960) Arteriovenous aneurysm of the vein of Galen. Arch Neurol 5:605–612

Hoffman HJ, Chuang S, Hendrick B, Humphreys RP (1982) Aneurysms of the vein of Galen. J Neurosurg 57:316–322

Hoffman JH, Mohr G, Kusunoki T (1976) Multiple arteriovenous malformations of spinal cord and brain in a child. Case report. Childs Brain 2:317–324

Hook O, Johanson C (1988) Intracranial arteriovenous aneurysms. A follow-up study with particular attention to their growth. Arch Neurol Psychiatry 80:39–54

Hooper R (1961) Hydrocephalus and obstruction of the superior vena cava in infancy: clinical study of the relationship between cerebrospinal fluid pressure and venous pressure. Pediatrics 28:792–799

Horton JA, Dawson RC (1988) Retinal wada test. AJNR 9:1167

Hubert P, Choux M, Houtteville JP (1989) Cavernomes cérébraux de l'enfant et du nourrisson. Neurochirurgie 35:104–140

Hudgins WR (1988) What is radiosurgery? Letter to the editor. Neurosurgery 23(2):272

Iplikcioglu AC, Benli K, Bertan B, Ruacan S (1986) Cystic cavernous hemangioma of the cerebellopontine angle: case report. Neurosurgery 19:641–642

Iwasa H, Indei I, Sato F (1983) Intraventricular cavernous hemangioma. Case report. J Neurosurg 59:153–157

Izukawa D, Lach B, Benoit B (1987) Intravascular papillary endothelial hyperplasia in intracranial cavernous hemangioma. Neurosurgery 21:939–941

Jaeger JR, Forbes RP, Dandy WE (1937) Bilateral congenital arteriovenous communication aneurysm. Trans Am Neurol Assoc 63:173–176

Jafar JJ, Johns MM, Mullan SF (1986) Effects of mannitol on cerebral blood flow. J Neurosurg 64(5):754–759

Janny P, Chazal J, Colnet G (1981) L'hypertension intracrânienne bénigne. Etude clinique, physiopathologique et nosographique. Neurochirurgie 27:79–88

Jellinger K, Minauf M, Garzuly F, Neumayer E (1968) Angiodysgenetische nekrotisierende Myelopathie. Arch Psychiatr Nervenkr 211:377–404

Jellinger K (1986) Vascular malformations of the ventral nervous system: a morphological overview. Neurosurg Rev 9:177–216

Jimenez JL, Lasjqunias P, Terbrugge K (1989) The transcerebral veins: Normal and nonpathologic angiographic aspects. Surg Radiol Anat 11:63–72

John ER, Chabot RJ, Prichep LS, Ransohoff J, Epstein F, Berenstein A (1989) Real-time intraoperative monitoring during neurosurgical and neuroradiological procedures. J Clin Neurophysiol 6(2):125–158

Johnson RT (1975) Radiotherapy of cerebral angiomas: with a note on some problems in diagnosis. In: Pia HW, Gleae JRW, Grote E, Zienski J (eds) Cerebral angiomas: advances in diagnosis and therapy. Springer, Berlin Heidelberg New York, pp 256–259

Johnston H (1973) Reduced CSF absorption syndrome. Reappraisal of benign intracranial hypertension and related conditions. Lancet 2:418–420

Johnston IH, Whittle IR, Besser M, Morgan MK (1987) Vein of Galen malformation: diagnosis and management. Neurosurgery 20:747–758

Jomin M, Lesoin F, Lozes G (1985) Prognosis for arteriovenous malformations of the brain in adults based on 150 cases. Surg Neurol 23:362–366

Jungreis CA, Horton JA (1989) Pressure changes in arterial feeder to cerebral AVM as guide to monitoring therapeutic embolization. AJNR 10:1057

Jungreis CA, Berenstein A, Choi IS (1987) Use of an open-ended guidewire: steerable microguidewire assembly system in surgical neuroangiographic procedures (t). AJNR 8:237

Kalyanaraman K, Jagannathan K, Ramamurthi B (1971) Vein of Galen malformation with atypical manifestations: a case report. Dev Med Child Neurol 13:625–629

Kangure MS, ApSimon HT (1989) Vessel rupture during calibrated leak balloon AVM embolization...some additional mechanisms (a). AJNR 8:970

Kaplan G, Roswit B, Krueger EG (1952) Results of radiation therapy in vascular anomalies of the central nervous system. Radiology 555–558

Kayama T, Suzuki S, Sakurai Y, Nagayama T, Ogawa A, Yoshimoto T (1986) A case of Moyamoya disease accompanied by an arteriovenous malformation. Neurosurgery 18:465–468

Kee DB, Wood JH (1987) Influence of Blood rheology on cerebral circulation. In: Wood JH (ed) Cerebral blood flow. Physiologic and clinical aspects. McGraw-Hill, New York, pp 173–185

Kendall BE, Russell J (1966) Haemangioblastomas of the spinal cord. Br J Radiol 39:817–823

Kerber C (1976) Balloon catheter with a calibrated leak. A new system for superselective angiography and occlusive catheter therapy. Radiology 120:547–550

Kerber CW, Flaherty LW (1980) Teaching and research simulator for therapeutic embolization. AJNR 1:167

Kikuchi T, Strother CM, Boyar M (1987) New catheter for endovascular interventional procedures. Radiology 165:870–871

Kinal ME (1962) Hydrocephalus and the dural venous sinuses. J Neurosurg 19:195–201

King CR, Lovrein EW, Reiss J (1977) Central nervous system arteriovenous malformations in multiple generations of a family with hereditary hemorrhagic telangiectasias. Clin Genet 12:372–381

Kjellberg RM, Hanamura T, Davis KR et al. (1983) Bragg peak proton beam therapy for arteriovenous malformations of the brain. N Engl J Med 309:269–274

Kjellberg RN, Poletti CE, Robertson GH, Adams RD (1978) Bragg peak proton treatment of arteriovenous malformations of the brain. In: Carrea R, LeVay D (eds) Neurological surgery with emphasis on non-invasive methods of diagnosis and treatment. Excerpta Medica, Amsterdam, pp 188–193

Knudson RP, Alden ER (1979) Symptomatic arteriovenous malformation in infants less than 6 months of age. Pediatrics 64(2):238–241

Kobayashi H, Kawano H, Ito H, Hayashi M, Yamamoto S (1984) Hemangiomas calcificans in the fourth ventricle. Neurosurgery 14:737–739

Kondor T, Tamaki N, Takeda N, Suyama T et al. (1988) Fatal intracranial hemorrhage after balloon occlusion of an extracranial vertebral arteriovenous fistula. J Neurosurg 69:945–948

Koussa A, Chiras J, Poirier B, Carpena JP, Bories J (1985) Aspect tomodensitométrique et angiographique des angiomes veineux due cerveau. A propos de 15 cas. Neurochirurgie 31:161–168

Krayenbuhl H, Siebenman R (1965) Small vascular malformations as a cause of primary intracerebral hemorrhage. J Neurosurg 22:7–20

Krayenbuhl H, Yasargil MG (1972) Klinik der Gefäßmißbildungen und Gefäßfisteln. In: Ganshirt E (ed) Der Hirnkreislauf. Thieme, Stuttgart, pp 465–511

Krayenbuhl H, Yasargil MG, McClintock HG (1969) Treatment of spinal cord vascular malformation by surgical excision. J Neurosurg 30:427–435

Krayenbuhl HA (1977) Angiographic contribution to the problem of enlargement of cerebral arteriovenous malformations. Acta Neurochir (Wien) 36:215–242

Kricheff II, Madayag M, Braunstein P (1972) Transfemoral catheter embolization of cerebral and posterior fossa arteriovenous malformations. Radiology 103:107–111

Kushner J, Alexander E Jr (1970) Partial spontaneous regressive arteriovenous malformation. Case report with angiographic evidence. J Neurosurg 32:360–366

Laine E, Jomin M, Clarisse J, Combelles G (1981) Les malformations artério-veineuses cérébrales profondes. Classification topographique. Possibilités thérapeutiques à propos de 46 observations. Neurochirurgie 27:147–160

Lakke JPWF (1970) Regression of an arteriovenous malformation of the brain. J Neurol Sci 11:489–496

Lamas E, Lobato R, Esparza J, Escudero L (1977) Dural posterior fossa arteriovenous malformation producing raised sagittal sinus pressure. J Neurosurg 46:804–810

Lantos G, Fein JM, Knep S (1984) Cortical artery aneurysm formation after extracranial to intracranial bypass surgery. J Neurosurg 60:636–639

Lasjaunias P, Berenstein A (1987a) Functional vascular of the craniofacial area. Springer, Berlin Heidelberg New York (Surgical neuroangiography, vol 1)

Lasjaunias P, Berenstein A (1987b) Endovascular treatment of the craniofacial area. Springer, Berlin Heidelberg New York (Surgical neuroangiography, vol 2)

Lasjaunias P, Burrows P, Planet C (1986a) Developmental venous anomalies: the so-called venous angiomas. Neurosurg Rev 9:233–244

Lasjaunias P, Chiu M, Terbrugge K (1986b) Neurological manifestations of intracranial dural arteriovenous malformations. J Neurosurg 64:724–730

Lasjaunias P, Manelfe C, Chiu MC (1986c) Angiographic architecture of intracranial AVMs and fistulas: pretherapeutic aspects. Neurosurgical Rev 9:245–263

Lasjaunias P, Terbrugge K, Chiu MC (1986d) Coaxial balloon-catheter device for treatment of neonates and infants. Radiology 159:269–271

Lasjaunias P, Terbrugge K, Lopez-Ibort L (1987a) The role of dural anomalies in vein of Galen aneurysms: report of six cases and review of the literature. AJNR 8:185–192

Lasjaunias P, Terbrugge K, Piske R, Lopez-Ibor L, Manelfe C (1987b) Dilatation de la veine de Galien. Formes anatomo-clinique et traitement endovasculaire à propos de 14 cas explorés et/ou traités entre 1983 et 1986. Neurochirurgie 33:315–333

Lasjaunias P, Piske R, Terbrugge K, Willinsky R (1988a) Cerebral arteriovenous malformations and associated arterial aneurysms. Acta Neurochir (Wien) 91:29–36

Lasjaunias P, Terbrugge K, Choi IS (1988b) Transmesencephalic arteries and veins. Angiographic aspects in tectal vascular lesions. Acta Neurochir (Wien) 92:138–143

Lasjaunias P, Rodesch G, Pruvost P (1989a) Treatment of vein of Galen aneurysmal malformation. J Neurosurg 70:746–750

Lasjaunias P, Rodesch G, Terbrugge K (1989b) Vein of Galen aneurysmal malformations. Report of 36 cases managed between 1982 and 1988. Acta Neurochir (Wien) 99:26–37

Lasjaunias P, Terbrugge K, Rodesch G, Willinsky R, Burrows P, Pruvost P (1989c) Vraies et fausses lésions veineuses cérébrales. Pseudo-angiomes veineux et hémangiomes caverneux. Neurochirurgie 35:132–139

Lasjaunias P, Garcia-Monaco G, Terbrugge K (1991a) Deep venous drainage in great cerebral vein (vein of Galen) absence and malformations. Neuroradiology 33:234–242

Lasjaunias P, Garcia-Monaco R, Rodesch G (1991 b) Vein of Galen malformation. Endovascular management of 43 cases. Childs Nerv Syst 7:360–367

Latchaw RE, Gold LH (1979) Polyvinyl foam embolization of vascular and neoplastic lesions of the head, neck and spine. Radiology 131(3):669–679

Lazar ML (1974) Vein of Galen aneurysm: successful excision of a completely thrombosed aneurysms in an infant. Surg Neurol 2:22–24

Lee DH, Wriedt CH, Kaufmann JCE, Pelz DM, Fox AJ, Vinuela F (1989) Evaluation of three embolic agents in pig rete. AJNR 10:773

Lees F (1962) The migrainous symptoms of cerebral angiomata. J Neurol Neurosurg Psychiatry 25:45–50

Lehman JS, Chynn KY, Hagstrom JWC, Steinberg I (1966) Heart failure in infancy due to arteriovenous malformations of the vein of Galen. AJR 98:653–659

Lejeune JP, Combelles G, Christiaens JL (1969) Formes familiales des cavernomes. Neurochirurgie 35:111–112

Leksell L (1971) Stereotaxis and radiosurgery. An operative system. Thomas, Springfield

Leo JS, Lin JP, Kircheff II (1979) Pseudoaneurysm formation secondary to spontaneous thrombosis of a massive cerebral arteriovenous malformation. Neuroradiology 17:115–119

Levine J, Misko JC, Seres JL, Snodgress RG (1973) Spontaneous angiographic disappearance of a cerebral arteriovenous malformation. Third reported cases. Arch Neurol 28:195–196

Levine OS, Jameson AG, Nelhaus G (1962) Cardiac complications of cerebral arteriovenous fistulas in infancy. Pediatrics 30:563–575

Levy RP, Fabbrikant JI, Frankel KA, Phillips MH, Lyman JT (1989) Stereotactic heavy-charged-particle Bragg Peak radiosurgery for the treatment of intracranial arteriovenous malformations in childhood and adolescence. Neurosurgery 24(6):841–852

Lindegaard KJ, Bakke SJ, Grolimund P, Aaslid R, Huber P, Nornes H (1985) Assessment of intracranial hemodynamics in carotid artery disease by transcranial Doppler ultrasound. J Neurosurg 63:890

Lipton RB, Nerger AR, Lesser ML, Lantos G, Portenoy RK (1987) Lobar us thalamic and basal ganglion hemorrhage: clinical and radiographic features. J Neurol 234:86–90

Litvak J, Yahr M, Ransohoff J (1960) Aneurysms of the great vein of Galen and midline cerebral arteriovenous anomalies. J Neurosurg 17:945–954

Lobato RD, Perez C, Rivas JJ et al. (1988) Clinical, radiological, and pathological spectrum of angiographically occult intracranial vascular malformations. Analysis of 21 cases and review of the literature. J Neurosurg 68:518–531

Lobo-Antunes J, Yahr MD, Hilal SK (1974) Extrapyramidal dysfunction with cerebral arteriovenous malformations. J Neurol Neurosurg Psychiatry 37:259–268

London D, Enzemann D (1981) The changing angiographic appearance of an arteriovenous malformation after subarachnoid hemorrhage. Neuroradiology 21:281–284

Long DM, Seljesko Y EL, Chou SN et al. (1974) Giant arteriovenous malformations in infancy and childhood. J Neurosurg 40:304–312

Luessenhop AJ (1984) Natural history of cerebral arteriovenous malformations. In: Wilson CB, Stein BM (eds) Intracranial arteriovenous malformations. Williams and Wilkins, Baltimore, pp 12–23

Luessenhop AJ (1987) AVM grading in assessing surgical risk. J Neurosurg 66:637

Luessenhop AJ, Gennarelli TA (1977) Anatomical grading of supratentorial arteriovenous malformations for deforming operability. Neurosurgery 1:30–35

Luessenhop AJ, Presper JH (1975) Surgical embolization of cerebral arteriovenous malformations through internal carotid and vertebral arteries. Long-term results. J Neurosurg 42:443–451

Luessenhop AJ, Rosa L (1984) Cerebral arteriovenous malformations. Indications for and results of surgery, and the role of intravascular techniques. J Neurosurg 60:14–22

Luessenhop AJ, Spence WI (1960) Artificial embolization of cerebral arteries: report of use in a case of arteriovenous malformation. JAMA 172:1153–1155

Luessenhop AJ, Gibbs M, Velasquez AC (1962) Cerebrovascular response to emboli. Observations in patients with arteriovenous malformations. Arch Neurol 7:264–274

Luessenhop AJ, Kachmann R, Shevlin W et al. (1965) Clinical evaluation of artificial embolization in the management of large cerebral arteriovenous malformations. J Neurosurg 23:400–417

Lumsden CE (1947) A case of aneurysm of the vein of Galen. J Pathol Bacteriol 59:328–331

Malis LI (1982b) Arteriovenous malformations of the brain. In: Youmans JR (ed) Neurological surgery, vol III. Saunders, Philadelphia, pp 1786–1806

Margolis G, Odom G, Woodhall B (1961) Further experiences with small vascular malformations as a cause of massive intracerebral bleeding. J Neuropathol Exp Neurol 20:161–167

Mawad ME, Hilal SK, Michelson WJ et al. (1984) Occlusive disease associated with cerebral arteriovenous malformations. Radiology 153:401–408

Mayberg M, Zimmerman CH (1988) Vein of Galen aneurysm associated with dural AVM and straight sinus thrombosis. J Neurosurg 68:288–291

Mazza C, Scienza R, Dalla Bernardin B, Beltramello A, Bontempini L, Dapian R (1989) Malformations caverneuses cérébrales (cavernomes) de l'enfant. Neurochirurgie 35:106–108

McCormick WF (1962) The pathology of vascular arteriovenous malformations. J Neurosurg 24(7):807–816

McCormick WF, Nofzinger JD (1966) "Cryptic" vascular malformations of the central nervous system. J Neurosurg 24:865–875

McCormick WF, Rosenfield DB (1973) Massive brain hemorrhage. A review of 144 cases and an examination of their causes. Stroke 4:946–954

McCormick WF, Hardman JM, Boulter TR (1968) Vascular malformations (angiomas) of the brain with special reference to those occuring in the posterior fossa. J Neurosurg 28:241–251

McKenzie I (1953) The clinical presentation of the cerebral angioma. A review of 50 cases. Brain 76:184–214

Mehta BA, Sanders WP, Malik G, Burke TH, Spickler EM, Patel SC (1984) Detroit cocktail, new embolic agent for preoperative embolization of cerebral AVM (a). AJNR 10:902

Menezes AHJ, Graf CJ, Jacoby CG, Cornell SH (1981) Management of vein of Galen aneurysms. Report of 2 cases. J Neurosurg 55:457–462

Merland JJ, Reizine D (1987) Treatment of arteriovenous spinal cord malformations. Semin Int Radiol 4:281–290

Michelsen WJ (1979) Natural history and pathophysiology of arteriovenous malformations. Clin Neurosurg 26:307–313

Mickle JP, Quisling RG (1986) The transtorcular embolization of vein of Galen aneurysms. J Neurosurg 64:731–735

Milhorat TH, Clark R, Hammock MK (1970) Experimental hydrocephalus, part 2: gross pathological findings in acute and subacute experimental hydrocephalus in the dog and monkey. J Neurosurg 32:390–399

Minakawa T, Tanaka R, Koike T, Takeuchi S, Sasaki O (1989) Angiographic follow-up study of vertebral arteriovenous malformations with reference to their enlargement and regression. Neurosurgery 24(1):64–74

Miyasaka K, Wolpert SM, Prager RJ (1982) The association of cerebral aneurysms, infundibula and intracranial arteriovenous malformations. Stroke 13:196–203

Mohr JP (1984) Neurological manifestations and factors related to therapeutic decisions. In: Wilson CB, Stein BM (eds) Intracranial arteriovenous malformations. Williams and Wilkins, Baltimore, pp 12–23

Moody RA, Poppen JL (1970) Arteriovenous malformations. J Neurosurg 23:503–511

Morello G, Borghi GP (1973) Cerebral angiomas. A report of 154 personal cases and a comparison between the results of surgical excision and conservative management. Acta Neurochir (Wien) 28:135–155

Morgan MK, Johnston I, Besser M, Baines D (1987) Cerebral arteriovenous malformations, steal and the hypertensive breakthrough threshold. J Neurosurg 66:563–567

Morgan MK, Johnston IH, De Silva M (1985) Treatment of ophthalmofacial-hypothalamic arteriovenous malformations (Bonnet-Dechaume-Blanc syndrome). J Neurosurg 63:794–796

Mullan S, Brown FD, Patrona WJ (1979a) Hyperemic and ischemic problems of surgical treatment of arteriovenous malformations. J Neurosurg 51:757–764

Mullan S, Kawanaga NJ, Patronas WJ (1979b) Microvascular embolization of cerebral arteriovenous malformations. A technical variation. J Neurosurg 51:621–627

Muraszko K, Wang HH, Pelton G, Stein BM (1970) A study of the reactivity of feeding vessels to arteriovenous malformations: correlation with clinical outcome. Neurosurgery 26(2):190–199

Nakayama Y, Tanaka A, Yoshinaga S (1989) Multiple intracerebral AVMs: report of 2 cases. Neurosurgery 25:281–286

Nehls DG, Pittman HW (1982) Spontaneous regression of arteriovenous malformations. Neurosurgery 11(6):776–780

Nelson G (1984) Arteriovenous malformations as a cause of congestive heart failure in the newborn and infant. Eur J Pediatr 142:248–300

Newton TH, Cronqvist S (1969) Involvement of dural arteries in intracranial arteriovenous malformations. Radiology 93:1071–1078

Nishizaki T, Tamaki N, Matsumoto S, Fujita S (1986) Consideration of the operative indications for posterior fossa venous angiomas. Surg Neurol 25:441–445

Norlen G (1949) Arteriovenous aneurysms of the brain: report of 10 cases of total removal of the lesion. J Neurosurg 6:475–494

Norman MG, Becker LE (1974) Cerebral damage in neonates resulting from an arteriovenous malformation of the vein of Galen. J Neurol Neurosurg Psychiatry 37:252–258

Nornes H (1984) Quantitation of altered hemodynamics. In: Wilson CB, Stein BM (eds) Intracranial arteriovenous malformations. Williams and Wilkins, Baltimore, pp 32–43

Nornes H, Grip A (1980) Hemodynamic aspects of cerebral arteriovenous malformations. J Neurosurg 53:456–464

Nornes H, Grip A, Wikeby P (1979a) Intraoperative evaluation of cerebral hemodynamics using direction Doppler technique, part 1: arteriovenous malformations. J Neurosurg 50:145–151

Nornes H, Lundar T, Wikeby P (1979b) Cerebral arteriovenous malformations: results of microsurgical management. Acta Neurochir (Wien) 50:243–257

Noterman J, Georges P, Brochti J (1987) Arteriovenous malformation associated with multiple aneurysms in the posterior fossa: a case report with a review of the literature. Neurosurgery 21(3):387–391

Numaguchi Y, Kishikawa T, Fukui M, Sawada K, Kitamura K, Matsuura K, Russel WJ (1979) Prolonged injection angiography for diagnosis intracranial cavernous hemangiomas. Radiology 131:137–138

O'Brien MS, Schechter MD (1970) Arteriovenous malformation involving the galenic system. AJR 110:50–55

O'Donnabhain D, Duff DF (1989) Aneurysm of the vein of Galen. Arch Dis Child 64:1612–1617

Occhiogrosso M, Carella A, D'Aprile P, Vailati G (1983) Brain-stem hemangioma calcificans. Case report. J Neurosurg 59:150–152

Okamoto S, Handa H, Hashimoto N (1984) Location of intracranial aneurysms associated with cerebral arteriovenous malformations: statistical analysis. Surg Neurol 22:335–340

Okudera T, Ohta T, Huang YP (1984) Embryology of the cranial venous system. In: Kapp J, Schmiedek H (eds) The cerebral venous system and its disorders. Grune & Stratton, New York

Olin MS, Eltomey AA, Dunsmore RH (1982) Thrombosed vein of Galen aneurysm. Neurosurgery 10:258–262

Omojola MF, Fow AJ, Vinuela FV, Drake CG (1982) Spontaneous regression of intracranial arteriovenous malformations. Report of 3 cases. J Neurosurg 57:818–822

Omojola MF, Fox AJ, Vinuela F et al. (1985) Stenosis of afferent vessels of intracranial arteriovenous malformations. AJNR 6:791–793

Ondra SL, Troupp H, George ED, Schwab K (1990) The natural history of symptomatic arteriovenous malformations of the brain: a 24 year follow up assessment. J Neurosurg 73:387–391

Oscherwitz D, Davidoff LM (1947) Midline calcified intracranial aneurysm between occipital lobes: report of a case. J Neurosurg 4:539–541

Osler WA (1901) A family form of recurring epistaxis associated with multiple telangiectasia of the skin and mucuous membranes. Johns Hopkins Hosp Bull 12:33–337

Otten P, Pizzolato GP, Rilliet B, Berney J (1989) A propos de 131 cas d'angiomes caverneux (cavernomes) du S.N.C. repérés par l'analyse retrospective de 24 535 autopsies. Neurochirurgie 35:82–83

Padget DH (1948) The development of the cranial arteries in the embryo. Contrib Embryol 32:205–262

Padovani R, Tognetti F, Proietti D et al. (1982) Extrathecal cavernous hemangioma. Surg Neurol 18:463–465

Papatheodorou CA, Gross SW, Hollin S (1961) Small arteriovenous malformations of the brain. Arch Neurol 5:666–672

Parkinson D, Bachers G (1980) Arteriovenous malformations. Summary of 100 consecutive supratentorial cases. J Neurosurg 53:285–299

Parkinson D, West M (1977) Spontaneous subarachnoid hemorrhage first from an intracranial and then from a spinal arteriovenous malformations: case report. J Neurosurg 47:965–968

Pascual-Castroviejo I, Pascual Pascual JI, Blazquez MG, Lopez Martin V (1977) Spontaneous occlusion of an intracranial arteriovenous malformation. Childs Brain 3:169–179

Paterson JH, McKissock W (1956) A clinical survey of intracranial angiomas with special reference to their mode of progression and surgical treatment: a report of 110 cases. Brain 79:233–266

Peeters FLM (1982) Angiographically demonstrated large vascular malformation in a patient with a normal angiogram 23 years before. A case report. Neuroradiology 23:113–114

Pellettieri L (1980) Surgical versus conservative treatment of intracranial arteriovenous malformations: a study in surgical decision making. Acta Neurochir [Suppl] (Wien) 29:1–86

Perret G, Nishioka H (1966) Report on the cooperative study of intracranial aneurysms and subarachnoid hemorrhage. Section VI. Arteriovenous malformations. An analysis of 545 cases of cranio-cerebral arteriovenous malformations and fistulae reported to the cooperative study. J Neurosurg 25:467–490

Pertuiset B, Ancri D, Clergue F (1982) Preoperative evaluation of hemodynamic factors in cerebral arteriovenous malformations for selection of a radical surgery tactic with special reference to vascular autoregulation disorders. Neurol Res 4:209–233

Pertuiset B, Ancri D, Arthuis F, Basset JY, Fusciaradi J, Nakano H (1985) Shunt-induced haemodynamic disturbances in supratentorial arteriovenous malformations. J Neuroradiol 12:165–178

Pevsner PH (1977) Microballoon catheter for superselective angiography and therapeutic occlusion. AJR 128:225–230

Pevsner PH, Doppman JL (1980) Therapeutic embolization with a microballoon catheter system. AJNR 1:171

Picard L, Moret J, Lepoire J (1984) Endovascular treatment of intracerebral arteriovenous angiomas. J Neuroradiol 11:9–28

Pile-Spellman JMD, Baker KF, Lisczak TM, Sandrew BB et al. (1986) High-flow angiopathy: cerebral blood vessel changes in experimental chronic arteriovenous fistula. AJNR 7:811

Pomposelli FB, Lamparello PJ, Riles TS, Craighead CC, Giangola G, Imparato AM (1988) Intracranial hemorrhage after carotid endartarectomy. J Vasc Surg 7(2):248–255

Pollock A, Laslett PA (1958) Cerebral arteriovenous fistula producing cardiac failure in the newborn infant. J Pediatr 53:731–736

Pool JL, Potts DG (1965) Aneurysms and arteriovenous anomalies of the brain, diagnosis and treatment. Harper and Row, New York, p 43

Pool JL (1968) Excision of cerebral arteriovenous malformations. J Neurosurg 29

Poppen JL, Avman N (1960) Aneurysms of the great vein of Galen. J Neurosurg 17:238–244

Powers AD, Smith RR (1989) Hyperperfusion syndrome after carotid endartarectomy. Transcutaneal doppler evaluation. Neurosurgery 26(1):56–60

Powers WJ, Grubb RL Jr, Baker RP, Mintun MA, Raichle ME (1985) Regional cerebral blood flow and metabolism in reversible ischemia due to vasospasm. Determination by positron emission tomography. J Neurosurg 62:539

Pribil S, Boone SC, Waley R (1983) Obstructive hydrocephalus at the anterior third ventricle caused by dilated veins from an arteriovenous malformation. Surg Neurol 20:487–492

Probst FP (1980) Vascular morphology and angiographic flow patterns in Sturge-Weber angiomatosis: facts, thoughts and suggestions. Neuroradiology 20:73–78

Prosenz P, Heiss WD, Kvicala V, Tschabitscher H (1971) Contribution to the hemodynamics of the arterial venous malformations. Stroke V 2:279–289

Quisling RG, Mickle PJ (1989) Venous pressure measurements in vein of Galen aneurysms. AJNR 10:411–417

Rao VRK, Mandalam KR, Gupta AK, Kumar S, Joseph S (1989) Dissolution of isobutyl-2-cyanoacrylate on long term follow-up. AJNR 10:135

Raybaud CA, Strother CM, Hald JK (1989) Aneurysm of the vein of Galen: embryonic considerations and anatomical features relating to pathogenesis of the malformation. Neuroradiology 31:109–128

Rendu H (1896) Epistaxis répétéez chez un sujet porteur de petits angiomas cutanés et muqueux. Bull Soc Med Hop (Paris) 13:131

Rigamonti D, Pappas CTE, Spetzler RF, Johnston PC (1990) Extracerebral cavernous angiomas of the middle fossa. Neurosurgery 27(2):306–310

Rizzoli H (1983) Comment. Neurosurgery 13:5, 580

Rodesch G, Lasjaunias P, Terbrugge K (1988) Lésions vasculaires artério-veineuses intra-craniennes de l'enfant. Place des techniques endovasculaires à propos de 44 cas. Neurochirurgie 34:293–303

Roman G, Fischer M, Perl DP et al. (1978) Neurological manifestations of hereditary hemorrhagic telangiectasia (Rendu-Osler-Weber disease). Report of 2 cases and review of the literature. Ann Neurol 4:130–144

Rosenblum BR, Bonner RF, Oldfield EH (1987a) Intraoperative measurement of cortical blood flow adjacent to cerebral AVM using laser Doppler velocimetry. J Neurosurg 66:396

Rosenfeld JV, Fabinyi GCA (1984) Acute hydrocephalus in an elderly woman with an aneurysm of the vein of Galen. Neurosurgery 15:852–854

Rosman NP, Shands KN (1978) Hydrocephalus caused by increased intracranial venous pressure: a clinicopathological study. Ann Neurol 3:445–450

Ross DA, Walker J, Edwards MSB (1986) Unusual posterior fossa dural arteriovenous malformations in a neonate: case report. Neurosurgery 19:1021–1024

Rubinstein LJ (1981) Tumors of the central nervous system, vol 6. Armed Forces Institute of Pathology, Washington, pp 235–256

Rubinstein LJ (1972) Tumors of the central nervous system. Atlas of tumor pathology, 2nd series. Armed Forces Institute of Pathology, Washington Fasc (8)

Rudolph AM (1970) The changes in the circulation after birth: their importance in congenital heart disease. Circulation 41:343–359

Rufenacht D, Merland JJ (1986a) A polyethylene microcatheter with a latex balloon as an implant for permanent vascular occlusions. A way for the treatment of distal intracranial or intraspinal large AV fistulas or aneurysms. Valk J (ed) Neuroradiology 1985/1986. Elsevier, Amsterdam

Rufenacht D, Merland JJ (1986b) Detachable latex balloon with valve-mechanism for the permanent occlusion of large brain AV fistulas of cerebral arteries. Valk J (ed) Neuroradiology 1985/1986. Elsevier, Amsterdam

Rufenacht D, Merland JJ (1986c) Modifications of a supple catheter avoiding the need of a balloon for flow-guidance. In: Valk J (ed) Neuroradiology 1985/1986. Excerpta Medica, Amsterdam, pp 311–314

Rufenacht D, Merland JJ (1986d) More precision in superselective angiography: flow independent guidance of soft catheters (a). AJNR 8:959

Ruscalleda J, Peiro A (1986) Prognostic factors in intraparenchymatous hematoma with ventricular hemorrhage. Neuroradiology 28:34–37

Russel B, Rengachary SS, McGregor D (1986) Primary pontine hematoma presenting as a cerebellopontine angle mass. Neurosurgery 19:129–133

Russel DS (1954) The pathology of spontaneous intracranial hemorrhage. Proc R Soc Med 47:689–693

Russel DS, Nevin S (1940) Aneurysm of the great vein of Galen causing internal hydrocephalus. J Pathol Bacteriol 51:375–385

Russel DS, Newton TH (1964) Aneurysm of the vein of Galen. AJR 92:756–760

Russel DS, Rubinstein LJ (1971) Pathology of tumours of the nervous system, 3rd edn. Arnold, London

Russell EJ, Berenstein A (1981) Meningeal collateralization to normal cerebral vessels associated with intracerebral arteriovenous malformations: a functional angiographic study. Radiology 139(3):617–622

Russell EJ, Berenstein A (1984) Somatosensory evoked potential monitoring for intraoperative radiology. Symposium on neuroimaging. Neurol Clin 2(4):873–902

Rutka JT, Zawadski MB, Wilson CB, Rosenblum ML (1988) Familial cavernous malformation. Diagnostic Potential of Magnetic Resonance Imaging. Surg Neurol 29:467–474

Sahs AI, Perret GE, Locksley HB et al. (1969) Intracranial aneurysms and hemorrhage, a cooperative study. Lippincott, Philadelphia

Sainte-Rose C, Lacombe L, Pierre-Khan A (1984) Intracranial venous sinus hypertension: cause or consequence of hydrocephalus in infants? J Neurosurg 60:727–736

Saito Y, Kobayashi N (1981) Cerebral venous angiomas clinical evaluation and possible etiology. Radiology 139:87–94

Sang H, Kerber C (1983) Ventricular obstruction secondary to vascular malformations. Neurosurgery 5:572–574

Schiffer J, Bibi C, Avidan D (1984) Cerebral arteriovenous malformation: papilledema as a presenting sign. Surg Neurol 22:524–526

Schlachter LB, Fleischer AS, Faria MA, Tindall GT (1980) Multifocal intracranial arteriovenous malformations. Neurosurgery 7:440–444

Schlesinger B (1940) The tolerance of the blocked galenic system against artificially increased intravenous pressure. Brain 63:178–183

Scott BB, McGillicuddy JE, Seeger JF, Kindt GW, Giannotta SL (1978) Vascular dynamics of an experimental cerebral arteriovenous shunt in the primate. Surg Neurol 10:34–38

Scott JA, Berenstein A, Blumenthal D (1986) Use of the activated coagulation time as a measure of anticoagulation during interventional procedures. Radiology 158:849–850

Seidenwurm D, Hyman A, Kowalski H, Berenstein A (1991) Vein of galen malformation correlation of arteriography, magnetic resonance imaging and computed tomography. AJNR 12:347–354

Seljeskog EL, Rogers HM, French LA (1968) Arteriovenous malformation involving the inferior sagittal sinus in an infant. Case report. J Neurosurg 29:623–628

Shenkin HA, Spitz EB, Grant FC et al. (1948) Physiologic studies of arteriovenous anomalies of the brain. J Neurosurg 5:165–172

Shi Y, Chen X (1986) A proposed scheme for grading intracranial arteriovenous malformations. J Neurosurg 65:484–489

Shimoji T, Murakami N, Shimizu A, Sato K, Ishii S (1984) Cavernous hemangioma with bone formation in a child: case report. Neurosurgery 14(3):346–349

Simard JM, Garcia-Bengochea F, Balliner WE, Mickle JP, Quisling RG (1986) Cavernous angioma: a review of 126 collected and 12 new clinical cases. Neurosurgery 18(2):162–172

Siqueira EB, Murray KJ (1972) Calcified aneurysms of the vein of Galen: report of a presumed case and review of the literature. Neurochirurgia 3:106–112

Smith DR, Donat JF (1981) Giant arteriovenous malformation of the vein of Galen: total surgical removal. Neurosurgery 8:378–382

Somach FM, Shenkin HA (1966) Angiographic end-results of carotid ligation in the treatment of carotid aneurysm. J Neurosurg 24:966–974

Spetzler RF, Martin NA (1986) A proposed grading system for arteriovenous malformations. J Neurosurg 65:476–483

Spetzler RF, Selman WR (1984) Pathophysiology of cerebral ischemia accompanying arteriovenous malformations. In: Wilson CB, Stein BM (eds) Intracranial arteriovenous malformations. Williams and Wilkins, Baltimore, pp 24–31

Spetzler RF, Wilson CB (1975) Enlargement of an arteriovenous malformation documented by angiography. J Neurosurg 43:767–769

Spetzler RF, Wilson CB, Weinstein P, Mehdorn M, Townsend J, Telles D (1978) Normal perfusion pressure breakthrough theory. Clin Neurosurg 25:651–672

Spetzler RF, Martin RNA, Carter LP, Flam RA, Raudzens PA et al. (1987) Surgical management of large AVMs by staged embolization and operative excision. J Neurosurg 67:17–28

Spetzler RF, Zabramski JM, Flom RA (1989) Management of juvenile spinal AVMs by embolization and operative excision. J Neurosurg 70:628–632

Stehbens WE, Sahgal KK, Nelson LN, Shaber RM (1973) Aneurysm of vein of Galen and diffuse meningeal angioectasia. Arch Pathol 95:333–335

Steiger HJ, Markwalder TM, Reulen HJ (1987) Clinicopathological relations of cerebral cavernous angiomas: observations in eleven cases. Neurosurgery 21:879–884

Steiger HJ, Markwalder RV, Reulen HJ (1989) Y a-t-il une relation entre manifestation clinique et l'image pathologique des cavernomes cérébraux? Neurochirurgie 35:84–88

Stein BM (1979) Arteriovenous malformations of the brain and spinal cord. In: Hoff J (ed) Practice of surgery. Harper and Row, Hagerstown, pp 1–40

Stein BM (1985) Comment. Neurosurgery 16:303

Stein BM, Wolpert SM (1977) Surgical and embolic treatment of cerebral arteriovenous malformations. Surg Neurol 7:359–369

Stein BM, Wolpert SM (1980) Arteriovenous malformations of the brain. I. Current concepts and treatment. Arch Neurol 37:1–5

Stein BM, Fraser RAR, Wolpert S (1975) Embolization in the preparation for surgery of large cerebral arteriovenous malformations. J Neurol Neurosurg Psychiatry 38:407

Steiner L (1984) Treatment of arteriovenous malformations by radiosurgery. In: Wilson CB, Stein BM (eds) Intracranial arteriovenous malformations. Williams and Wilkins, Baltimore, pp 29–314

Steiner L (1985) Radiosurgery in cerebral arteriovenous malformations. In: Fein JM, Flamm ES (eds) Cerebrovascular surgery, vol IV. Springer, Berlin Heidelberg New York, pp 1161–1215

Steiner L (1986) Radiosurgery in arteriovenous malformations in the brain. In: Flamm E, Fein J (eds) Textbook of cerebrovascular surgery. Springer, Berlin Heidelberg New York

Steiner L (1987) Stereotactic radiosurgery with a cobalt 60 gamma unit in the surgical treatment of intracranial tumors and arteriovenous malformations. In: Schmidek HH, Sweet WH (eds) Operative neurosurgical techniques: indications, methods and results, 2nd edn. Grune and Stratton, Orlando, pp 515–529

Steiner L, Leksell L, Forster DMC et al. (1972) Stereotactic radiosurgery for cerebral arteriovenous malformations. Report of a case. Acta Chir Scand 138:459–462

Steiner L, Greitz T, Backlund EO, Leksell L et al. (1979) Radiosurgery in arteriovenous malformations of the brain. Undue effects. In: Szikla G (ed) Stereotactic cerebral irradiations. Amsterdam, Elsevier, pp 257–269

Steinheil SO (1928) Über einen Fall von Varix aneurysmaticus im Bereich der Gehirngefäße. Cited by Dandy WE Arteriovenous aneurysm of the brain. Arch Surg 17:190–243

Steinmeier R, Schramm J, Muller HG, Fahlbusch R (1989) Evaluation of prognostic factors in cerebral arteriovenous malformations. Neurosurgery 24(2):193–200

Stimac GK, Solomon MA, Newton TH (1986) CT and MR of angiomatous malformations of the choroid plexus in patients with Sturge-Weber disease. AJNR 7:623–627

Strand T, Asplund K, Eriksson S, Hagg E, Lithner F, Wester P (1984) A randomized controlled trial of hemodilution therapy in acute ischemic stroke. Stroke 15:980–989

Stroobandt G, Harmant-van Ruckevorsel K, Mathurin P, De Nijs C, De Ville de Goyet J (1986) Hydrocephalie externe et interne par malformation artério-veineuse chez un nourrisson. Neurochirurgie 32:81–85

Sturge WA (1879) A case of partial epilepsy, apparently due to a lesion of one of the vaso-motor centers of the brain. Trans Clin Soc London 12:162–167

Sukoff MH, Barth B, Moran T (1972) Spontaneous occlusion of a massive arteriovenous malformation. Case report. Neuroradiology 4:121–123

Sundt TM (1979) Blood flow regulation in normal and ischemic brain. Current concepts. Upjohn

Sundt TM, Sharbrough FW, Piepgras DO, Kearns TP et al. (1981) Correlation of cerebral blood flow and electroencephalographic changes during carotid endarterectomy – with results of surgery and hemodynamics of cerebral ischemia. Mayo Clin Proc 56:533–543

Sutherland GR, King M, Drake CG, Peerless SJ, Vezina WC (1988) Platelet aggregation within cerebral arteriovenous malformations. J Neurosurg 68:198–204

Svien HJ, McRae JA (1964) Arteriovenous anomalies of the brain. Fate of patients not having definitive surgery. J Neurosurg 23:23–28

Tada T, Sugita K, Kobayashi S, Watanabe N (1986) Supra- and infratentorial arteriovenous malformations with an aneurysmal dilatation: a case report. Neurosurgery 19:831–834

Tagle P, Huete I, Mendez J, Del Villard S (1986) Intracranial cavernous agniomas: presentation and management. J Neurosurg 64:720–723

Takashima S, Becker LE (1980) Neuropathology of arteriovenous malformations in children. J Neurol Neurosurg Psychiatry 43:380–385

Takeuchi S, Kikuchi H, Karasawa J, Naruo Y et al. (1987) Cerebral hemodynamics in arteriovenous malformations: evaluation by single-photon emission CT. AJNR 8:193–197

Tamaoka A, Sakuta M, Yamada H (1987) Hemichorea-hemiballism caused by arteriovenous malformations in the putamen. J Neurol 234:124–125

Tanaka Y, Furuse M, Iwasa H, Masazawa T, Saito K, Sato F, Mizuno Y (1986) Lobar intracerebral hemorrhage: etiology and a long-term follow-up study of 32 patients. Stroke 17:51–57

Tardieu M, Malherbe V, Garcia-Monaco R, De Victor D, Zerah M, Lasjaunias P (1990) Les malformations anévrysmales de la veine de Galen. Pediatrie 45 [Suppl]:223–230

TerBrugge K, Lasjaunias P, Chiu MC, Marotta TR, Tatton W, Glen J (1989) Rhesus monkey as animal model for training in interventional neuroradiology. AJNR 10:1203

TerBrugge K, Scotti G, Ethier R, Melancon D, Tchang S, Milner C (1977) Computed tomography in intracranial arteriovenous malformations. Radiology 122:703–705

Theron J, Newton TH, Hoyt WF (1974) Unilateral retinocephalic vascular malformations. Neuroradiology 7:185–196

Thomson JLG (1959) Aneurysm of the vein of Galen. Br J Radiol 32:680–684

Troost BT, Mark LE (1979) Resolution of classic migraine after removal of an occipital lobe AVM. Ann Neurol 5(20):199–201

Troost BT, Newton TH (1975) Occipital lobe arteriovenous malformations. Clinical and radiologic features in 26 cases with comments on the differentiation from migraine. Arch Ophthalmol 93:250–256

Tyndel FJ, Bilbao JM, Hudson A, Colapinto EV (1985) Hemangioma calcificans of the spinal cord. Can J Neurol Sci 12:321–322

Ueda S, Saito A, Inomori S et al. (1987) Cavernous angioma of the cauda equina producing subarachnoid hemorrhage. Case report. J Neurosurg 66:134–136

Valavanis A, Wellauer J, Yasargyl AG (1983) The radiological diagnosis of cerebral venous angioma. Cerebral angiography and computed tomography. Neuroradiology 24:193–199

Ventureyra ECG, Bajdedo A (1984) Galenic arteriovenous malformation with precocious puberty. Surg Neurol 21:45–48

Ventureyra ECG, Choo SH, Benoit BG (1980) Super giant globoid intercranial aneurysm. J Neurosurg 53:411–416

Verdura J, Shafron M (1969) Aneurysm of vein of Galen in infancy. Surgery 65:494–498

Vidyasagar C (1979) Persistent embryonic veins in arteriovenous malformations of the posterior fossa. Acta Neurochir (Wien) 48:67–82

Vinuela F, Drake CG, Fox AJ et al. (1982) Giant intracranial varices secondary to high-flow arteriovenous fistulae. J Neurosurg 66:198–203

Vinuela F, Fox AJ, Debrun G et al. (1983a) Progressive thrombosis of brain arteriovenous malformations after embolization with isobutyl-2-cyanoacrylate. AJNR 4:1233–1238

Vinuela F, Fox AJ, Kan S et al. (1983b) Balloon occlusion of a spontaneous fistula of the posterior inferior cerebellar artery. J Neurosurg 58:287–289

Vinuela F, Nombela L, Roach MR, Fox AJ, Pelz DM (1985) Stenotic and occlusive disease of the venous drainage system of deep brain AVMs. J Neurosurg 63(2):180–184

Voigt K, Beek U, Beinshagen G (1973) A complex cerebral vascular malformation studied by angiography: multiple aneurysms angiomas and arterial ectasia. Neuroradiology 5:117–123

Wada JT, Rasmussen S (1960) Intracarotid injection of sodium amytal for the lateralization of cerebral speech dominance. J Neurosurg 17:266–282

Walsh FB, King AB (1942) Occular sign of intracranial saccular aneurysms: experimental work on collateral circulation through the ophthalmic artery. Arch Ophthalmol 27:1–33

Waltimo O (1973a) The change in size of intracranial arteriovenous malformations. J Neurol Sci 19:21–27

Waltimo O (1973b) The relationship of size, density and localization of intracranial arteriovenous malformations to the type of initial symptom. J Neurol Sci 19:13–19

Wang AM, Morries JH, Fisher EG, Peterson R, Lin JCT (1988) Cavernous hemangioma of the thoracic spinal cord. Neuroradiology 30:261–264

Waybright EA, Selhorst JB, Rosenblum WI, Suter CG (1978) Blue rubber bled nevus syndrome with CNS involvement and thrombosis of a vein of Galen malformation. Ann Neurol 3:464–467

Weber F, Cantab MB (1907) Multiple hereditary developmental angiomata (telangiectasia) of the skin and mucuous membrane associated with recurring hemorrhages. Lancet II:160–162

Weber FP (1922) Right-sided hemi-hypertrophy resulting from right-sided congenital spastic hemiplegia, with a morbid condition of the left side of the brain, revealed by radiograms. J Neurol Psychopathol 3:134–139

Weir BKA, Allen PBR, Miller JDR (1968) Excision of thrombosed vein of Galen aneurysm in an infant. Case report and technical notes. J Neurosurg 29:619–622

Wilkins RH (1985) Natural history of intracranial vascular malformations. A review. Neurosurgery 16:421–430

Willinsky R, Lasjaunias P, Comoy J, Pruvost P (1988) Cerebral microarteriovenous malformations (mAVMs). Review of 13 cases. Acta Neurochir (Wien) 91:37–41

Willinsky R, Lasjaunias P, Terbrugge K, Pruvost P (1988) Brain arteriovenous malformations: Analysis of the angioarchitecture in relationship to hemorrhage. J Neuroradiol 15:225–237

Willinsky R, Lasjaunias P, Terbrugge K, Burrows P (1990a) Multiple cerebral arteriovenous malformations. Review of our experience from 203 patients with cerebral vascular lesions. Neuroradiology 32:207–210

Willinsky R, Lasjaunias P, Terbrugge KN, Hurth M (1990b) Angiography in the investigation of spinal dural arteriovenous fistula. A protocol with application of the venous phase. Neuroradiology 32:114–116

Willinsky R, Terbrugge K, Lasjaunias P, Montanera W (1990c) The variable presentations of craniocervical and cervical dural arteriovenous malformations. Surg Neurol 34:118–123

Wilson CB, Roy M (1964) Calcification within congenital aneurysms of vein of Galen. AJR 91:1319–1326

Wilson CB, U HS, Dominique J (1979) Microsurgical treatment of intracranial vascular malformations. J Neurosurg 51:446–454

Wisoff JH, Berenstein A, Choi IS (1990) Management of vein og Galen malformations. Concepts Pediatr Neurosurg 10:137–155

Wolfe HR, France NE (1949) Arteriovenous aneurysms of the great vein of Galen. Br J Surg 37:76–78

Wolpert SM, Stein BM (1975) Catheter embolization of intracranial arteriovenous malformations as an aid to surgical excision. Neuroradiology 10:73–85

Wolpert SM, Barnett FJ, Prager RJ (1981) Benefits of embolization without surgery for cerebral arteriovenous malformation. AJNR 2:535

Wood JH (1987) Cerebral blood flow. Physiologic and clinical aspects. McGraw-Hill

Wyburn-Mason R (1943a) Arteriovenous aneurysm of midbrain and retina, facial naevi and mental changes. Brain 66:163–203

Wyburn-Mason R (1943b) The vascular abnormalities and tumours of the spinal cord and its membranes. Kimpton, London

Yamada S, Cojocaru T (1987) Arteriovenous Malformations. In: Wood JH (ed) Cerebral blood flow. Physiologic and clinical aspects. McGraw-Hill, New York, pp 580–590

Yamada S (1982) Arteriovenous malformations in the functional area: surgical treatment and regional cerebral blood flow. Neurol Res 4:283–322

Yamasaki T, Handa H, Yamashita J, Moritake K, Nagasawa S (1984) Intracranial cavernous angiomas angiographically mimicking venous angioma in an infant. Surg Neurol 22:461–466

Yasargil MG (1978) Operative treatment of spinal angioblastomas. In: Pia HW, Djindjan R (eds) Spinal angiomas: advances in diagnosis and therapy. Springer, Berlin Heidelberg New York

Yasargil MG, Antic J, Laciga R et al. (1976) Arteriovenous malformations of the vein of Galen. Microsurgical treatment. Surg Neurol 16:195–200

Yasargil MG (1987) Pathologic considerations. In: Yasargil MG (ed) Microneurosurgery, AVM of the brain: history, embryology, pathologic considerations, hemodynamics, diagnostic studies, microsurgical anatomy, vol 3A. Thieme, New York, pp 49–211

Yatsu FM, Pettigrew LC, Grotta JC (1987) Medical therapies for acute ischemic stroke. In: Wood JH (ed) Cerebral blood flow. Physiologic and clinical aspects. McGraw-Hill, New York, pp 603–612

Yi L, Ke-Wei H (1985) Thrombosis of the galenic system veins in the adults. Chin Med J 95:365–369

Yokota A, Oota T, Matsukado Y, Okudera T (1978) Structures and development of the venous system in congenital malformations of the brain. Neuroradiology 16:26–30

Young B (1979) Hydrocephalus and elevated intracranial venous pressure. Case report. Childs Brain 5:73–80

Zampella EJ, Aronin PA, Odrezin GT (1988) Conservative management of thrombosed vein of Galen malformations. Report of two cases and review of the literature. Pediatr Neurosci 14:264–271

Zanetti P, Sherman F (1972) Experimental evaluation of a tissue adhesive as an agent for the treatment of aneurysms and arteriovenous anomalies. J Neurosurg 36:72–79

Zellem RT, Buchheit WA (1985) Multiple intracranial arteriovenous malformations: case report. Neurosurgery 17:88–93

Zerah M, Garcia-Monaco R, Rodesch G, Terbrugge K, Tardieu M, De Victor D, Lasjaunias P (1992) Hydrodynamics in vein of Galen malformation. Child's Nervous Syst 8:1–7

Subject Index

Numbers preceded by an F refer to figure numbers, those preceded by a T refer to table numbers

Made in the USA
Coppell, TX
09 June 2021